Special Tests

For Mosby:

Senior Commissioning Editor: Ninette Premdas
Project Development Manager: Katrina Mather
Project Manager: Morven Dean
Design: Judith Wright
Illustration Manager: Bruce Hogarth

Special Tests

The procedure and meaning
of the commoner tests in hospital

Fifteenth Edition

David MD Evans MD FRCP FRC Path
Formerly Consultant Pathologist to the South Glamorgan Health Authority
based at Llandough Hospital, Hon. Clinical Teacher, University of Wales
College of Medicine, Cardiff

Christopher D Evans MB, BS, FRCP
Consultant Dermatologist, Lanarkshire Acute Hospitals NHS Trust, based at
Monklands Hospital, Airdrie

Robert A Evans MB, BS, FRCS
Consultant Otolaryngologist, Bro Morgannwg NHS Trust, based at Princess of
Wales Hospital, Bridgend

Mosby
An Affiliate of Elsevier Science

MOSBY
An imprint of Elsevier Science Limited

Fifteenth edition 2003

ISBN 0 7234 3289 9

British Library Cataloguing in Publication Data
A catalogue record for this book is available from the British Library

Library of Congress Cataloging in Publication Data
A catalog record for this book is available from the Library of Congress

Note
Medical knowledge is constantly changing. Standard safety precautions must be followed, but as new research and clinical experience broaden our knowledge, changes in treatment and drug therapy may become necessary or appropriate. Readers are advised to check the most current product information provided by the manufacturer of each drug to be administered to verify the recommended dose, the method and duration of administration, and contraindications. It is the responsibility of the practitioner, relying on experience and knowledge of the patient, to determine dosages and the best treatment for each individual patient. Neither the Publisher nor the author assumes any liability for any injury and/or damage to persons or property arising from this publication.

ELSEVIER
SCIENCE

your source for books,
journals and multimedia
in the health sciences

www.elsevierhealth.com

The
Publisher's
policy is to use
**paper manufactured
from sustainable forests**

Printed in China

Contents

Preface   ix
Units of measurement   x
List of abbreviations   xi
Acknowledgements   xiv

1 Introduction   1

Activities of living   1
Tests   1
Preparing the patient and gaining consent   2
Laboratory investigations   3
Point of care and near patient testing   5

2 Tests related to the environment   7

Skin	Skin biopsy	8
Allergy	Skin tests used in allergy	9
	Blood tests used in allergy	9
Infection	Tests for infections	11
	Diagnostic skin tests	14
	Microbiological tests on blood	16
	Temperature	19
Imaging Techniques	X-ray examinations	20
	Ultrasound	20
	CT scan	21
	Magnetic resonance	21
	Foreign bodies	21
	Radiation monitoring	22
	Radioisotopes, Gallium scanning, PET scan	23

3 Tests related to communicating (1)   25

Speech	Speech tests	26
Sight	Sight tests	27
Hearing	Hearing tests	29
The Neuromuscular system	Tests for meningeal irritation	30
	Examination of cerebrospinal fluid (CSF)	30
	Examination of cranial nerves	33
	Reflex actions	34
	Coordination	35
	Sensation	36
	Malingering	36
	Detailed study of brain and spinal cord	38
	Peripheral nerves	40

| | Muscular system | 40 |
| | Mental development tests | 41 |

4 Tests related to communicating (2) — 43

Endocrine system	Thyroid gland investigation	45
	Parathyroid gland investigation	49
	Adrenal gland investigation	50
	Pituitary gland investigation	56

5 Tests related to breathing — 61

Respiratory system	Upper respiratory tract investigations	61
	Lower respiratory tract investigations	63
	Lung Function tests	67
	Blood gases and pH	73

6 Tests related to circulation — 77

Cardiovascular system	Blood pressure	77
	Cardiac function	79
	Imaging examination of the cardiovascular system	83
	Central venous pressure	85

7 Tests related to blood (1) — 87

Haematology	Blood counts and related investigations	88
	Bone marrow puncture	93
	Lymph node biopsy	93
	Investigations for haemorrhagic disorders	93
	Investigations for the haemolytic anaemias	98
	Other tests in haematology	101
Blood transfusion	Blood group tests	103
	Antenatal blood tests	104
	Essentials of blood transfusion	105

8 Tests related to blood (2) — 109

| Chemistry (Chemical pathology) | Chemical analysis of blood | 110 |

9 Tests related to eating and drinking — 123

Nutrition	Milk	124
	Vitamin deficiencies	125
Upper alimentary tract	Tests related to the mouth	128
	Tests related to the oesophagus	129
	Tests related to stomach and intestines	130
Liver	Imaging techniques for liver examination	137

	Routine liver function tests	*137*
	Additional liver function tests	*139*
Gall bladder and bile ducts		*141*
Pancreas	Tests of pancreatic function (secretion of pancreatic juice and insulin)	*142*
	Pancreatic and related tumours	*148*
Small intestine	Tests for intestinal absorption	*149*
Peritoneum	Other abdominal tests	*150*

10 Tests related to eliminating (1) *153*

Lower alimentary tract	Visual examination of rectum and colon	*153*
	X-ray examination of gut	*155*
	Examination of faeces	*156*

11 Tests related to eliminating (2) *159*

Urinary system	Urinalysis	*160*
	Routine examination of urine in the microbiology laboratory	*163*
	Microscopical examination of urine	*164*
	Renal function tests	*165*
	Radiology of the urinary tract	*168*
Excreted substances	Chemical analysis of urine	*170*

12 Tests related to mobilizing *175*

Skeletal system	X-ray and MRI examination of bone joints and tendons	176
	Other tests related to joints and bones	*178*
	Physiotherapy assessment	*179*

13 Tests related to sexuality *181*

Heredity	Sex chromatin and chromosome examination	*183*
Paternity	Blood groups and genetic fingerprinting	*184*
Prostate	Tumours: Cytology and biopsy	*185*
Infertility	Tests in females	*185*
	Tests in males	*186*
	Post-coital test	*186*
Gonads	Gonadal endocrine function investigations – urine, blood	*187*
Pregnancy	Pregnancy tests	*188*
	Placental and fetal monitoring	*189*
Neonatal screening	Phenylketonuria, congenital hypothyroidism, galactosaemia	*193*
Breast examination	Self-examination	*194*
	Breast biopsy	*195*

Female genital tract	Laparoscopy	*196*
	Radiography and ultrasound	*196*
	Uterine curettings	*196*
	Gynaecological cytology	*197*
	Colposcopy	*198*
	Discharges	*198*
Sexually transmitted diseases	Urethral discharge and related infections	*199*
	Blood tests for syphilis	200
	Other blood tests used in infections	201

14 Tests related to drug taking   *203*

Therapeutic drug monitoring		*204*
Overdose and poisoning	Drug overdose	*206*
	Poisoning	*206*
Drug addiction and substances of abuse	Alcohol	*208*
	Cannabis	*208*

15 Tests related to dying   *209*

Tests for brain death	Preconditions	*209*
	Diagnostic tests	*210*
	Other considerations, including organ donation	*211*
Investigating the cause of death	Informing the coroner	*211*
	Obtaining relatives' permission	*212*
	Scope and types of autopsy	*212*

Index	*215*

Preface to Fifteenth Edition

The ordering of diagnostic investigations such as pathology tests and X-rays, previously undertaken only by doctors, has been placed first of the ten key roles for nurses, central to the modernization and reform of the NHS.[1] It is the aim of this book to provide a clear picture of the range, nature and significance of these tests.

In the current medical climate it is essential to ensure that the *patient* is fully aware of the nature of any tests being undertaken. Informed written permission is necessary for all but the simpler tests, such as a blood pressure estimation, for which verbal agreement is sufficient. Details of the revised consent forms are included.

There are new sections on the following:

- General: 'point of care' and 'near patient' testing; management of 'high risk' specimens; radioisotope scanning of lung, thyroid, gallbladder, kidney and bone; gallium scanning; positron emission tomography (PET)
- Circulation: ambulatory cardiac monitoring, pulse oximetry and chemical markers for myocardial ischaemia
- Blood: coagulation factor assays; screening for disseminated intravascular coagulation; testing for autoantibodies; tumour markers; serum zinc estimation
- Alimentary system: salivary gland radiology, including sialogram; oesophageal scanning; assessment of peptic ulceration risk; monitoring control of diabetes mellitus; detection of gastrointestinal bleeding; identification of pancreatic tumours
- Reproductive systems: preimplantation genetic diagnosis (PGD) in IVF to ensure that a baby does not carry a gene for a life-threatening disorder; screening for prostatic cancer by prostatic specific antigen (PSA); testing for antispermatozoal antibodies as a cause for infertility; advances in placental and fetal monitoring; cordocentesis; neonatal monitoring for inborn errors of metabolism (congenital hypothyroidism, phenylketonuria and galactosaemia); chlamydia and herpes genitalis infections; development of liquid-based cytology (LBC) for cervical cytology
- Drugs: monitoring of drugs used in the control of heart failure, asthma, epilepsy, depression, schizophrenia, immunosuppression and infection by anaerobic organisms.

In addition, there are changes arising from the inclusion of nationally-accepted values for the numerous chemical substances found in blood, CSF and urine.

---

[1]Logan, B. Expanding nurses' roles: from vision to reality. *Clinical Medicine* (4): 292–293. London. Royal College of Physicians. 2002.

Units of Measurement

cm	centimetre: one hundredth of a metre $(m \times 10^{-2})$
dB	decibel: one tenth of a bel (unit of sound intensity)
dl	decilitre: one tenth of a litre $(l \times 10^{-1})$
fl	femtolitre: one thousandth of a millionth of a millionth of a litre $(l \times 10^{-15})$
g	gramme
h	hour(s)
IU	International Unit
kg	kilogram: one thousand grams $(g \times 10^{3})$
kPa	KiloPascal (unit of gas pressure; standard atmospheric pressure is approximately 101 kPa)
l	litre
m	metre
m	minute(s)
mEq	milli-equivalent: one thousandth of the equivalent weight in grammes
mg	milligramme: one thousandth of a gramme $(g \times 10^{-3})$
ml	millilitre: one thousandth of a litre $(l \times 10^{-3})$. For practical purposes this is equal to one cubic centimetre (cm^{3}).
mm	millimetre: one thousandth of a metre $(m \times 10^{-3})$
mm³	cubic millimetre
mmol	millimole: one thousandth of a mole
mol	mole: for molecular substances this is the molecular weight in grammes
mosmol/kg	osmotic pressure exerted by one millimole of a substance in one kilogramme
mPAS/s	millipascal/second (unit of viscosity, previously termed centipoise)
mU	milliUnit: one thousandth of a Unit
ng	nanogramme: one thousandth of a millionth of a gramme $(g \times 10^{-9})$
nm	nanometre: one thousandth of a millionth of a metre $(m \times 10^{-9})$. Nanometre is the unit of measurement of light wavelength.
nmol	nanomole: one thousandth of a millionth of a mole
osmol/kg	osmotic pressure exerted by one mole of substance in one kilogramme of solvent
pg	picogramme: one millionth of a millionth of a gramme $(g \times 10^{-12})$
pmol	picomole: one millionth of a millionth of a mole
sec	second(s)
U	unit (used in the measurement of IgE, p. 118)
µg	microgramme: one millionth of a gramme $(g \times 10^{-6})$
µm	micrometre: one millionth of a metre $(m \times 10^{-6})$
µmol	micromole: one millionth of a mole
<	less than
>	greater than

Abbreviations

ACTH	Adrenocorticotrophic hormone
ADH	Antidiuretic hormone
AFP	Alpha-fetoprotein
αHBD	Alphahydroxybutyrate dehydrogenase
ALA	Amino laevulinic acid
ALT	Alanine aminotransferase
AMP	Adenosine monophosphate
ANF	Antinuclear factor
APTT	Activated partial thromboplastin time
AST	Aspartate transferase
BAO	Basal acid output
BCG	Bacille Calmette–Guérin
βHCG	beta subunit human chorionic gonadotrophin
BR	British ratio
BUN	Blood urea nitrogen
CEA	Carcinoembryonic antigen
CH	Congenital hypothyroidism
CK	Creatine kinase
CPK	Creatine phosphokinase
CRP	C-reactive protein
CSSD	Central Sterile Supply Department
CSU	Catheterized sample of urine
CVP	Central venous pressure
CVS	Chorionic villous sampling
DAT	Differential agglutination test
DDAVP	des-amino d-arginine vasopressin
DIC	Disseminated intravascular coagulation
DLE	Disseminated lupus erythematosus
DST	Dexamethasone suppression test
DVT	Deep vein thrombosis
DXA	Dual-energy X-ray absorptiometry
ECG	Electrocardiogram, electrocardiograph
EDTA	Ethylene-diamine-tetraacetic acid
EEG	Electroencephalogram, electroencephalograph
ELISA	Enzyme-linked immunosorbent assay
ELT	Euglobin lysis time
EMU	Early morning urine
EP	Erythropoietic porphyria
ERCP	Endoscopic retrograde cholangiopancreatography
ERV	Expiratory reserve volume
ESR	Erythrocyte sedimentation rate
ETR	Effective thyroxine ratio
FEV_1	Forced expiratory volume in 1 second
FNA	Fine needle aspiration

FRC	Functional residual capacity
FSH	Follicle-stimulating hormone
FTAT	Fluorescent treponemal antibody test
FVC	Forced vital capacity
G6PD	Glucose-6-phosphate dehydrogenase
GFR	Glomerular filtration rate
γGT	gammaglutamyl transferase
GH	Growth hormone
GHb	Glycosylated haemoglobin
GOT	Glutamic oxalacetic transaminase
GTT	Glucose tolerance test
HANE	Hereditary angioneurotic edema
hCG	Human chorionic gonadotrophin
HDL	High-density lipoprotein
HGH	Human growth hormone
HIDA	Hydroxy iminodiacetic acid
HPF/hpf	High power field (microscopy measure)
HPL	Human placental lactogen
HSV2	Herpes simplex virus type 2
IC	Inspiratory capacity
INR	International normalized ratio
IRV	Inspiratory reserve volume
ITT	Insulin tolerance test
IV	Intravenous
IVF	In-vitro fertilization
IVP	Intravenous pyelography
IVU	Intravenous urography
KLB	Klebs–Löffler bacillus
LBC	Liquid based cytology
LDH	Lactic dehydrogenase
LDL	Low-density lipoprotein
LH	Luteinizing hormone
LMP	Last monthly period
MCD	Mean cell diameter
MCH	Mean cell haemoglobin
MCHC	Mean cell haemoglobin concentration
MCV	Mean cell volume
MSH	Melanocytic stimulating hormone
MSU	Midstream urine
NBT	Nitroblue tetrazolium
NPT	Near patient test
NSE	Neurone-specific enolase
PA	Pernicious anaemia
PAO	Peak acid output
PBG	Porphobilinogen
PBI	Protein-bound iodine

PCI	Prothrombin consumption index
pCO_2	Carbon dioxide pressure
PCV	Packed cell volume
PET	Positron emission tomography
PFR	Peak flow rate
PGD	Pre-implantation genetic diagnosis
PKU	Phenylketonuria
pO_2	Oxygen pressure
POCT	Point of care tests
PP	Pancreatic polypeptide
PPD	Purified protein derivative
Ppoma	Tumour secreting pancreatic polypeptide
PRIST	Paper radioimmunosorbent test
PSA	Prostatic specific antigen
RAST	Radioallergosorbent test
RPCFT	Reiter protein complement fixation test
RV	Residual volume
SAS	Supraregional Assay Service
SCA	Sickle cell anaemia
SCAT	Sheep cell agglutination test
SLE	Systemic lupus erythematosus
TA test	Thyroglobulin antibody test
TAB	Killed organisms of typhoid, paratyphoid A and B
TBG	Thyroid-binding globulin
TCFT	Thyroid complement fixation test
TGT	Thromboplastin generation test
TIT	Treponema immobilization test
TLC	Total lung capacity
TPHA	*Treponema pallidum* haemagglutination test
TPR	Temperature, pulse and respiration
TRH	Thyrotropin releasing hormone
TSH	Thyroid stimulating hormone
UHT	Ultra high temperature
VC	Vital capacity
VDRL	Venereal disease reference laboratory
VIP	Vasoactive intestinal polypeptide
VMA	Vanillylmandelic acid
WR	Wassermann reaction
ZE	Zollinger–Ellison syndrome.

Acknowledgements

In preparing this 15th edition we wish to thank Dr David Perkins of Charing Cross Hospital for providing us with the list of normal values of the various chemical substances found in the body, compiled by him on behalf of the Royal College of Physicians for reference in the MRCP examination; Dr Stephanie Matthews, chemical pathologist at Llandough Hospital for guidance concerning their estimation; and Dr Ragnheidn Olafsdottir, cytopathologist at Llandough Hospital, for information on liquid based cytology. We are also indebted to Mrs Alison Bowers for her meticulous scrutiny of the text, and to Dr Peter Evans for his help in programming the computer, which greatly facilitated the whole process of revision.

CHAPTER ONE

Introduction

Activities of living | Tests | Preparing the patient and gaining consent | Procedures for laboratory tests

Index of tests	Page
Biopsy	8
Collection of blood samples	5
Collection of infected material	5
Collection of urine	5
Frozen section	4
Needle biopsy	4
Point of care testing (POCT), near-patient testing and quality control	5
Preparing the patient and gaining consent	2
Request for investigation	3
Specimen labelling	3
Tests, special tests and investigations	1

Activities of living

Patients are people; each individual has his own life pattern. In recognition of this, Roper et al. (1996) have developed a model for nursing based on activities of living.[1] The tests used for investigating and monitoring disease may be approached in a similar way, as tests related to:

- Environment
- Communicating
- Breathing
- Circulation
- Blood
- Eating and drinking
- Eliminating
- Mobilizing
- Sexuality
- Drug taking
- Dying.

Tests, special tests and investigations

A routine clinical examination includes a number of tests, viz. inspection, palpation, percussion and auscultation. When such tests are insufficient to fully diagnose or assess the condition from which the patient is suffering, special tests are needed.

Their nature, the procedures involved and the significance of the test results are the essence of this book. The term 'investigation' often includes a number of tests which are required to define the condition from which a patient is suffering, e.g. 'thyroid gland investigation' (p. 45). The investigation of the nervous system and special senses includes tests which are on the borderline between routine clinical examination and special tests and, where relevant, these are included.

Preparing the patient and gaining consent

It is important to tell the patient why the test should be undertaken and how the result is likely to help. Its nature should be described in clear and simple terms before gaining consent for the test to be done. For the simpler tests, such as measurement of blood pressure (p. 77), verbal consent or implicit agreement is usually sufficient. Written consent is required if the procedure is complex, lengthy or risky. Consent forms are defined in the next section. If there is a refusal this must be recorded.[2] Some tests require special preparation, e.g. barium enema (p. 155), when it is advisable to give the patient an instruction sheet. He/she must also be told where the test is to be done, what time to attend and when the results will be available. In the case of certain tests, e.g. for HIV (AIDS, p. 201), special counselling is necessary, both at the time of testing and, particularly if positive, when the result becomes known. With any test, the meaning of the results should be explained, and reassurance given as to their significance.

Consent forms

The Department of Health has reviewed all previous consent forms and replaced them with the following:[3]

Consent form 1: Patient agreement to investigation and treatment, to be used where *the patient will be anaesthetized or sedated*. This form needs to be signed by the patient, a healthcare professional who has appropriate knowledge of the proposed procedure and, if relevant, by an interpreter. The term 'patient' includes children under 16 if they have 'sufficient understanding and intelligence to enable them to understand fully what is proposed'.

It includes procedures planned in advance, when patients are reminded that they may change their minds between giving consent and the actual procedure. If the patient withdraws consent, this is recorded on the form.

Consent form 2: Parental agreement to investigation or treatment for a child or young person, to be used for *children who are not considered competent* and where parents, or those who have parental responsibility, are agreeing to the procedure on their behalf. The child may also sign the back of the form if he/she wishes (but if sufficiently competent to fully understand the procedure, consent form 1 should be used).

Consent form 3: Patient/parental agreement for investigation or treatment, *where consciousness is not impaired*, to be used for procedures where the patient is expected to remain alert throughout and where an anaesthetist is not involved in their care.

Consent form 4: For adults who are *unable to consent* to investigation or treatment, to be used if a healthcare professional considers that a patient is unable to consent and that the proposed procedure is in the patient's best interests. The clinician is required to sign the form, giving reasons and taking final responsibility. There are also spaces for a relative, spouse or carer to sign.

About the consent form (new guidance for patients). This detailed leaflet tells patients about to undergo procedures what the healthcare professional should tell patients about a proposed procedure. It also contains questions that patients might wish to ask (including asking about the clinician's success rate for the said procedure or its alternatives).

Laboratory investigations

The following procedure for specimens and their accompanying request form is an essential part of each investigation.

Specimen labelling

Collect each specimen into the correct container and immediately label with the patient's full name, identifying particulars and date. A single forename and surname, as in 'Mary Jones', may not distinguish between two patients on the same ward. Any confusion, particularly concerning blood transfusion, can be fatal.

Send specimen to the laboratory without delay. Normally this should be early in the day.

Request for investigation

An appropriate request form must accompany each specimen and provide the following information:

- Patient's surname, forename, sex, age (or date of birth) and hospital registration number if available. The patient's address should also be given with all requests for blood grouping and cross-matching.
- Hospital and ward; or address and telephone number of practice or clinic. **NB:** If a patient moves to another ward, steps must be taken to ensure that the new ward is shown on the request form or that the laboratory is notified.
- Nature of specimen with date and time of collection.
- Examination required.
- Provisional diagnosis and clinical summary, with stress on information relevant to the investigation.
- Signature of clinician making request and date.

Requests should not be made by telephone except in dire emergency. In such emergency the patient's name must be spelt or lettered over the telephone. The telephone message must be confirmed by a request form (mandatory for blood transfusion requests).

Examination of tissue (histology)

Biopsy

A biopsy involves collecting some tissue from a patient for histological examination (cutting a thin section of the tissue and examining it under a microscope). This frequently enables a correct diagnosis to be made. It is of particular value in determining whether a tumour is malignant or not; the treatment to be adopted often depends on the result of the histological examination. The nature of the test must be explained to the patient and written consent obtained by the clinician undertaking the biopsy.

Refer to the following pages for details of different types of skin biopsy (p. 8), lymph node biopsy (p. 93), gastric biopsy (pp. 132–133), liver biopsy (p. 140), duodenal biopsy (p. 133), bladder biopsy cystoscopy, (p. 170) and breast biopsy (p. 195–196). After the lesion has been excised the tissue is placed in the container with at least ten times its volume of fixative (usually 10% formol saline, often buffered). Occasionally a fresh unfixed specimen is required, collected into a dry container. In either case the container is accurately labelled and sent, with a completed request form, to the histopathology laboratory. Samples of fixed tissue are dehydrated and mounted in a wax block from which thin sections are cut, stained and examined microscopically. A report is usually available in 24–48 hours, but may take longer.

Frozen section

A more rapid method is available using a freezing process which provides a result within 5–10 minutes. This method can be used during the course of an operation; for example, a portion of a tumour from the breast can be examined at the commencement of an operation, and on receipt of the report some minutes later the extent of the operation can be determined. The pathologist is notified in advance to ensure that he or she is available. The tissue for examination is placed in a dry container and sent to the histology laboratory as quickly as possible. Then the pathologist selects an appropriate small block of tissue. The technician freezes the tissue on to a holder (chuck). He then cuts sections using a microtome which are placed inside a refrigerated cabinet (cryostat). The sections are put on slides, stained rapidly and then examined by the pathologist, who telephones the result to the operating theatre. Frozen sections are also used to demonstrate fats (lipids) and enzymes which would be destroyed by the ordinary processing methods.

Needle biopsy

There are several types of needle biopsy: Trucut needle biopsy or Biopty gun; marrow puncture and fine needle aspiration.

Trucut or Biopty gun

The Trucut needle is large enough to provide a small cylinder of tissue for histology. The Biopty gun (Bard, Europe Div.) is similar but quicker and easier to use. The nature of the test must be explained to the patient and written consent obtained by the clinician undertaking the test. Biopsy procedure for the liver is described on p. 140. A similar technique is used for pleura (p. 75), kidney (p. 167), breast (p. 195) and spleen. When used for breast it can be painful, even with local anaesthetic. FNA (see below, p.5) is therefore often preferred.

Marrow puncture

The marrow puncture needle is strong enough to penetrate through cortical bone and provide samples of bone marrow (p. 93).

Fine needle aspiration (FNA)

Fine needle aspiration differs from the above in that the needle used is so fine that it causes little pain and so no local anaesthetic is required. Its simplicity and ready acceptance by patients, with the possibility of obtaining a diagnosis at first attendance, make it a valuable outpatient procedure. The technique used for breast lumps is described on p. 195.

Collection of blood sample

Blood samples are required for many laboratory tests, in microbiology (pp. 16–19), haematology (p. 89) and chemical pathology (p. 109). Finger-prick samples are collected by laboratory staff and venous samples by venepuncturists. Blood must be taken into the appropriate container for the test: a plain container for clotted blood; otherwise one with the right anticoagulant for the test, as given in this book or, if available, in the local laboratory handbook.

Collection of infected material

Details of the collection of infected material, including high risk specimens, are given on pp. 11–13.

Collection of other types of specimen

Collection of urine samples is described on p. 160 and cervical swabs on p. 197. For the collection of the many other types of specimen, see index or go to appropriate chapter.

Point of care testing (POCT), near patient testing (NPT) and quality control

The use of stick tests and special instruments has made a wide range of tests possible at the point of care (POCT), viz. in the ward, clinic side room, operating theatre, emergency room (ER) and general practitioner centre. There are two main applications of POCT: the acute clinical crisis, where speed of delivery is paramount, and chronic diseases, where POCT enables the clinician to monitor therapy and check compliance.[4] Examples are tests for sugar and ketones in urine (pp. 144–145), other abnormal substances in urine (pp. 161–163), blood sugar (p. 146), bilirubin (p. 138), urea (pp. 165–166), cholesterol (p. 110), triglycerides (p. 119), creatinine (p. 113), gammaglutamyl transferase (p. 117), aminotransferases (p. 116) and uric acid (p. 121). The term 'near patient testing' (NPT) has been used where tests of this type are carried out either in the patient's home or in a clinic, e.g. the detection of *H. pylori* antibodies in patients with dyspepsia[5] (p. 132), the assessment of C-reactive protein[6] (Nyocard) (p. 112) as a quick alternative to the ESR (p. 89) and the measurement of blood sugar (p. 118) in the control of diabetes mellitus.[7] It is clear that the terms POCT and NPT have a similar significance. Both provide a quick result while the patient waits. If necessary the treatment is then modified.

The value of such tests depends on the care with which they are performed and also on quality control. Even a carefully performed test is useless if the reagents are inactive. *Quality control* is needed to ensure that the reagents are working and that the instruments are reading correctly. For this, the laboratory can provide control samples to test the reagents and instruments on a regular daily basis. Without such control the results may be misleading and endanger a patient's health or life.

Reference

1. Roper, N, Logan, W W, Tierney, A J. *The Elements of Nursing*, 4th edn. New York. Churchill Livingstone. 1996.

2. UKCC. *Guidelines for professional practice*. London. United Kingdom Central Council for Nursing, Midwifery and Health Visiting. 1996.

3. Medical Defence Union. *News. The Journal of the MDU*. MDU, 230, Blackfriars Road, London. 2002: 18 (1, May): 4–5.

4. Price, C. Point of care testing: focusing on the patient. *Education in pathology*. London. Royal College of Pathologists. 2002: 117: 21.

5. Delaney, B C, Kenkre, J E, Hobbs, F D R. A whole blood near patient test for antibodies to *Helicobacter pylori;* effect on the management of dyspepsia in primary care. *Family Practice* 1995: 12: 263–264.

6. Kenkre, J E, Hobbs, F D R, Carter, Y H. Evaluation of a C-reactive protein assay (Nyocard) as a near patient test in primary care. Clin Rheumatol. 1994: 13: 359–360.

7. Grieve, R, Beech, R, Vincent, J, Mazurkiewicz, J. Near patient testing in the diabetes clinic: appraising the costs and outcomes. Health Technol Assess. 1997: 1: 39–45.

CHAPTER TWO

Tests related to the environment

Skin | Allergy | Infection | Temperature | Radiation | Imaging techniques

Index of tests	Page		
Abortus fever	16	Infected fluids	11
Abscesses	11	Influenza	13
AIDS	17	Kveim test	14
Air contamination	10	Late allergy (extrinsic allergic alveolitis)	9
Allergy	9	Legionnaire's disease	18
Antibiotic assay	12	Leptospira antibodies	18
Aspergillosis	17	Magnetic resonance imaging (MRI)	21
Bilharziasis	18	Microbiological tests on blood	16
Blanket contamination	10	Mantoux test	15
Blood cultures	16	Moniliasis	17
Blood tests for syphilis	18	MRSA	11
Blood tests used in allergy	9	Needle stick injuries	12
Brucellosis	16	Patch test	15
Candidiasis	17	Positron emission tomography (PET)	23
Casoni test	14	Primary atypical pneumonia antibodies	19
Cat-scratch fever test	14	Psittacosis	19
Coccidioidin test	14	Q fever	19
Coccidioidomycosis	17	Radiation monitoring and radioisotopes	22
Computerized tomography (CT) scan	21	Rickettsial infections	13
Cryptococcosis	17	Rubella antibodies	18
Diagnostic skin tests	14	Schick test	15
Diphtheria	15	Schistosomiasis	18
Discharges	11	Skin biopsy	8
Eye swabs	12	Skin fungal infections	13
Foreign bodies	21	Skin tests used in allergy	9
Fungal infections of skin	13	Staphylococcal antibodies	19
Gallium scanning	23	Sterility of dressings	10
German measles antibodies	18	Streptococcal ASO titre	18
Hepatitis	16	Swabs	11
High-risk specimens	12	Tests for infections	11
Histoplasmin test	14	Toxoplasma antibodies	19
Histoplasmosis	17	Transport media	11
Hydatid disease	18	Trichina antigen test	15
Imaging techniques	20	Trypanosomiasis	19
Immediate allergy	9	Tuberculin skin reactions	15
Infection	10	Typhoid	12

Index of tests	Page		
Ultrasound	20	Widal reaction for typhoid, etc.	16
Undulant fever	16	Wounds	11
Viral hepatitis	17	X-ray examinations	20
Virus infections	13		

Environment and the human body

The *skin* may suffer from its constant contact with the environment. Most tests on the skin are undertaken by the dermatologist, often with the help of the histopathologist. *Allergy* is due to certain substances in the environment to which some individuals are unduly sensitive; tests are performed by the dermatologist, the chest physician and the immunologist. *Infections* are caused by environmental exposure to microorganisms; freshly collected specimens are sent without delay to the microbiology laboratory, who may also be consulted concerning further appropriate tests and measures to be adopted to prevent spread of infection. *Temperature* is frequently the result of infection; its recording is often the responsibility of the nurse. *Radiation* is a potential environmental hazard, but it also provides the basis for many *imaging techniques* which are an essential part of much medical investigation; these are undertaken by the radiologist and radiographer.

Skin

The continuous contact between skin and environment is responsible for a number of its disorders.

Skin biopsy

This is of great value in the diagnosis of many skin diseases. The written consent of the patient must first be obtained, normally by the dermatologist who performs the procedure. An early untreated lesion is usually chosen. For all but the smallest biopsies 1% lidocaine (lignocaine) is injected round the biopsy site, after cleaning the skin with a topical antiseptic such as chlorhexidine (e.g. Hibitane). The excised biopsy material is placed in fixative provided by the local laboratory (e.g. 10% formol saline, often buffered). A plaster dressing is applied to the site after biopsy.

1. *Elliptical surgical biopsy* is one of the most commonly used techniques. Equipment required includes sterile disposable scalpel, eyeless needle with suture, needle-holder, fine-toothed forceps and scissors. A small lesion is totally excised in the ellipse of skin. If the lesion is large, the biopsy is taken at right angles to the margin and includes some normal skin.

2. *Punch biopsy* provides a small disc of skin about 5 mm in diameter. The punch is a small hollow cylinder with a cutting edge, usually attached to a plastic handle, often disposable.

3. *Curettage* with a sharp-edged disposable curette followed by cautery is often used for the treatment and confirmatory diagnosis of small lesions such as *viral warts, seborrhoeic* and *solar keratosis* and *basal cell carcinomas* ('rodent ulcers'). Although the material provided is fragmented, the pathologist is usually able to establish a diagnosis but cannot determine whether the lesion is completely removed.

4. *Shave biopsy* is obtained by shaving off the lesion flush with the surface of the skin, using a blade such as a No. 11 scalpel blade. Although it usually provides a satisfactory cosmetic result it often fails to remove the lesion completely and so recurrence is likely.

Allergy

Skin tests used in allergy

Allergy is a sensitivity to certain substances. Common conditions resulting from allergen exposure include *hay fever* and *contact dermatitis*.

Prick tests or *Scratch tests* are used to investigate *asthma*. Reagents are also available to test for *allergies* to some foods, animal hair and house dust mite. The reagents are applied to the forearm with a dropper and the skin gently pricked or scratched with a needle. A positive result shows within 20 minutes as a red weal and flare. False reactions are common. Precautions to avoid cross-infection are vital and resuscitation facilities must be available.

Patch tests are used for investigating *contact dermatitis*. Common allergens include nickel (in jewellery, watch buckles and coins), fragrance and chrome (in leathers and bricklayers' cement). The reagents are available as patches arranged along adhesive strips. The strips are applied to the back and the area examined at 48 hours and 96 hours. A positive result shows as redness or blisters at the site of a particular reagent. Lifestyle advice may help the patient avoid further exposure.

Blood tests used in allergy
Immediate allergy

About 5 ml of clotted blood is required. The main antibody involved is reaginic antibody (IgE). Serum levels may be estimated by PRIST (Paper RadioImmunoSorbent Test). Values greater than 80 may be demonstrated by RAST (Radio AllergoSorbent Test) against specific allergens such as house dust mite, pollens, fungi, etc. (see also Immunoglobulins, p. 118).

Late allergy (extrinsic allergic alveolitis)

About 5 ml of clotted blood is required. Diseases in which late allergy is involved include :

- *Farmer's lung* from the fungus *Micropolysporon faeni* in mouldy hay.
- *Birdhandler's lung* from the serum and droppings of pigeons, budgerigars and other such birds.
- *Humidifier fever* from *amoeba* in humidifier water.

Less common examples are :

- *Poultryhandler's lung* from chickens, ducks and geese.
- *Maltworker's lung* from *Aspergillus clavatus*.

- Late allergy to inhaled antigens is associated with precipitating antibodies, and these are detected by the 'double gel diffusion test' (see aspergillosis, p. 17).

Infection

Air contamination

The degree of air contamination by organisms can be measured by a slit sampler. This sucks in air at a controlled rate over a rotating blood agar plate. The organisms stick to the surface and after incubation the bacterial colonies are counted. It is becoming a standard method of checking the degree of air contamination in the ward and operating theatre.

Culture plates (settle plates), exposed to the air, are also used to determine the number of bacteria-carrying particles settling on the surface over a known time interval. By counting the number of colonies on the plates after incubation, the number of bacteria-carrying particles which have settled on a unit area in a given period can be estimated.

Sterility of dressings

Five tests are in common use to check whether an autoclave is functioning adequately.

1. *Spore strips* containing spores of *Bacillus stearothermophilius* can be inserted in the dressing pack prior to sterilization. At the completion of sterilization, the spare strip should be sterile when subsequently cultured in the laboratory.

2. A *small tube (Browne's tube)* containing a red liquid may be placed in a dressing pack prior to sterilization. Different tubes are used for different types of appliance. After sufficient time at the required temperature the liquid turns green. Amber ('caution') implies inadequate sterilization. Old tubes may change colour after inadequate heat exposure or even without any exposure to heat. So it is important to use only fresh tubes.

3. The *Bowie–Dick test* for high vacuum sterilization is frequently used. A batch of a dozen surgical towels is taken and to one of the central towels two strips of special tape (made by 3M, the Minnesota Mining and Manufacturing Co.) are stuck in the form of a St Andrew's cross. After sterilization the brown bands which develop on the tape must be present at the site of the intersection.

4. *Paper which changes colour*, e.g. Klintex autoclave test paper, is not so reliable but does provide evidence that the drum has been exposed to heat.

5. *Thermocouple.* The insertion of a thermocouple into the material being sterilized is a very reliable method of measuring the temperature. It is not convenient for the daily routine but should be used on commissioning a new autoclave, after repairs and also at regular intervals.

Blanket contamination

For this test sterile salt agar in a Petri dish is provided by the laboratory. Immediately before sampling, the cover of the Petri dish is removed. The base of the Petri dish containing the salt agar is inverted over the blanket. Six sweeps are made across the surface of the blanket. The edge of the Petri dish roughs up the blanket and any organisms tend to be brushed up on to the surface of the agar. The cover is replaced. The Petri dish is labelled and returned to the laboratory. The test, previously used to check blanket sterility, is now mainly used to detect whether a person is a carrier of staphylococci to the extent of contaminating the blankets.

Tests for infections

Blood tests used in the diagnosis of infections are described under microbiological tests on blood (p. 16).

Wounds, abscesses, discharges and infected fluids

Before starting treatment of a septic condition it is important to send a specimen of the infected material to the laboratory so that the causative organism may be identified and tested for sensitivity to antibacterial drugs. Pus should be collected into a sterile container, if present in sufficient quantity. If not, a *sterile swab* should be taken. Exceptionally, e.g. with discharges from *actinomycotic* sinuses, it may be necessary to send the dressings to the laboratory in an appropriate sterile receptacle. For *vaginal* and *urethral discharges* see p. 198, for *urinary infection* p. 163 and for *throat infections* p. 62. For *septicaemia*, blood cultures are required (p. 16). In *meningitis* the cerebrospinal fluid is examined (p. 30).

Staphylococcus aureus which has developed multiple resistance to antibiotics (MRSA, methicillin resistant *S. aureus*) requires special mention. It has become common and has caused a number of surgical units to be shut down. As with other types of staphylococci, it can be carried on skin, hair, clothing and other articles; the nasal cavity often acts as a reservoir. Nasal carriers may be detected by taking a nasal swab (see p. 62).

Type of swab to use

The swabs commonly used in most hospitals are (a) serum coated, (b) charcoal, (c) alginate and (d) commercial swabs. Serum coated cotton wool swabs are the ones generally used, e.g. for nasal, throat, wound, pus swabs, etc. Charcoal swabs are used for suspected *gonococcal* infection but must not be used for eye infections of the newborn (*ophthalmia neonatorum*) for which a platinum loop is usually used (see eye swabs, p. 12). Alginate swabs are used almost entirely for laryngeal swabs when *tuberculosis* is suspected. Many microorganisms die very quickly (especially gonococci and the anaerobic organisms, e.g. bacteroides, etc.) if they are allowed to dry or are exposed to air for more than a very short time. So transport medium should be used if any delay is anticipated. Commercial swabs, such as Transwab (Medical Wire and Equipment Co.) for aerobes and anaerobes, incorporate transport medium and charcoal, making them multipurpose swabs.

NB: It is better to send pus in a sterile container rather than swabs whenever possible. Similarly, a specimen of stool in a universal container is better than a stool swab.

Transport media

These should be used if there is a possibility of any delay between taking the specimen from the patient and sending it to the laboratory:

- virus transport medium
- Stuart's medium
- Trichomonas medium
- other transport media.

Virus transport medium is a balanced salt solution containing antibiotics used for throat swabs, mouth washings, etc. when virus infection is suspected. *Stuart's medium* is excellent for most bacteriological infections. It is a clear, thick fluid containing reducing substances to prevent anaerobic bacteria dying. *Trichomonas medium* is a dark brown fluid used for isolating trichomonas and candida (monilia) from vaginal swabs, etc. Other transport media include *cytomegalovirus (CMV) medium* which is similar to virus transport medium but contains a special sugar (sorbitol) and should be used when transporting urine or throat swabs for suspected CMV infections, mainly in infants. See also transport outfits for urine, p. 164.

High-risk specimens
When collecting or handling specimens from patients who are HIV-positive or hepatitis B antigen-positive or who have other transmissible infections, e.g. *MRSA* (see p. 11), *typhoid* or *bacillary dysentery*, take the following precautions. Protective clothing such as disposable gown and gloves should be worn. For a case of open *tuberculosis*, a mask should be worn. Do not squirt fluid through a fine needle as this produces an aerosol. Avoid spillage. Treat any spilt fluid immediately with strong hypochlorite, 2% activated glutaraldehyde, one of the chlorine-releasing agents or peroxygen compounds. Place specimen containers in individual plastic bags marked with coloured 'High-Risk' stickers. Put a similar sticker on the request form. Use sticky tape to seal the bags, not staples, ensuring that neither container nor bag can leak. Dispose of needles and syringes safely into 'sharps' boxes specially provided. Do not attempt to resheath needles (see needle stick injuries, below). Report any accident or mishap immediately.

NB: For highly infectious diseases, e.g. haemorrhagic virus diseases such as *Lassa fever*, some of the above recommendations may need to be modified in the light of the isolation unit's own code of practice.

Needle stick injuries
If the skin is accidentally punctured by a contaminated injection needle, the following actions should be taken. The wound must be made to bleed and washed with soap and water. *The subject must then report* to the occupational health or accident and emergency department, and *must also complete an incident form*.

Assay of antibacterial drugs
Occasionally it is of value to collect samples of blood or other fluids to estimate the level of antibacterial substances present; 5 ml of blood, or other fluid, should be collected into a sterile container. This procedure is necessary when testing new drugs. when the presence of kidney damage could lead to toxic blood levels, and when monitoring effectiveness of antibiotics during long periods of treatment for certain infections, e.g. *bacterial endocarditis*.

Eye swabs
These are taken prior to operations on the eye and also in cases of infections of the eye. It is best for the swab to be taken by the laboratory staff at the bedside. A platinum loop is used which is sterilized by flaming and then plunged into sterile saline. The upper lid is held firmly to prevent blinking and the lower lid everted. The swab is then taken from the conjunctiva over the lower anterior surface of the sclera.

It is most important that the swab does not touch the eyelids. Sutcliffe medium is inoculated with the swab and it is then spread directly onto a 'chocolate' blood agar plate, which is then incubated for 48 hours or more. If organisms such as *Staphylococcus aureus* or *beta-haemolytic Streptococcus* are present, any ophthalmic operation must be postponed until the infection is cleared.

Fungal infections of skin, including ringworm

Skin scrapings and damaged hairs from the affected area should be sent to the laboratory in a dry sterile container or folded matte black paper (available from the X-ray department), where the fungus can be identified by microscopy and culture.

Wood's glass is a coloured filter placed in front of an ultraviolet (UV) lamp, used sometimes in the diagnosis of *ringworm* or the confirmation of its cure. If the light is shone on to a suspected area, hairs affected by *ringworm* show up in a fluorescent manner. It is not an infallible test.

Virus and rickettsial infections

Viruses and rickettsiae can be isolated by culture, but more often their presence is inferred by the demonstration of increasing amounts of antibody in the patient's blood. In certain virus and rickettsial infections microscopy is of value in demonstrating inclusion bodies inside the patient's cells.

Culture

Viruses can be grown only in living tissue, usually in the form of a tissue culture or in the developing membranes of a chick embryo. They will not grow like bacteria in simple culture broths. *Poliomyelitis* virus, for example, can be isolated from faeces using a tissue culture of monkey kidney epithelium; *influenza* virus can be isolated in a chick embryo from throat washings of a patient. This is of great value in identifying the type of virus in an epidemic but is too slow for routine diagnosis.

Rickettsiae, such as that which causes *typhus* fever, can also be grown in a developing chick embryo, but are usually first isolated by inoculating the blood of a fresh case into the peritoneal cavity of a guinea pig.

Antibody demonstration

Two samples are required, each about 5 ml of clotted blood, the first early in the disease, the second late or during convalescence. The second sample shows at least a four-fold increase in titre of antibody against a particular virus or rickettsia if this has caused the disease. *This is the most widely used diagnostic method in virology.*

The blood from a patient with *typhus* contains antibody which agglutinates a strain of proteus (Weil–Felix reaction).

Microscopy

Viruses cannot be seen as separate particles by the ordinary microscope, only by the electron microscope. Rickettsiae are slightly larger and are just visible under the ordinary light microscope, especially if present in large numbers. In certain virus and rickettsial diseases, bodies visible under the ordinary microscope appear inside the cells and are known as inclusion bodies. They may be seen in smears from the eyelids in *acute trachoma* or in *swimming-pool conjunctivitis*, also in brain sections from dogs with *rabies*.

Electron microscopy

In some centres it is becoming a practical proposition to make a diagnosis of the type of virus causing an infection by recognition of its shape under the electron microscope. This is commonly performed on stool specimens to identify viruses causing infective diarrhoeas (see p. 156).

Diagnostic skin tests

In the following intradermal skin tests a positive result implies sensitivity to a particular protein, either from an infecting organism or else some other foreign protein. A test in which a positive result has a different implication is the Schick test, described on p. 15.

NB: Apart from tests for allergy (p. 9) and Tuberculin skin reactions (p. 15), diagnostic skin tests are now rarely used.

Casoni test

This is a test for hydatid disease. It is no longer performed in the United Kingdom.

Sterile hydatid fluid is injected intradermally. A weal occurring in 20 minutes is a positive response.

The test is positive in some 90% of cases of hydatid disease. It does, however, remain positive for many years after a hydatid cyst has been removed.

Cat-scratch fever test

Antigen prepared from an affected lymph node of a known case of this disease is obtainable (but not often available) from the Public Health Laboratory and 0.2 ml is injected intradermally. A positive result is a firm red area at least 1 cm in diameter appearing in 48 hours and persisting sometimes for several weeks. It implies present or previous *cat-scratch fever*. An alternative test for *cat-scratch fever* is lymph node biopsy (p. 93).

Coccidioidin test

Coccidioidin is the antigen prepared from the fungus *Coccidioides immitis* which causes *coccidioidomycosis*, and 0.2 ml of the antigen preparation is injected intradermally. A positive result is a firm red area at least 1 cm in diameter within 48–72 hours. It implies present or previous *coccidioidal infection*. See also p. 17.

Frei test for lymphogranuloma venereum

See p. 201.

Histoplasmin test

Histoplasmin is the antigen prepared from the fungus *Histoplasma capsulatum* which causes *histoplasmosis*. The skin test is performed as for coccidioidin (above). A positive result implies present or previous infection. See also p. 17.

Kveim test

This is a test for *sarcoidosis*. The Kveim antigen, available from the Public Health Laboratory, is injected intradermally. Several weeks later a small swelling appears at the site. A biopsy specimen of the swelling is taken into formalin for histology. In a positive result there are microscopic changes typical of *sarcoidosis*. This implies that the patient has *sarcoidosis*.

Trichina antigen test

This is a test for *trichiniolsis*, a condition in which the muscles are invaded by the larvae of a parasite, *Trichinella spiralis*. The test is carried out as for coccidioidin (above). A positive result implies that the patient has trichinosis. See also p. 19.

Tuberculin skin reactions

A positive tuberculin skin reaction indicates that the subject has at some time been infected by the tubercle bacillus. Although it is really a test for sensitivity to tuberculin, it is taken to indicate that the person has some degree of immunity against *tuberculosis*. It does not indicate whether or not active infection is present. A negative reaction indicates an absence of immunity to *tuberculosis*. This is usually because the person has not been exposed to *tuberculous infection* and is therefore susceptible; it may very occasionally be found in a person with active infection who is without any immunity.

Immunity may be conferred by inoculation with BCG (*bacille Calmette–Guérin*), a harmless form of the tubercle bacillus. If successful, the tuberculin reaction which was previously negative becomes positive within 6 weeks of immunization.

Mantoux test

This is the most reliable tuberculin skin reaction and the one in common use. A small quantity of tuberculin is injected intradermally, using old tuberculin or tuberculin purified protein derivative (PPD) in a dilution of 1 in 1000. An intradermal injection of 0.1 ml is given on the flexor surface of the forearm. Normal saline may be used as a control at another site. If the test is positive a red area appears at the site of injection, reaching its maximum at 48 hours. If no reaction occurs, the test is repeated using tuberculin diluted 1 in 100. In patients who may have active *tuberculous infection*, the first test should be done using tuberculin at a dilution of 1 in 10 000 to avoid the possibility of a serious general reaction. A variant of the Mantoux test is the multiple puncture technique (Heaf test). Instead of using a syringe, a special instrument with a number of points is used to introduce the tuberculin intradermally. Another alternative is the Tine test.

Patch test for tuberculin sensitivity

This is more convenient for babies, but is not so reliable and may give false negative reactions. A small patch containing tuberculin is stuck on the skin, usually on the back, for 48 hours. A control area is included in the patch. After 48 hours the result is read. A positive result is similar to that for the Mantoux test.

Diphtheria

Schick test

This test is used to ascertain whether a person is *susceptible* to diphtheria: 0.2 ml of the diluted diphtheria toxin, specially prepared for the Schick test, is injected intradermally into the flexor surface of the forearm. A control injection of heated toxin into the other arm is used as a comparison.

If in 24–48 hours there is a red area about 2.5 cm wide, the reaction is positive and the person is susceptible to diphtheria. If there is no red area, or if there is a slight reaction, equal in both arms, the test is negative and the person is not susceptible to diphtheria.

The test is also used in doubtful cases of diphtheria, the majority of such cases giving a positive test. Later in the disease the test becomes negative. The test is also of value in examination of persons who are contacts in a diphtheria epidemic: they may be thus divided into those who may develop the disease, and those who probably will not.

Persons found to be susceptible to diphtheria may be protected against it by means of immunizing injections. The latter are now given routinely to children, diphtheria immunization being a component of triple vaccination.

Microbiological tests on blood
Blood cultures
The circulating blood is normally sterile and any isolated organisms gaining entrance to the circulation are rapidly destroyed by the body's defences. In *bacteraemia*, living organisms are present in the bloodstream and in *septicaemia* they multiply. Septicaemia may be suspected in cases of septic illness with recurrent high temperature and rigors. The presence of bacteria in the bloodstream may be confirmed by blood culture, which should be taken *before giving any antibacterial drugs*.

For this purpose about 10 ml of blood are taken from a vein after the skin has been disinfected with 70% alcohol, e.g. Medi-Swab. The blood is transferred aseptically into bottles containing suitable broth culture media. These are then placed in an incubator for up to a fortnight or longer. Repeated cultures may have to be done to obtain a positive result in cases of *septicaemia*.

Blood cultures are especially useful in the diagnosis of *puerperal sepsis, endocarditis, typhoid fever* in the early stages, and all cases of *pyrexia* of undetermined origin.

1. **Widal reaction for typhoid and paratyphoid**
2. **Tests for brucellosis (abortus and undulant fevers)**

A person with any of the above infections usually develops corresponding antibodies 7–10 days after the onset of the disease. The antibodies are called agglutinins because of their ability to agglutinate or clump suspensions of bacteria causing the infection. The strength of the antibody increases during the disease. This rising titre is demonstrated by the increasing dilution of the patient's serum at which the antibody can be detected.

In people who have previously been vaccinated with TAB (killed organisms of typhoid, paratyphoid A and B) the corresponding antibodies will be found in the serum, but a rising titre on repeat test is strong evidence of active infection. In a suspected case of any of these diseases 5 ml of clotted blood are collected in a dry tube and sent to the laboratory, where the serum is tested as described.

The Vi test
This is a special type of agglutination test, used mainly to demonstrate the typhoid carrier state. Additional serological tests (antiglobulin and complement fixation tests) are useful in the diagnosis of *brucellosis*.

Other blood tests used in infections
Hepatitis B (serum hepatitis)
The 5 ml of clotted blood required must be collected with great care, preferably into a vacuum container, and the needle discarded safely (see p. 12). Laboratory tests are undertaken against antigen and antibody.

Antigen

The presence of surface (S) antigen and of core (e) antigen indicates infection by *hepatitis B* (an industrial disease). Blood containing the 'e' antigen is of high infectivity.

Antibody

Hepatitis B antibody in the blood (≥100 IU) is evidence of immunity. In the blood of a person inoculated against hepatitis B it indicates successful immunization. If present in the blood of a hepatitis patient it is evidence of recovery and of reduced infectivity. The mode of infection and time taken to develop antibodies are similar to *AIDS* (see p. 201), but the chances of infected material transmitting infection are about seven times greater for hepatitis than for AIDS.

Viral hepatitis A, C, D, E, etc.

Viruses for hepatitis A–E have already been identified, and screening for these is now part of routine microbiological testing. Collection of blood requires the precautions described above for hepatitis B. Epidemiology and other studies indicate the existence of several 'non-A–E' hepatitis agents, probably for hepatitis F and G and perhaps beyond.

Aspergillosis

About 5 ml of clotted blood is required. The demonstration of serum antibodies to the fungus *Aspergillus fumigatus* assists in the diagnosis. The patient's serum and antigens from *A. fumigatus* are allowed to diffuse towards each other in agar gel ('double gel diffusion'). A line of precipitation where the two meet indicates the presence of antibody to *A. fumigatus*. A positive result is of great value in interpreting the finding of fungus in the sputum, indicating infection and not just contamination. Heavy lines of precipitation distinguishes *aspergilloma* (a fungal ball) from *allergic bronchopulmonary aspergillosis*.

Candidiasis (moniliasis)

About 5 ml of clotted blood is required. Systemic *Candida albicans* infection may be diagnosed by the demonstration of antibodies in the patient's serum. The method used is agar gel diffusion as for *aspergillosis* (see above), using instead antigens from *Candida albicans*.

Coccidioidomycosis

About 5 ml of clotted blood is required. The demonstration of serum antibodies to the fungus *C. immitis* assists diagnosis. See also coccidioidin skin test (p. 14).

Cryptococcosis

About 5 ml of clotted blood is required. In the initial stages antibodies are detected against *Cryptococcus neoformans* cells by agglutination. Later *Cryptococcus* antigen may be detected in serum using latex particles coated with antibody. This test is more frequently carried out on cerebrospinal fluid.

Histoplasmosis

About 5 ml of clotted blood is required. The demonstration of serum antibodies to the fungus *Histoplasma capsulatum* assists in the diagnosis of this infection. See also histoplasmin skin test (p. 14).

Hydatid disease

About 5 ml of clotted blood is required. Immunological diagnosis of hydatid disease can be made by the demonstration of antibodies in the patient's serum.

Legionnaire's disease

About 5 ml of clotted blood is required. Antibodies to the causative organism, *Legionella pneumophila*, may not be demonstrable until 3–4 weeks after infection. During the acute phase the organism can be cultured from sputum, using a special type of agar medium.

Leptospira antibodies

About 10 ml of clotted blood is required. The patient's serum may be tested in three ways:

1. agglutination and lysis of live leptospira
2. agglutination of dead formalized leptospira
3. complement fixation test.

The tests become positive at about the tenth day in *Weil's disease* (due to *Leptospira icterohaemorrhagiae*) and infection by the dog leptospira (*L. canicola*).

Rubella (german measles) antibodies

About 5 ml of clotted blood is required. *Rubella infection* in the first three months of pregnancy can cause congenital abnormalities, e.g. heart disease in the fetus. So it is routine practice for blood to be sent for rubella antibody (and syphilis serology) testing at the first antenatal attendance of each pregnancy. An antibody level of at least 15 IU/ml indicates immunity. Less than 15 IU/ml indicates lack of immunity and the mother is warned of the danger to the fetus of exposure to *rubella*. A rising titre, associated with a corresponding IgM level (see p. 118) indicates active infection. *Rubella* during the first 3 months of pregnancy is considered to warrant therapeutic abortion.

Streptococcal ASO (antistreptolysin 'O') titre

About 5 ml of clotted blood is required. Patients infected with *Streptococcus haemolyticus* develop antibodies, particularly against the 'O' haemolysin, reaching their maximum 2–4 weeks after infection. An ASO titre of 200 or above implies recent streptococcal infection. Under the age of 5 years a lower titre may be significant. It is of value in determining the cause of *rheumatic fever, erythema nodosum, nephritis* and allied conditions in patients from whom Group A streptococci have not been recovered, e.g. because of antibiotic therapy. **NB:** ASO titres do not rise in every case, thus causing false-negative results. False-positive results can also occur due to cholesterol-like substances in the blood.

Schistosomiasis (bilharziasis)

About 5 ml of clotted blood is required. Demonstration of serum antibodies to schistosomes is of value in the diagnosis of chronic infections when microscopy of urine (see p. 165), faeces (see p. 157) and bladder tissue (see p. 170) has proved negative.

Staphylococcal antibodies

About 5 ml of clotted blood is required. Two antibody tests, anti-alpha-haemolysin and antileucocidin, especially the former, are of value in ascertaining whether hidden *staphylococcal infection* is present, e.g. *osteomyelitis.*

Toxoplasma antibodies

About 5 ml of clotted blood is required. Toxoplasma antibodies are usually detected by means of a dye test. The demonstration of an antibody indicates infection with toxoplasma, either present or past. Active infection may be inferred either from a high antibody titre of over 1/256 or from a rising titre when the test is repeated after an interval of 2 weeks. About a third of normal adults have a titre of 1/8 to 1/128, indicating past infection. Evidence of an active infection is also provided by the blood IgM (see p. 118).

Antibodies in primary atypical pneumonia

Most patients with primary atypical pneumonia develop antibodies which can be detected by a complement fixation test. The condition is often due to *Mycoplasma pneumoniae* but can also be caused by *influenza, psittacosis, Q fever* and *legionnaire's disease* (see also p. 18). Two samples of about 5 ml of clotted blood are required, one early in the disease and one late or during convalescence. A rising titre is diagnostic.

Antibody tests in other infectious diseases

Two 10 ml samples of clotted blood, one taken as early as possible during the disease and the second about a fortnight later, provide similar diagnostic information in many infectious diseases including *virus infections* (see p. 13) and many parasitic infections, e.g. *trypanosomiasis, cysticercosis, fascioliasis* (liver fluke), *filariasis, leishmaniasis* (including *kala-azar*) and *trichiniasis* (see also p. 15). Evidence of infection is also provided by IgM and IgG (p. 118).

Temperature

In most hospitals and clinics, temperatures are taken with an aural thermometer which is placed gently in the patient's external auditory meatus for a few seconds and registers the temperature automatically. It is more accurate, safer and easier to use than a mercury thermometer, particularly for young children. Taking an adult's temperature by means of a mercury clinical thermometer placed under the tongue usually presents no problems. An infant's temperature cannot be taken orally. Using a mercury thermometer in the axilla or groin takes about 8 minutes and tends to be very inaccurate, usually under-reading. Measuring the temperature rectally is far more reliable, takes only 1–3 minutes with a mercury thermometer (10–20 seconds with an electronic thermometer) and, if undertaken properly, carries very little risk. With the infant lying on its back, the nappy is undone, both ankles are firmly grasped in one hand so as to flex and abduct the hips, revealing the anus. With the other hand the examiner holds the thermometer between finger and thumb, 2–3 cm from the bulb. Lubricated with a little vaseline or K-Y jelly and held at about 30° to the horizontal, the bulb end of the thermometer is gently inserted for a minute or two, with the flexed legs held firmly in the other hand. Usually the infant is quite relaxed in this position, which is similar to that for nappy changing. The normal rectal temperature is 36.5–37.5 °C. After use the thermometer is washed, dried and disinfected, e.g. with a spirit swab.

Imaging techniques

X-ray examinations

The ability of X-rays to pass through skin and soft tissues is of considerable diagnostic value; damage to tissue has been minimized in modern equipment by greatly reducing the amount of radiation required. However, in view of the sensitivity of fetal tissues to radiation, X-ray examination of the female pelvis or abdomen should be avoided if pregnancy is a possibility (as in the second half of the menstrual cycle).

X-rays are invisible to the human eye but have the ability of exciting a fluorescent screen or acting on a photographing emulsion to produce a visible image on the screen or a permanent record on an X-ray film, the radiograph (*plain radiography*). Fluoroscopic screening enables organs to be visualized directly (*fluoroscopy*). This is chiefly of value for examining movements such as the act of swallowing and the peristalsis of the stomach.

X-rays can penetrate matter, and the penetration depends on the thickness and density of the parts examined. Thus bones will appear as dense opaque structures, soft tissues will be more transparent and air contained in the lungs or abdomen will be completely transparent. Breast screening for cancer is by means of *breast imaging* (see *mammography*, p. 194). Contrast media, which are radioopaque, can be introduced into various organs to make their outlines clearly visible on screen or radiograph. Barium sulphate emulsions taken by mouth or administered as an enema are used to opacify the gastrointestinal tract (*upper* and *lower GI contrast studies*). Iodine- containing solutions injected intravenously are excreted in the urine to outline the renal tracts (*intravenous urography*, p. 168). Similar solutions can be injected directly into veins, arteries (*angiography* or *vascular contrast studies*, pp. 83, 169) or by catheter into the heart to demonstrate its anatomy and function (*cardiac catheterization* or *angiocardiography*, pp. 83–84). The injection of various radioisotopes, e.g. technetium, enables organs such as the brain, bones, thyroid, liver and spleen to be defined by scanning (*nuclear medicine*). Modern apparatus is designed to reduce radiation to the patient while increasing the clarity of the image. Nevertheless X-rays do have harmful biological effects and excessive use should be avoided (see p. 22, radiation monitoring and pp. 189–190, placental and fetal monitoring).

Dental (including *paediatric dental*) radiographs play an important part in dental practice, e.g. in demonstrating unerupted teeth or the site of root infections (see teeth, p. 128).

Ultrasound (U/S)

Ultrasound is an alternative to X-rays which avoids the use of ionizing irradiation. High frequency sound waves, inaudible to the human ear, can penetrate tissue and outline internal organs. An image is produced on a TV screen and recorded on Polaroid film. Liver, gall bladder, spleen, kidneys, uterus and ovaries are much more clearly demonstrated by ultrasound than by straight X-ray. Ultrasound has virtually replaced X-rays for examination of the abdomen and pelvis during pregnancy (*obstetric U/S* p. 190).

Computerized tomography (CT) scan (CAT scan)

Another important development which provides detailed images of the inside of the skull and also of the whole body is computerized tomography (CT) scan (**Fig. 2.1**). This provides an X-ray image of a transverse slice through the patient at any required level in the body (*CT body*). This can be used to define the extent of a tumour, for example in the chest (p. 84), in the abdomen (p. 151) or lesions affecting the spinal cord or the brain (p. 38). It is also used to provide high-resolution, three-dimensional images of soft tissues, joints and fractures (p. 176).

Magnetic resonance imaging (MRI)

This is an imaging technique which enables a picture of the internal organs of the body to be constructed by computer, using magnetic resonance information generated by powerful magnetic fields. It has the great advantage over X-rays that, like ultrasound, it involves no radiation exposure and requires no preparation of the patient, apart from explaining the procedure. Although the equipment is expensive, many centres have access to MRI for appropriate cases. See also brain and spinal cord scans p. 38, pituitary gland p. 56, and soft tissues p. 176.

Foreign bodies

The diagnostic value of X-rays and the patient preparation required are described in the appropriate sections. It is, however, convenient to consider foreign bodies here since they can affect any organ in the body. They can be demonstrated radiologically if opaque to X-rays. If non-opaque, ultrasound or magnetic resonance (see above) may be used. Methods of X-ray examination include:

1. Straight radiographs.
2. Stereoradiography. The stereoscope is an instrument whereby two X-ray photographs taken from slightly different positions enable a three-dimensional X-ray picture to be obtained. This procedure may help in the localization of a foreign body.

Fig. 2.1   Computerized tomography scanner.

3. Sinogram. In some cases contrast medium may be injected down a chronic sinus and an X-ray examination carried out to ascertain its extent.
4. Computerized tomography (CT scan, see p. 21). This is being used more frequently as the equipment required becomes more readily available in hospitals.

Alimentary tract
Articles may be swallowed by children or adults. If by adults it may be by accident or by intention (attempted suicide and in mental disorders). Such articles may be coins, portions of dentures, pieces of bone, buttons, pins, safety-pins, cutlery, buckles, etc.

The size of the article may indicate whether removal is advisable or not. If there is a probability of the object passing through the alimentary tract without injury, a series of radiographs can be taken to follow its progress.

Foreign bodies may also be introduced into the rectum occasionally.

Aural and nasal cavities
Foreign bodies may be introduced here by children. An X-ray may be advisable in some cases of chronic discharge.

Respiratory system
Small foreign bodies which are inhaled may pass into the larynx and thence to the bronchi. Such articles may be teeth, portions of dentures, small beads, fragments of toys, etc. X-ray examination may localize the object prior to bronchoscopy.

Urogenital system
Foreign bodies may be introduced into the bladders of children and occasionally of adult females.

Radiation monitoring
The use of X-rays and radioactive substances in hospitals is rigidly controlled. Radiation safety is the responsibility of the hospital manager but almost invariably he or she has a radiation protection adviser (a physicist) and departmental radiation protection supervisors.

Radiology departments
Within the departments the radiologists and radiographers are responsible for patients and staff. Patients who have received an X-ray examination or treatment are no radiation hazard to anyone.

Radioisotopes
Most radioisotopes used in medical diagnosis have a short half-life (they disappear quickly) and so they present no hazard after the day of administration. With a few simple precautions and common sense they need not present any danger to hospital workers, the tests being performed in the department of nuclear medicine. When discussing matters with patients who have recently received radioisotopes nurses should not stay too close to their patients; for example, they should talk to them holding the foot of the bed and should not lean over their bodies in a display of concern. The administration of radioactive substances can only be undertaken by a doctor holding a DHSS certificate authorizing him to do so. This doctor is responsible for explaining the nature of the test to the patient before obtaining the patient's written permission for the test to be done. There must also be a clearly defined drill of precautions to be

taken in the event of an incident such as spillage. This drill should be in writing, readily available, preferably displayed, and should include the telephone number of the local department of medical physics.

The main rule that all staff should follow is not to contaminate themselves. Impermeable gloves and aprons should be worn. Disposable paper towels (not expensive cotton ones) should be used. Depending on the level of activity, they can be disposed of via the normal sluice or stored for disposal. Advice on this is available from the department of medical physics or the radiographer concerned.

Following the administration of most radioisotopes an appreciable fraction of the dose given is excreted in the urine. So, if bedpans are handled, gloves and aprons must be worn. Toilets should be checked to ensure that the patients have been adequately careful with their personal hygiene. If the workload is sufficiently high, those responsible may, in some instances, consider it desirable for nurses to wear personal monitors or personal dosimeters. These are usually films in special badges but sometimes they are delicate electronic instruments. They are worn either on the lapels or at waist (gonadal) level.

In only a few cases is it cost-effective to supply wards with contamination monitors. These are usually instruments held in departments of medical physics and based on either Geiger or scintillation counters. They give a visible and audible indication of the amount of contamination present. There will always be a few clicks because there is and always has been radiation in the environment. The regulations specify the contamination levels at which various decontamination procedures should be undertaken and what precautions to take. Again the physicist can help if there is any problem. See also radioactive iodine tests (p. 47)

Gallium scanning

Using a tracer dose of the radioisotope gallium it is possible to detect foci of infection and also several different types of tumour. These include *lymphoma, hepatoma* and *carcinomas of gut, kidney, uterus and testis.* Prior to the test it is desirable to give a laxative or enema to reduce gallium uptake by the bowel. At 4–6 hours after the gallium injection the patient has a whole-body scan in the department of nuclear medicine, where the technologist passes a radionuclide detector slowly over the body, usually with additional scans at 24, 48 and 72 hours. The test is contraindicated by pregnancy, because of the risk of damaging the fetus.[1]

Positron emission tomography (PET, PET scan)

The number of centres at which PET is available is increasing throughout the world. It can detect and localize small foci of tissue abnormality such as tumour or infarction (p. 39), often not demonstrable by other methods.[2] It is also being used to elucidate the abnormal brain function in conditions such as *Parkinson's disease* and *schizophrenia,*[3] and to assess the effect of drugs on various tissues. The patient is given a small dose of the radioactive substance appropriate to the tissue under investigation. This emits positrons from the relevant site and these in turn cause gamma rays to be emitted. The site of emission is pinpointed by using an array of detectors outside the body. PET is at present very expensive because of the cost of equipment and staff training involved, but it is becoming an important diagnostic tool.[2] Like gallium scanning (above), it is contraindicated by pregnancy.

Reference

1. Pagana, K D, Pagana, T J. Gallium scan. In: Pagana, K D, Pagana, T J (eds). *Mosby's Diagnostic and Laboratory Test Reference*. St Louis. Mosby Year Book. 1992: 360–361.

2. Pagana, K D, Pagana, T J. Positron-emission tomography. In: Pagana, K D, Pagana, T J (eds). *Mosby's Diagnostic and Laboratory Test Reference*. St Louis. Mosby Year Book. 1992: 575–577.

3. Grasby, P M. Imaging the neurochemical brain in health and disease. *Clinical medicine*, Journal of the Royal College of Physicians of London. London. Royal College of Physicians. 2002: 2 (1): 67–73.

CHAPTER THREE

Tests related to communicating (1)

Speech | Hearing | Neuromuscular system

Index of tests	Page		
Abdominal reflex	35	Magnetic resonance imaging (MRI)	38
Adult mental function	41	Malingering	36
Angiography	39	Meningeal irritation	30
Articulation disturbance	26	Mental age	41
Audiometry	29	Muscle power	40
Auditory nerve	34	Muscular electrical reactions	40
Brain biopsy and smear	40	Myelography	40
Brain scans	38	Nerve conduction	40
Cerebrospinal fluid examination	30	Oculomotor nerves	33
Cisternal puncture	31	Olfactory nerve	33
Clonus response	35	Optic discs	33
Colour tests	27	Optic nerve	33
Computerized tomography (CT) scan	38	Otoscopy	29
Coordination	35	Pain sensation	36, 37
Corneal reflex	34	Palatal reflex	35
Cranial nerves	33	Patella clonus	35
Deep reflexes	35	Perimeter or field analyser tests	28
Developmental screening tests	41	Plantar reflex	35
Discrimination sense	36	Position sense	36
Distraction tests	29	Psychometry	41
Electrical response audiometry	30	Pupil reflexes	33
Electroencephalography	38	Reflex actions	34
Electromyography	41	Refraction tests	28
Encephalography	39	Rinne's test	29
Facial nerve	33	Semicircular canal tests	34
Glossopharyngeal nerve	34	Sensation	36
Griffiths tests	41	Sight tests	27
Hearing tests	29	Spinal accessory nerve	34
Heat and cold sensation	36	Spinal reflexes	35
Intelligence quotient (IQ)	41	Stanford–Binet tests	41
Intraocular pressure	29	Superficial reflexes	34
Knee jerk	35	Tendon reflexes	35
Language disturbance	26	Test types	28
Laryngoscopy	27	Touch sensation	36
Lumbar puncture	30	Trigeminal nerve	33

Index of tests	Page		
Vagus nerve	34	Vibration sense	36
Ventriculography	40	Voice assessment	26
Vestibular tests	34		

Introduction

Communication involves speech, sight, hearing and the neuromuscular system. Ability to understand is affected by mental development. Speech tests are mainly carried out by the speech therapist; laryngoscopy, rhinoscopy and hearing tests by the ENT surgeon; most tests on the neuromuscular system by the neurologist; mental development tests by the medical psychologist; and imaging by the radiologist. In many tests the cooperation of the patient is essential and the nurse plays an important part in achieving this.

Speech

Speech tests

Disturbances of speech can be divided into those affecting language, voice and articulation.

Tests for language disturbance

Language disturbance includes dysphasia and aphasia. Tests are used by speech therapists to assess what kind of language dysfunction exists, e.g. whether of comprehension (receptive) or of expression (expressive or executive) or both (global or mixed). Ability to read, write and calculate is also tested. There are also language attainment tests for children, e.g. Peabody and English vocabulary scales.

Voice assessment

At the present time this is generally assessed by auditory perception, which is necessarily subjective. If an abnormality is suspected the patient is referred to an ENT specialist, e.g. for rhinoscopy (p. 61), otoscopy (p. 29), and laryngoscopy (p. 27).

Tests for the disturbance of articulation

Defects of articulation take the form of distortions, substitutions, omissions and transpositions of sounds. They may be caused by:

- Neuromuscular disturbance (dysarthria), detected by neurological examination
- Structural defect such as cleft palate, detected by examination of the oral cavity
- Mental deficiency, detected by developmental screening tests (p. 41)
- Emotional disturbance, usually detected by case history
- Imitation of speech, also usually detected by case history
- Hearing loss, detected by screening tests and audiometry (pp. 29–30).

In order to assess articulation in children an articulation attainment test (e.g. Renfrew) may be used.

Laryngoscopy

Examination of the larynx may be carried out in three ways:

1. Indirect laryngoscopy, using a mirror
2. Using a modern rigid or flexible laryngoscope
3. Direct laryngoscopy, using rigid instruments with the patient's neck extended.

Indirect laryngoscopy

The patient is seated on a chair in a darkened room. A beam of light is directed from a reflecting mirror on the operator's forehead into the patient's mouth. The laryngeal mirror is warmed to prevent condensation, care being taken that it does not burn the patient. This is introduced into the mouth just beneath the uvula and adjusted so that the epiglottis and larynx can be viewed. It is chiefly of value for examining the vocal cords for paralysis, infections and growths.

Rigid or flexible laryngoscope

A rigid Hopkins Rod with a 70° or a 90° viewing angle and built-in illumination can be held in the mouth instead of a mirror. It provides a more close-up view than a mirror. Alternatively, the larynx may be examined with a flexible fibreoptic nasolaryngoscope (shorter and thinner than a fibreoptic bronchoscope); this is passed through the nose, after the latter has been anaesthetized with a 5% cocaine spray, to project beyond the end of the soft palate so that it provides a clear view of the larynx.

Direct laryngoscopy

A laryngoscope fitted with light is introduced over the back of the tongue, with the patient's neck extended over a pillow. A direct view of the larynx can be obtained in this way. This method is most commonly used by anaesthetists introducing laryngeal tubes during anaesthesia. For a more thorough examination, after the patient is anaesthetized, a rigid laryngoscope (like a straight hollow tube) allows direct inspection of the larynx, with the operating microscope if required. If a *tumour* is suspected a laryngeal biopsy may be performed: a small portion of tissue is collected from the lesion using laryngeal biopsy forceps, placed in a container with at least ten times its volume of 10% formol saline and sent with completed request form to the histopathology laboratory. A report on the type of lesion present (e.g. tumour or inflammation) will ideally be received by the ward within 24–48 hours.

Sight

Sight tests

Before eyesight tests are performed the eyes should be carefully examined, using an ophthalmoscope (see optic discs, p. 33).

Colour tests

Colour blindness is tested by using Ishihara charts. These are composed of coloured dots arranged in such a way that the numbers visible in the patterns are altered by colour blindness. This condition is much commoner in men than women, affecting one man in eight.

Perimeter or field analyser tests

A perimeter is a fixed upright to which is attached a movable curved arm on which objects can be moved to test lateral vision. In certain ocular diseases and *cerebral tumours* the visual fields are considerably diminished. This is a routine test in cases of *cerebral tumour*, and the results are recorded in the form of a circle (**Fig. 3.1a,b**). The irregular shaded portion shows average normal vision. The unshaded central portion shows extent of vision in a particular case, with greatly restricted visual fields due to a *pituitary tumour*. The visual fields are now often measured by ophthalmologists and opticians using a field analyser. Its principle is similar to the perimeter but it is more sophisticated and easier to use.

Refraction tests

In certain types of eye, vision is defective because the lens cannot correctly focus an image on the retina. This is corrected by means of glasses. In refraction tests various types of lens are used until the right combination to give optimum vision is found. Refraction tests are carried out by opticians and ophthalmologists.

Test types

A common test of vision is that of 'test types'. This consists of a white card on which are printed black letters of varying size – a large letter at the top and letters in rows of decreasing sizes underneath. The top large letter should be readable at a distance of 60 metres, the second row at 36 metres, and so on to the seventh row, which should be readable at 6 metres. The patient is placed at a distance of 6 metres from the card and has to read off as many lines as possible with each eye in turn. The result is expressed as 6/6, 6/36, 6/60, etc.:

6/6.   Normal vision

6/36. Patient can only read at 6 metres what he should read at 36

6/60. Patient can only read at 6 metres what he should read at 60.

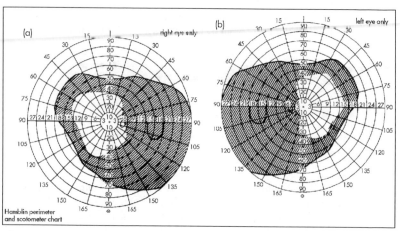

Fig. 3.1 Perimeter test: (a) right, (b) left

Intraocular pressure

Pressure within the eyeball is most conveniently measured by a Tonometer, using the indirect method. The instrument emits a small jet of air against the eyeball and measures the degree of corneal indentation, from which the intraocular pressure is determined. The raised pressure characteristic of *glaucoma* can thus be detected at an early stage, enabling it to be treated before vision deteriorates or any symptoms occur. This can now be undertaken by opticians at the time of an eye test for spectacles, when the retina is also examined for any abnormalities (see optic discs, p. 33).

Eye swabs

See page 12.

Hearing

Hearing tests

Distraction tests

Health visitors test the hearing of every 9-month-old baby as part of their development assessment. The baby sits on the parent's knee facing the 'distracter' who quietly plays with a toy to hold the baby's attention. The tester presents a sound (rattle or warble tones) from one side and out of the baby's field of view. A positive result is when the baby turns its head to find the sound stimulus. By repeating the test from alternate sides, with progressively quieter sounds of different frequencies, the hearing threshold of a normal baby can be quickly assessed. A normal baby responds to sound as quiet as a whisper (35 dB).

Clinical tests

Voice tests, from loud voice to whisper, and tuning fork tests (Rinne and Weber) give a rough guide to the hearing threshold.

Rinne's test

A tuning-fork is struck and is held to the external auditory meatus. When the patient ceases to hear it, it is placed on the mastoid process and the patient indicates if he can hear it. Normally he cannot, but in *middle-ear deafness* he can.

Weber's test

This is a comparison of the bone conduction of the two ears. A tuning fork is struck, and placed on the vertex of the skull, and the patient indicates in which ear he hears it louder. In *middle-ear deafness*, it is louder in the affected ear; in *nerve deafness* it is fainter.

Audiometry

The accurate assessment of hearing (audiometry) is usually carried out in an otolaryngology (ENT) department. The first step is careful examination of the external ears (otoscopy). Most people over the age of 5 years can perform a pure tone audiogram.

Otoscopy

The eardrum and external auditory meatus can be examined with an electric auriscope or else with an aural speculum, head mirror and lamp. Using either, the auricle (ear) is pulled gently backwards and upwards before inserting the speculum. It may be necessary to remove wax from the ears before audiometry can be performed.

Audiometric tests

Hearing is assessed accurately by an audiometer, an electrical apparatus enabling sounds of varying intensity and pitch to be applied to each ear. The result, expressed on a graph as an audiogram, indicates the degree and type of any hearing loss that may be present. A normal adult can hear sounds quieter than a whisper (20 dB).

Objective tests

Electrical response audiometry (ERA), electrocochleography (ECOcG), brainstem response audiometry (BERA, BSER) and cortical evoked response audiometry (CERA) are performed by measuring the electrical responses from different parts of the hearing pathway: from cochlea, brainstem and auditory cortex, allowing assessment of hearing threshold without the patient having to make a subjective response. A population screening programme to detect deafness in the newborn is being introduced.

The neuromuscular system

Tests for meningeal irritation

Neck rigidity

With the hand placed behind the patient's head the neck can normally be flexed until the chin touches the sternum. Flexion of the neck is greatly limited in meningeal irritation.

Kernig's sign

The patient lies flat on his back on the bed and the thigh is flexed. An attempt is then made to straighten the leg by extending the knee. Normally this can be carried out, but in meningeal irritation the muscles of the thigh pass into a state of contraction and that leg cannot be extended. The above tests are positive in the majority of cases of *meningitis*, in *subarachnoid haemorrhage* and in *meningism*.

Examination of cerebrospinal fluid (CSF)

The examination of cerebrospinal fluid is an essential part of the investigation of many diseases of the nervous system, including possible subarachnoid haemorrhage when the CT scan (see p. 38) is normal. It may also be used to lower the pressure in benign intracranial hypertension. About 5 ml are required for complete examination, 1 ml being placed in a fluoride tube for glucose estimation. The fluid is obtained by lumbar puncture.

Lumbar puncture (LP)

For this procedure the nurse prepares a sterile trolley containing towels, swabs, spirit, iodine, local anaesthetic with syringe and needles and the lumbar puncture instruments from an LP pack provided by the CSSD. Underneath the trolley there should be four sterile universal containers numbered 1–4 and a glucose vial for CSF. The patient should be lying on his side with the knees and chin closely approximated. Both the head and buttocks should be at the same level. The puncture is usually made between the spines of the 3rd and 4th lumbar vertebrae after cleaning and anaesthetizing the skin.

Pressure of cerebrospinal fluid

This is estimated by a manometer, which is a calibrated glass tube, attached to the lumbar puncture needle by means of a rubber tube. The height of the fluid in the tube above the level of the needle gives the pressure of the cerebrospinal fluid. Normally this pressure is 75–150 mm of cerebrospinal fluid and is affected by pulse and respiration. Pressure significantly above 150 mm indicates an increased intracranial pressure, often due to *cerebral tumour* or *infection*.

The estimation of the pressure by observing the rate of flow through the lumbar puncture needle is not reliable.

Queckenstedt's test

Compression of both jugular veins with the manometer in position causes a sharp rise in the cerebrospinal fluid pressure, followed by a sharp fall when the pressure is released. Coughing produces a similar rise and fall. When the flow of the cerebrospinal fluid is obstructed, for instance by a *spinal tumour*, this rise and fall is diminished in amount and rate. Where the obstruction is complete, no rise occurs.

NB: This test must not be used if there is raised intracranial pressure.

Cisternal puncture

In cases where lumbar puncture is not practicable, cerebrospinal fluid can be obtained by cisternal puncture.

The back of the patient's neck should be shaved and full aseptic precautions are necessary as for lumbar puncture. The patient is seated with the head well flexed and held by an assistant. The skin is anaesthetized and a lumbar puncture needle is introduced through the foramen magnum into the cisterna magna. This method is used in cases of *complete spinal block*.

Routine investigation of CSF

Normally the cerebrospinal fluid is clear and colourless. A yellowish tinge of the fluid (xanthochromia) is suggestive of *haemorrhage* or *spinal block*.

Coagulum on standing

This occurs in *meningitis* (*tuberculous, syphilitic* or *septic*). Massive clotting takes place in *spinal block* (Froin's syndrome), due to the great increase in protein.

Presence of blood

If blood is present at the commencement of the flow and later disappears, it is often due to the accidental injury of a blood vessel by the needle. If blood is mixed with the fluid throughout the whole specimen, it is suggestive of *haemorrhage into the cerebrospinal space*, e.g. *subarachnoid haemorrhage*.

Turbidity

This may be due to pus, blood or bacteria.

Cells

The number of cells is counted in a counting chamber under the microscope. As Table 3.1 indicates, the number normally present is 0–5 per mm^3. In syphilitic conditions the number is from 10 to 100 per mm^3. In *tuberculous meningitis* the number is from 20 to 400, mainly lymphocytes. In *pyogenic meningitis* large numbers are present, up to 2000 or more, mainly polymorphs. The presence of excessive numbers of cells in the cerebrospinal fluid with neighbouring septic conditions (e.g. mastoiditis) indicates the possibility of the onset of *septic meningitis*.

Bacteria

These are present in meningitis. They are detected by stained film and culture: meningococci in *cerebrospinal meningitis*; tubercle bacilli in *tuberculous meningitis; other organisms in septic meningitis*, e.g. pneumococci, streptococci and *H. influenzae*.

Chloride

This is normally 120–130 mmol/litre (120–130 mEq/litre). The chloride is normal in early *tuberculous* and *pyogenic meningitis*, only becoming reduced late in the disease (see Table 3.1).

Glucose

This is normally 2.8–5.0 mmol/litre (50–90 mg/100 ml). It is greatly reduced in *meningococcal* and *septic (pyogenic) meningitis*. It is less reduced in *tuberculous meningitis* (under 2.8 mmol/litre) (see Table 3.1).

Lactate

This is normally 1–2 mmol/litre. It is raised in *bacterial meningitis* but usually normal in *viral meningitis*. In cases of meningitis, values <3.5 mmol/litre are indicative of bacterial infection and values of >3.0 mmol/litre of viral infection. It is more reliable than glucose and protein at differentiating between *bacterial* and *viral meningitis*. Rapid measurement of lactate is of particular value when diagnosis is difficult, e.g. in partially treated cases of bacterial infection when the bacteria cannot be demonstrated, or in early *viral meningitis* when there may be a predominance of polymorphs.[1]

Protein

This is normally 200–400 mg/litre (20–40 mg/100 ml) of cerebrospinal fluid. It is raised in many diseases of the central nervous system, especially so in *tumours* and *infections* of all kinds (see Table 3.1, below).

Test for cryptococcal infection

It is possible to detect cryptococci in the CSF by direct microscopy. The presence of cryptococcal antigen (see p. 17) also indicates infection of the central nervous system by this organism.

Tests for syphilis

The VDRL and TPHA (see p. 200) are frequently carried out.

Drug concentration

See assay of antibacterial drugs, p. 12.

Table 3.1 CSF findings

	Cells per mm³	Chlorides mmol/litre	Protein g/litre	Glucose mmol/litre
Normal	0–5	120–130	0.2–0.4	2.8–5.0
General paralysis	10–100	Normal	Up to 1.0	Normal
Cerebrospinal syphilis	10–100	Normal	Slightly increased	Normal
Tuberculous meningitis	Up to 400	85–110	Up to 2.5	0.5–2.8
Pyogenic meningitis	Up to 2000	110–120	Up to 5.0	0–1.4
Tabes dorsalis	0–10	Normal	Slightly increased	Normal
Multiple sclerosis	0–10	Normal	Slightly increased	Normal

Examination of cranial nerves

In certain diseases of the central nervous system, e.g. *cerebral tumour* and other conditions, it is necessary to test the various cranial nerves to see if they are functioning normally.

1st, olfactory

Small bottles are used containing articles with a powerful smell, e.g. scent, peppermint, etc.

2nd, optic

Part of the optic nerve, the optic disc, can be viewed directly. Vision can be tested for colour, extent of field (perimetry) (p. 28) and acuity (refraction test and test types, p. 28). Pupil reflexes (see below) also involve the optic nerve.

Optic discs

The optic disc is the only part of the nervous system which is visible on clinical examination. An ophthalmoscope is required to view the interior of the eye and the examination is rendered easier by darkness.

Raised intracranial pressure causes swelling of the optic disc (papilloedema). *Hypertension* and *diabetes mellitus* cause distinctive changes in the retinal blood vessels, which may be associated with retinal exudate and small haemorrhages as the severity of the condition increases.

Pupil reflexes

Reaction to light

If a light is flashed in the eye the pupil will contract. A similar reaction is given if the eye is covered and then uncovered.

Reaction to accommodation

The patient is asked to look at a distant object, and then to look immediately at an object held just in front of his nose. Normally the pupil will contract on looking at the nearer object. Variations in the pupil reflexes take place in diseases of the central nervous system, especially space-occupying lesions in the skull.

3rd, 4th and 6th, oculomotor nerves

These are responsible for the movements of the eyeball. If paralysed, there is defective movement of the eyeball on following the movement of a finger, also a squint and double vision (diplopia) at certain angles. When the 3rd nerve is affected, ptosis or drooping of the eyelid is also present.

5th, trigeminal

This supplies sensation to the face and also supplies muscles of mastication. Its function is tested by (a) testing the face for loss of sensation; and (b) asking the patient to clench his teeth while one's hands are held over the muscles of the jaw – any lack of muscular contraction can then be felt.

7th, facial

This supplies the muscles of the face and if paralysed as in Bell's palsy, there is a distinct difference between the two sides of the face when a muscular movement is attempted, e.g. whistling, shutting the eyes tightly, showing the teeth.

8th, auditory

This nerve transmits information (a) for hearing, from the inner ear (cochlea), and (b) for balance, from the semicircular canals (vestibular apparatus).

Hearing

Simple hearing tests are described on p. 29. More accurate assessment is by audiometry (pp. 29–30).

Vestibular (semicircular canal) tests

Of these the caloric test is most often used. Tap water at 30°C is allowed to flow against the eardrum from an irrigation can 30 cm above the patient's head. A stopwatch is used to time the nystagmus (jerking movement of the eyes). It is repeated with water at 44°C. Abnormal responses are seen in *Ménière's syndrome* and in diseases of the 8th nerve and brain.

9th, glossopharyngeal

This supplies the posterior third of the tongue and the mucous membrane of the pharynx. It is tested by (a) taste sensation of posterior part of tongue, e.g. to bitters and (b) tickling the pharynx to see if the 'gag' reflex is present.

If the 9th nerve is paralysed, other nerves are usually affected.

10th, vagus

This supplies the palate, pharynx, larynx, heart and abdominal contents.

It is tested by (a) noting any deviation of the soft palate, (b) pronunciation of certain words requiring full use of nasopharynx, e.g. tub, egg, etc., and (c) observation of paralysis of the larynx through a laryngoscope.

One branch, the recurrent laryngeal, has a course in the upper part of the thorax, and the larynx may be paralysed in cases of *mediastinal tumour, aneurysm*, etc.

11th, spinal accessory

This supplies some of the muscles acting on the shoulder joint. If paralysed, the patient is unable to shrug the shoulder on the affected side.

This nerve may be damaged in extensive operations on the neck or by skull fracture.

12th, hypoglossal

This supplies the muscles of the tongue. The patient is asked to put his tongue out. If the right hypoglossal nerve is paralysed the tongue will be pushed over to the right. This might be caused by a *wound, tumour* or *carotid aneurysm*.

Reflex actions

A reflex action is an involuntary response to an external stimulus. The stimulus may be either superficial, e.g. stroking the skin, or deep, e.g. striking a tendon. Changes in the normal response take place in various diseased conditions of the central nervous system: the reflex may be absent, exaggerated or altered.

Some of the commoner reflexes will be mentioned.

Superficial reflexes

Corneal reflex

If the conjunctiva is touched, a reflex closure of the eyelids is produced. This reflex is used in estimating the degree of anaesthesia or unconsciousness.

Palatal reflex

On touching the soft palate it is elevated. This reflex is often absent in hysterical conditions.

Abdominal reflex

The skin of the abdominal wall is stroked, and this is followed by a contraction of the abdominal muscles.

Plantar reflex

The patient should be lying down with the muscles relaxed. The sole of the foot should be warm. The outer sole is stimulated by pressing firmly with a blunt object, e.g. Yale key or handle of a patellar hammer, and drawing it forward from the heel towards the toes. Normally a slight contraction of the muscles of the leg occurs, and in addition the toes are flexed on the sole of the foot. This is the 'normal flexor response'.

Babinski's sign is present when in the place of the normal flexor response there is an 'extensor response' and the big toe is turned upwards. When this sign is present it indicates definite disease of the central nervous system, involving the upper motor neurones (pyramidal tracts). In some conditions the reflex may be absent.

Deep, spinal or tendon reflexes

Knee jerk

If the patient can sit up he should cross one leg over the other. If lying in bed, the knee should be raised, and supported to relax the muscles. The reflex is obtained by striking the patellar tendon just below the patella with a patellar hammer. In a normal case the leg jerks forward.

In diseased conditions of the central nervous system the reflex may be absent or exaggerated. It is absent in lower motor neurone and sensory nerve disease, e.g. *poliomyelitis*, *neuritis* and *tabes dorsalis*. It is increased in upper motor neurone disease, e.g. *hemiplegia* and *multiple sclerosis*.

Tendon reflexes of a similar type are the ankle jerk, the elbow jerk, the biceps jerk and the wrist jerk.

Clonus response

This is the production of a series of contractions in response to a stimulus. The ankle clonus is the commonest example. The knee is bent slightly and is supported by one hand. With the other hand the anterior part of the foot is taken, and suddenly moved upwards, i.e. dorsiflexed; the foot is maintained in this position, and a series of contractions in the muscles in the calf of the leg is produced, causing clonic movements of the ankle.

Patellar clonus is produced with the leg extended, and suddenly pushing down the patella towards the foot. A series of clonic contractions of the muscles of the anterior part of the thigh is produced.

Clonus is only produced in the presence of disease of the central nervous system.

Coordination

By coordination, the cooperation of certain groups of muscles to carry out certain acts is meant. In diseases of the central nervous system this cooperation is often defective, and the patient has incoordination.

Coordination is tested in the following ways:

- Romberg's sign. The patient stands upright with his feet together and his eyes closed. This is normally possible. If Romberg's sign is positive he sways about and may fall.
- The patient is instructed to touch his nose with his finger, first with eyes open, and then with the eyes closed.
- The arms are widespread and the patient is instructed to bring his fingertips together, first with eyes open, then with them closed.
- The patient tries to walk along a straight line.
- The patient when lying in bed is asked to place one heel on the opposite knee and run it down the front of the leg to the ankle. As in previous tests this is first done with the eyes open, then with them closed. Incoordination is present in cases of *multiple sclerosis*, *tabes dorsalis*, *cerebral tumour*, and several other diseases of the nervous system.

Sensation

In many diseases of the nervous system sensation is affected, and this can be assessed in various ways.

Sensation to touch

The eyes are closed and the patient is tested with a wisp of wool. The contact may not be felt (anaesthesia) or may be felt excessively (hyperaesthesia). The patient may be unable to localize the area touched.

Sensation to pain

A sharp and blunt object are used, e.g. the point and head of a pin. The patient may not be able to differentiate them. Deep sensation to pain, e.g. by squeezing the muscles of the calf, may be diminished or increased.

Sensation to heat and cold

Small metal containers of hot and cold water are used, and the patient asked to differentiate between them when placed on certain spots. Areas are mapped out on the body where the sensation is abnormal, and the two sides of the body are compared.

Discrimination, vibration and position sense

Further tests of sensation are seeing if the patient can recognize various objects placed in his hand when the eyes are closed, and if the patient can feel the vibrations of a tuning fork when placed on the body surface. Position sense may be tested by altering the position of the patient's digit or limb when his eyes are closed, and seeing whether he can describe the altered position.

Malingering

Symptoms are described inaccurately and in a different manner on repeated questionings.

Anaesthetic areas

The patient is blindfolded and the areas mapped out. On retesting, the areas will differ considerably.

Pain

An assumed pain differs in description on repeated questioning. If asked to indicate the painful spot it will be found that this area can be pressed on without complaint of pain later in the examination. Movements alleged to be impracticable on account of pain are performed painlessly in another way – thus if he says he cannot stoop down, he can probably sit up in bed and lean well forward – an action which produces the same degree of movement.

Paralysis of a limb

The patient may resist passive movements. If the limb is held up there is a momentary pause before it drops. The reflexes are normal and there is no wasting.

Loss of sight

Special tests by an ophthalmic surgeon readily expose a case of malingering of this type.

Deafness

A provocative remark made in an ordinary tone, such as the ordering of a strong purgative, or the addition or removal of some article of diet, may demonstrate that the patient has heard. The matter can always be cleared up by an aural surgeon or audiometrician using special tests (pp. 29–30).

Dizziness

The Romberg test is performed (p. 36). In a genuine case the patient rocks or actually falls. If malingering is suspected, the attention of the patient is distracted, e.g. by asking him if he feels pinpricks. In a genuine case the unsteadiness still persists, while in a fraudulent case it usually ceases. If allowed to fall (the examiner having taken precautions to see that no injury can occur) the patient will slide to the ground rather than fall.

Artificial temperature

The patient may achieve this by placing the thermometer in hot liquid. Take the temperature under actual observation and, if necessary, with another thermometer.

Artificial oedema

Evidence of constriction of a limb may be present.

Haemoptysis

The mouth and throat are examined for a self-inflicted injury. Also the body surface for a cut or abrasion from which blood may be transferred to a handkerchief.

Skin conditions

Artificial lesions produced by fingernails, forks, household chemicals, dyes, etc., are found in areas easily accessible to the dominant hand, are longitudinal in form, and not usually found on the genital organs.

Mental symptoms

The symptoms do not conform to any of the recognized mental disorders. The symptoms are only present when an observer is at hand.

If any suspected case of malingering is indefinite, a strict regime of low diet, no smoking or reading will usually soon indicate whether the symptoms are genuine or not.

Detailed study of brain and spinal cord
Electroencephalography (EEG)

An electroencephalogram is a record of the electrical activity in the brain (**Fig. 3.2**). It is used in the investigation of the various forms of *epilepsy* and of *cerebral trauma* and *drug intoxication*, in the detection of *cerebral tumours, abscesses, infarction* and in the confirmation of *cerebral death* in comatose patients. It is also used to monitor blood flow to the brain during surgical procedures, e.g. on the carotid artery.[2]

Conscious patients should be reassured that the only electric current involved is that which the brain itself produces and told that a number of electrodes will be pasted to the surface of the head and that it is important to lie still while the recording is being made, with freedom to move about during breaks in the recording.[2]

Brain scans

Intravenous injection of radioisotopes (p. 22) is now frequently used to demonstrate space-occupying lesions in the brain, such as *tumours* or *haematomata*, reducing the need for other investigations. Ultrasound scans may also be used, e.g. to demonstrate a shift of the midline of the brain.

Computerized tomography (CT) scan

A CT scan (p. 21) provides an accurate, sometimes three-dimensional, image of tumours or cysts in the brain or spinal cord. In some centres it is considered that patients should fast overnight for a morning scan or after a light 08.00 breakfast for an afternoon scan, to minimize any danger of aspirating gastric contents when contrast medium is injected (which sometimes causes nausea). In other centres fasting is considered unnecessary, even when contrast medium is used.

Magnetic resonance imaging (MRI)

An excellent image of the brain and spinal cord can be obtained by magnetic resonance (**Fig. 3.3**). *Brain tumours, zones of demyelination, meningeal thickening* and even the early (preclinical) changes of *Alzheimer's disease* can be visualized. The images produced enable a lesion to be accurately localized without the use of contrast medium. In certain cases contrast medium may be needed to enhance the image of an area of the brain where an abnormality is suspected. No exposure to X-rays is involved and MRI is now preferred to encephalography and ventriculography (see also p. 21).

Fig. 3.2   Electroencephalography (EEG)

Angiography

Abnormal conditions of the cerebral vessels, e.g. *aneurysms*, can be demonstrated by injecting a contrast medium, such as sodium diatrizoate, rapidly into the carotid artery in the neck. This procedure is not free from risk and is often replaced by CT scan or MRI (p. 38). However, in certain types of neurosurgery angiography is used in addition to CT scan and MRI. It is also being used increasingly for detecting stenosis of blood vessels which can then be treated surgically by endarterectomy. Having given informed consent (see pp. 2,3), the patient is fasted for 6 hours before angiography.

Positron emission tomography (PET)

Where available, PET (p. 23) can be used to detect and localize small foci of tissue abnormality such as tumour or infarction in the brain, and foci of biochemical activity using radioactive glucose.[3] It is also being used to elucidate the abnormal brain function in conditions such as *Parkinson's disease* and *schizophrenia*,[4] and to assess the effect of drugs.

Encephalography

A lumbar puncture is performed with the patient in a sitting posture, and some cerebrospinal fluid is allowed to escape. About 50–90 ml of air are then injected through the lumbar puncture needle. This ascends to the cavities in the brain, and their outline will be seen on a radiograph, an encephalogram. Photographs are taken with the patient lying down, and the head in special positions.

Fig. 3.3 Magnetic resonance image showing a tumour in the brain stem (arrow A) with associated oedema (arrow B)

A method is also available in which only a small quantity of air, about 5–10 ml, is injected and photographs taken after tilting the head in various positions.

This procedure, used in cases of *cerebral tumour*, is being replaced by CT scan and MRI (p. 38).

Ventriculography

A small hole is bored through the skull in the parietal region, and a special cannula inserted through the cortex into the lateral ventricle. Some cerebrospinal fluid is allowed to escape, and then about 20–30 ml of air are injected. On X-ray examination an outline of the ventricle will be seen, a ventriculogram. This procedure, used in cases of *cerebral tumour*, is being replaced by CT scan and MRI (p. 38).

Myelography

The spinal cord can be examined by the injection of contrast medium into the space between the meninges and the cord (subarachnoid space). A lumbar puncture is performed (see p. 30). With the patient sitting, contrast medium is injected into the subarachnoid space. The patient is then placed on a tilting table and screened. If an obstruction or filling defect is demonstrated (e.g. due to a *tumour*), films are taken. This test is being replaced by CT and MR scans (p. 38).

Brain biopsy and smear

After making a burr hole in the skull, often in the course of a brain operation, a small sample of brain tissue may be taken into fixative for histology, or smeared on to a slide and fixed while still wet for cytology. This enables the presence and type of a *tumour* to be determined.

Peripheral nerves
Nerve conduction

Testing nerve conduction is of value in nerve injuries and peripheral neuropathy. The nerve is stimulated electrically through the skin (giving the patient a slight stinging sensation). The speed of nerve conduction is measured by placing electrodes at a measured distance from the point of stimulation. Damage to a nerve causes impaired conduction of electrical impulses.

Muscular system
Muscle power

The power of muscle groups can be assessed by asking the patient to push or pull against the resistance provided by the hands of the examiner.

Muscular electrical reactions

A normal muscle will contract on stimulation by an electric current. In cases of paralysis the contraction may be diminished or absent. By testing individual muscles the extent of paralysis can be ascertained, and to some extent the prospect of recovery estimated. The procedure is used in diseases of the nervous system, injuries to nerves, primary muscle disease and to assist in the differentiation of hysterical forms of paralysis.

Electromyography (EMG)

An electromyogram is a record of the electrical activity in a muscle, either at rest or during contraction. It is obtained by inserting a needle electrode into the muscle. Different patterns of activity are seen in health and disease.

Mental development tests

If an infant is late sitting up, walking, talking, and gaining control of the bladder and rectum it may or may not indicate mental subnormality, which will be more evident later. Sometimes indications may be present, e.g. *hydrocephalus*, *Down's syndrome*, etc. In some cases a diagnosis of mental subnormality cannot be made definitely until the child is 7 or 8 years old.

Developmental screening tests (Stycar and Denver)

These detect developmental delay as early in life as possible. The STYCAR (Sheridan Tests for Young Children and Retards) series also test hearing and vision. The Denver tests are designed for use by trained non-medical personnel.

Stanford–Binet tests

These are a series of tests graduated to the age of the individual from the age of 2 years upwards – thus normally:

1. Child of 3 knows its sex, can name simple everyday objects, etc.

2. Child of 5 can carry out simple consecutive directions, e.g. put the paper down and close the door, etc.

3. Child of 7 knows days of week, etc.

Griffiths' tests

For the age range 0–8 years these tests produce a developmental quotient for the following functions: locomotor, personal–social, hearing and speech, hand–eye coordination, performance and (over 2 years) practical reasoning.

Mental age

This is given by the ability to carry out numerous intelligence tests – thus a child of 14 might have a mental age of 8, i.e. only be able to carry out the tests capable of being done by a normal child of 8.

Intelligence quotient (IQ)

This is expressed as the ratio between the real age and the mental age based on a figure of 100. Thus if a child of 10 can only do the tests of a normal child of 5 the IQ is 50 (i.e. 1/2). If the IQ of a child in its teens is 50–70, it is definitely mentally subnormal, and will probably require continual care and supervision.

Adult mental function

Similar tests of mental function (psychometry) can be carried out on adults. Impaired performance may indicate dementia due to physical (organic) disease of the brain, such as *tumour* or *syphilis*, or due to severe mental disorder (*psychosis*).

Reference

1. Beetham, R. Investigation of cerebrospinal fluid. In: Marshall, W J and Bangert S K (eds). *Clinical biochemistry; metabolic and clinical aspects*. New York. Churchill Livingstone. 1955: 557–568.

2. Pagana, K D and Pagana, T J. Electroencephalography. In: Pagana, K D and Pagana, T J (eds). *Mosby's Diagnostic and Laboratory Test Reference*. St. Louis. Mosby Year Book. 1992: 288–291.

3. Pagana, K D and Pagana, T J. Positron-emission tomography. In: Pagana, K D and Pagana, T J (eds). *Mosby's Diagnostic and Laboratory Test Reference*. St Louis. Mosby Year Book. 1992: 575–577.

4. Grasby, P M. Imaging the neurochemical brain in health and disease. *Clinical medicine*, Journal of the Royal College of Physicians of London. London. Royal College of Physicians. 2002; 2 (1): 67–73.

CHAPTER FOUR

Tests related to communicating (2)

Endocrine system (chemical communication within the body)

Index of tests	Page		
Acromegaly	58	17-hydroxy-corticosteroids (17-OHCS) in urine	52
Addison's disease	53	Hyperparathyroidism	49
ADH (antidiuretic hormone) stimulation test	60	Hypoparathyroidism	50
Adrenal cortex	50	Hypopituitarism (Simmond's disease)	59
Adrenal cortical tumour	52	Insulin-induced hypoglycaemia stimulation test	58
Adrenal medullary tumour	55	Insulin stress test	58
Adrenocortical insufficiency	52	Insulin tolerance test (ITT)	58
Adrenocorticotrophic hormone (ACTH)	57	Joffroy's sign	49
Aldosterone in plasma	51	17-ketogenic steroids in urine	52
Anterior pituitary function assessment	56	17-ketosteroids in urine	52
Anterior pituitary hormones	56	Luteinizing hormone (LH)	56
Antidiuretic hormone (ADH)	59	Melanocytic stimulating hormone (MSH)	56
Aspiration cytology of thyroid	49	Moebius's sign	49
Biopsy of thyroid	49	Nephrogenic diabetes insipidus	60
Catecholamines in urine	55	11-oxygenation index	53
Chvostek's sign	50	17-oxosteroids (17-OS)	52
Clomiphene and gonadotrophin releasing hormone		Pancreatic secretion of insulin	60
(LH/FSH-RH) tests	58	Parathormone	50
Combined test of anterior pituitary function	58	Parathyroid biopsy	50
Congenital adrenal hyperplasia	52	Perimeter or field analyser tests	56
Cortisol (11-hydroxycorticosteroids, 11-HCS)		Phaeochromocytoma	55
in plasma	51	Pituitary function, anterior, posterior	56, 59
in urine	52	Pituitary tumour	56
Cushing's disease	59	Posterior pituitary function assessment	59
Cushing's syndrome	59	Pregnanetriol in urine	52
Dexamethasone suppression test	54	Primary adrenocortical insufficiency	53
Diabetes insipidus	59	Prolactin	57
Erb's sign	50	Protein-bound iodine (PBI)	46
Exophthalmos	49	Radioactive iodine tests	47
Follicle stimulating hormone (FSH)	57	Simmond's disease (hypopituitarism)	59
Free T_4 and free T_3 indices (FT_4I, FT_3I)	46	Steroid excretion test	52
Gigantism	57	Steroids in blood	51
Glucagon test	58	Steroids in urine	52
Gonadal endocrine function investigations	60	Stimulation tests	44
Growth hormone (GH)	57	Suppression tests	44
Human growth hormone (HGH)	57	Synacthen (ACTH) test	53

Index of tests	Page		
T$_4$ (thyroxin) estimation	45	Thyroid stimulating hormone (TSH)	46
T$_3$ (triiodothyronine) estimation	45	Total 17-oxogenic steroids (T–17OGS) in urine	52
Tetany	50	TRH (thyrotropin releasing hormone) test	47
Thyroid antibodies	48	Trousseau's sign	50
Thyroid function tests (thyroid profile)	45	Vanillylmandelic acid	55
Thyroid gland visualization	48	von Graefe's sign	49
Thyroid scan	47	Water deprivation test	59

Introduction

The endocrine system provides a means of chemical communication within the body. Each endocrine gland secretes hormones into the bloodstream which affect certain bodily functions. The pituitary gland affects all the other endocrine glands by means of controlling hormones and has been called 'the leader of the endocrine orchestra'; anatomically, it is attached to the hypothalamus, a part of the brain concerned with the emotions. It follows that there is both an anatomical and a chemical link between the endocrine system and the emotions that we feel often expressed in body language. Many of the tests involve the chemical estimation of hormones in blood or urine and are undertaken by the chemical pathologist or biochemist. The supervision of urine collection and the recording of any drugs taken by the patient is often a critical part of the test and is usually the responsibility of the nurse.

Endocrine system

Endocrine glands may secrete too much or too little hormone. Abnormal secretion may be due to a *primary* abnormality in the gland or be *secondary* to an abnormality of the controlling mechanism. If clinical examination and hormone assay give equivocal results, *dynamic tests* may be used. There are two groups:

1. *Stimulation tests* are used in the diagnosis of inadequate secretion by a gland. The trophic hormone which normally stimulates the gland (or its synthetic analogue) is administered. A normal response excludes a primary abnormality of the gland; failure to respond confirms it.

2. *Suppression tests* are used in the diagnosis of excessive secretion by a gland. A substance is administered which would suppress a normal gland. A normal response excludes a primary abnormality of the gland; failure to suppress secretion confirms it.

NB: With improvements in the techniques for measuring hormone levels, the need to use stimulation and suppression tests has been reduced.

Thyroid gland investigation

The thyroid gland secretes two hormones which together regulate the body's metabolism (the sum total of all the physical and chemical changes occurring in the body). The hormone with the highest blood level is thyroxine (T_4); the other hormone is triiodothyronine (T_3), which although present in much smaller amounts is four times more active in its physiological effect. The greater part of both hormones is in protein-bound form, the protein being mainly γ-globulin (thyroid-binding globulin, TBG), but some of each hormone is free (unattached to protein). It is the free form which enters cells and controls the body's metabolism. These active forms are measured as the 'free T_4 index' and the 'free T_3 index', which more accurately reflect thyroid gland effectiveness than the blood level of T_4 and T_3. The secretion of the thyroid hormones is controlled by thyroid stimulating hormone (TSH), secreted by the pituitary gland, and in turn controlled by thyrotropin releasing hormone (TRH), secreted by the hypothalamus. For *thyroid nodules or tumours* see calcitonin (p.111) and thyroid aspiration cytology and biopsy (p. 49).

Thyroid function tests (thyroid profile)
The following may all be estimated on 10 ml of clotted blood:
- T_4 (thyroxine) estimation
- T_3 (triiodothyronine) estimation
- T_3 (triiodothyronine) uptake and/or thiopac 3
- Free T_4 index (FT_4I) and free T_3 index (FT_3I)
- Thyroid stimulating hormone (TSH).

The procedure adopted is along the following lines. T_4 estimation is performed on all samples. If the T_4 is low, thyroid stimulating hormone (TSH) assay is performed. If the TSH is high it indicates that the primary failure is in the thyroid, i.e. *primary hypothyroidism*. With improvements in the accuracy of TSH measurement, this estimation can now be used as the first line test of thyroid function.[1] If the T_4 is high, measurements are undertaken from which the FT_3I and FT_4I are calculated. A high level of one or both these indices confirms a diagnosis of *hyperthyroidism*. If a diagnostic problem still exists after completion of the thyroid profile it should be discussed with the laboratory and further tests may be undertaken, e.g. radioactive iodine test (p. 47).

T₄ (thyroxine) estimation
The serum level of thyroxine, the principal thyroid hormone, can be measured by radioimmunoassay. It accounts for 90% of the protein-bound iodine (PBI, pp. 46–47), but its estimation is much less affected by outside factors than PBI. The results are reported in SI units, the normal range being 55–150 nmol/litre (4.5–15 μg/100 ml) or as thyroxine iodine (2–7 μg/100 ml). The level for free T_4 is 10–22 pmol/litre. It is reduced in *hypothyroidism*, rising on treatment; and raised in *hyperthyroidism*, falling on treatment.

T₃ (triiodothyronine) estimation
T_3 has four times the biological activity of T_4 but normally the ratio of T_4 to T_3 in blood is 50 to 1. However, in some cases of *thyrotoxicosis* it is mainly the T_3 that is increased and so its measurement is of practical value. The normal serum T_3 level is 1.3–3.2 nmol/litre. The level for free T_3 is 5–7 pmol/litre.

T₃ (triiodothyronine) uptake and/or thiopac₃

The test measures the capacity of serum protein to bind T_3. This indicates the number of free sites available to combine with the thyroid hormone. Using thiopac$_3$ the results are expressed as a percentage of the standard T_3 uptake, 92–117% being accepted as the normal. It is increased in *hypothyroidism* (because more sites are unoccupied) and reduced in *thyrotoxicosis*. It provides a valuable check on T_4 results which can be affected by certain conditions, e.g. pregnancy and the contraceptive pill.

Free T₄ index (FT₄I) and free T₃ index (FT₃I)

These indices provide a numerical description of the thyroid status. They provide values which are corrected for the serum proteins and are therefore more reliable than serum T_4 and T_3 levels, not being significantly affected by oral contraceptives or pregnancy. The normal FT_4I is 55–145 nmol/litre and the FT_3I is 1.4–3.7 nmol/litre. One or both indices are increased in *thyrotoxicosis* and reduced in *myxoedema*. A similar index used in some hospitals is the effective thyroxine ratio (ETR).

Thyroid stimulating hormone (TSH)

This hormone, produced by the pituitary gland, controls thyroid gland activity. It is estimated by radioimmunoassay. The normal range is 0.5–5 mU/litre. The level is always increased in untreated *primary hypothyroidism*, reflecting the pituitary's attempt to stimulate an inadequate thyroid gland into greater activity. A normal TSH level usually indicates that the patient is euthyroid (i.e. has normal thyroid function). An undetectably low level of TSH occurs in *overt thyrotoxicosis*, in *subclinical thyrotoxicosis* (where thyroid hormone secretion is not yet excessive) and in patients treated with excessive doses of replacement thyroid hormone. The suppression of TSH secretion by the pituitary gland sometimes persists in treated *thyrotoxicosis* even after the thyroid hormone levels have returned to normal. A low or undetectable TSH level also occurs, especially in the elderly, during corticosteroid or dopamine therapy and during fasting.[1]

Thyroid binding globulin (TBG)

In the blood, most of both thyroid hormones is bound to carrier proteins, the most important being TBG. This is measured by immunoassay, the normal plasma level being 13–28 mg/litre. *Pregnancy*, oestrogen-containing contraceptives and *hydatidiform mole* are associated with raised levels. Low levels occur in *Cushing's disease*, *acromegaly* and other conditions including severe illness.[1]

Thyroglobulin

Within the thyroid gland, thyroid hormones are stored in vesicles filled with colloid and are in the form of a glycoprotein called thyroglobulin. A protein-splitting enzyme splits off the hormones before they are secreted into the bloodstream, where they mainly combine with γ-globulin. Normally only very small amounts of thyroglobulin are present in the blood. In patients who have had *thyroid cancer*, a raised level may indicate a recurrence.[1]

Protein-bound iodine (PBI)

Since the thyroid hormones are mainly in the protein-bound form, measurement of the PBI provides a convenient way of assessing the level of circulating thyroid hormone. However, if the level of protein in the blood is low, as in the *nephrotic syndrome*, a misleadingly low level is found. A misleadingly high PBI occurs in pregnancy, with steroid contraceptives and with certain other drugs, e.g. phenothiazine or clofibrate.[2] For this test 10 ml of clotted blood must be collected into a special container. The average normal PBI is 3–8 μg per 100 ml. It is reduced in *hypothyroidism*, rising on treatment; and raised in *hyperthyroidism*, falling on treatment. This test has been virtually replaced by direct measurement of the thyroid hormones.

The TRH (thyrotropin releasing hormone) test

TRH is a substance (tripeptide) produced by the hypothalamus which controls the secretion of TSH (thyroid stimulating hormone) by the pituitary gland. After 5 ml of clotted blood has been collected for control TSH estimation, 200 μg synthetic TRH in 2 ml saline is injected rapidly intravenously. Further blood samples are taken 20 and 60 minutes later for TSH assay. The test is of value in cases of *hyperthyroidism* where the serum T_4 and T_3 levels are borderline. The diagnosis of hyperthyroidism is confirmed by finding a rise of less than 2 mU above the control level at 20 and 60 minutes. In *primary hypothyroidism* the basal level is raised and the response to TRH exaggerated and prolonged. If thyroid failure is secondary to *pituitary disease* the TSH response is usually absent or impaired. If the cause of the thyroid failure lies in the hypothalamus, the TSH level at 20 minutes may be normal but the 60 minute level is higher, whereas in normal subjects it falls below the 20 minute peak.

Radioactive iodine tests
Urine excretion method

For general management, see radioisotopes, p. 22. After the patient has fasted for at least 2 hours he is given a measured dose of radioactive iodine (^{131}I). Urine is carefully collected into three separate Winchester bottles during the periods: 0–8 hours, 8–24 hours, and 24–48 hours. Alternative methods of collection are used in some hospitals, e.g. a separate container for each specimen passed, noting the time of each collection. The amount of radioactive iodine excreted is measured by means of a Geiger–Muller counter. In *thyrotoxicosis* a larger proportion of the iodine than normal is concentrated in the thyroid and so less than normal is excreted in the urine. In *myxoedema* the reverse occurs.

On the results of the above test, certain cases may be selected for further laboratory tests. A thyroid scan directly measures the uptake of radioactive iodine by the thyroid. The protein-bound radioactive iodine can also be measured.

Thyroid scan

The uptake of radioactive iodine by different parts of the thyroid gland is mapped out, using a Scintiscan or Gammascan. This distinguishes the overall increase in thyroid activity of *Graves' disease* from *toxic nodular goitre* where 'hot' areas (of high activity) are surrounded by 'cold' areas (of low activity). A cold nodule may be indicative of *thyroid cancer*. An even more detailed picture of both structure and function of the thyroid gland is obtainable with positron emission tomography (PET, see p. 23). NB: If the patient is pregnant, a radioisotope thyroid scan should if possible be avoided, and an ultrasound scan or MRI used instead (see p. 48).

Thyroid gland visualization

This is achieved by straight X-ray, CT scan, thyroid scan (see above), ultrasound scan and magnetic resonance imaging (MRI).

Straight X-ray and CT scan

On a straight X-ray, the thyroid gland shows up as a soft shadow. This can be of value, e.g. in demonstrating a *retrosternal goitre*. Foci of calcification can also be clearly seen. A CT scan (see p. 21) can provide a three-dimensional picture.

Ultrasound scan

An ultrasound scan of the neck enables cystic and solid lesions of the thyroid gland to be distinguished. No preparation is required and exposure to X-rays is avoided, of particular value during pregnancy.

Magnetic resonance imaging (MRI)

MRI (p. 21) provides a much clearer picture of the thyroid tissues than straight X-ray, CT scan or even an ultrasound scan, and, like the latter, avoids exposure to irradiation.

Other tests of thyroid function

Blood creatinine (p. 113) is raised in *hyperthyroidism* and lowered in *myxoedema*. Blood cholesterol (p. 111) is raised in myxoedema. The resting pulse rate is raised in hyperthyroidism.

Tests for thyroid antibodies

Patients with *autoimmune thyroiditis* produce antibodies against (1) their thyroid gland products, and (2) their own thyroid tissue itself.

Antibodies against thyroid gland products

Anti-thyroid peroxidase (AntiTPO)

This is a commonly used test for autoimmune thyroiditis. The blood level of AntiTPO antibody is raised in nearly all cases of Hashimoto's disease, in 85% of patients with thyrotoxicosis and in 10% of asymptomatic individuals.

Thyroglobulin antibody (TA) test

The patient's serum is tested against latex particles coated with thyroglobulin. Antibody causes the particles to stick together in visible clumps

Antibodies against thyroid tissue

Thyroid precipitin test

The serum is tested against thyroid tissue extract in agar gel on a slide. The presence of antibody is shown by a line of precipitation in the agar.

Immunofluorescent test for thyroid antibody

This test is very sensitive and in some cases is the only way of demonstrating thyroid antibody. The principle of a fluorescent test is described on p. 103.

   For the above tests 10 ml of clotted blood is required. The tests are of value in demonstrating the presence of antibodies characteristic of *autoimmune thyroid disease*. They are also sometimes found in other autoimmune diseases, e.g. *pernicious anaemia*, and occasionally in healthy people.

Special signs associated with hyperthyroidism (exophthalmic goitre)
Exophthalmos
This is an abnormal protrusion of the eyeball.

von Graefe's sign
The patient is asked to look up and down by following a finger. The movement of the eyelid lags behind the movement of the eyeball.

Joffroy's sign
The patient is asked to depress the head and then look up towards the ceiling with the head in this position. There is an absence of wrinkling of the forehead.

Moebius's sign
On attempting to focus the eyes on a near object, the eyes do not converge.

Aspiration cytology of thyroid
Fine needle aspiration (p. 5) can provide the diagnosis of a thyroid lesion (e.g. *papillary carcinoma*, *Hashimoto's disease*), but may not always give a definitive diagnosis (e.g. follicular lesions).

Biopsy of thyroid (frozen section)
In spite of all the tests available it is often difficult to decide whether a thyroid nodule is benign or malignant. So it is common for the surgeon to take tissue for frozen section (p. 4) in the course of an operation. This usually provides the answer but one may have to wait a day or so for a paraffin section to be sure.

Parathyroid gland investigations

The four parathyroid glands, usually situated at the back of the thyroid gland, secrete parathormone, the hormone controlling the level of calcium in the blood. If the blood level of ionized calcium falls, increased parathormone secretion restores the level by reabsorbing calcium from the kidney tubules and mobilizing calcium from the bones. Excessive parathormone secretion removes too much calcium from the bones, causing them to become cystic, and calcium and phosphorus are lost in the urine (hyperparathyroidism, below). Too little parathormone cause the blood calcium to fall (hypoparathyroidism, p.50).

In disturbances of the parathyroid gland the following tests are of value: parathormone (p. 50), blood calcium (p. 110), phosphorus (p. 111), alkaline phosphatase (p. 111) and urine calcium (p. 171).

Hyperparathyroidism
In *hyperparathyroidism* the blood parathormone, blood calcium and calcium excretion are all increased, also the alkaline phosphatase if the bones are involved, but blood phosphorus is diminished provided there is no kidney failure.

Where the cause for a raised serum calcium is uncertain a cortisone test may be performed. If the calcium level does not fall after 10 days of cortisone treatment it implies that *hyperparathyroidism* is present. This is because cortisone reduces the gut's sensitivity to vitamin D so that the absorption of calcium is reduced. This lowers the serum calcium in patients not suffering from *hyperparathyroidism*.

Hypoparathyroidism

In *hypoparathyroidism*, sometimes associated with tetany (see below), the blood parathormone, blood calcium and calcium excretion are reduced, blood phosphorus is increased and the alkaline phosphatase is normal. The cyclic AMP (p. 113) rises to peak levels about 20 minutes after injection of parathormone. In *pseudohypoparathyroidism* it does not.

Tetany

In tetany there is an increased excitability of the nerves and muscles, associated with a low serum calcium (p. 110) and potassium (p. 115) and also alkalosis (73–74) and electrolytes, pp. 113–114.

Chvostek's sign

If the facial nerve is tapped where it crosses the jaw, a spasmodic contraction of that side of the face occurs.

Erb's sign

If a galvanic current is passed, strong muscular contractions are produced.

Trousseau's sign

Pressure round the circumference of the arm produces tetanic spasm, with flexion at the wrist and metacarpophalangeal joints.

Laboratory tests

The low serum calcium is characteristic. In cases of urgency plasma calcium should be estimated, 5 ml of blood being taken into a heparinized container; see also parathyroid gland investigation (p. 49) and *hypoparathyroidism* (above).

Parathyroid biopsy (frozen section)

During operation for parathyroid overactivity it is common for the surgeon to take tissue samples for frozen section (p. 4) to decide whether there is an adenoma of one parathyroid gland (which suppresses the other parathyroid glands) or whether there is overactivity of all four glands. Paraffin sections, produced a day or so later, are also examined to check on the frozen section findings.

Parathormone

Parathormone is the hormone secreted by the parathyroid glands. Its action is to raise the serum calcium. The normal plasma parathormone is 0.9–5.4 pmol/litre. It is increased in *tumours of the parathyroid gland* and *renal osteodystrophy*. It may be reduced as a result of accidental *surgical removal of the parathyroid glands* during thyroidectomy. Practical details should be obtained from the local laboratory and the local normal range checked.

Adrenal gland investigation

There are two adrenal (suprarenal) glands, each having an outer cortex and an inner medulla.

Adrenal cortex

The adrenal cortex secretes a number of steroid hormones which have differing functions, including maintenance of water and electrolyte balance (pp. 113–116), control of protein and carbohydrate metabolism, and involvement in the body's response to stress.[3] The estimation of the steroid hormones, in blood or in urine, particularly after appropriate stimulation or suppression, provides an index of cortical function. Blood is easier to collect but indicates cortical activity only at the time of collection. A 24-hour urine reflects the total daily cortical secretion but its accurate collection requires careful supervision (see p. 160). There are also tests to measure the response of the adrenal cortex to stimulation by ACTH (see pp. 53–54), and suppression by dexamethasone (see p. 54).

Overactivity of the adrenal cortex, occurring in *Cushing's syndrome* and *Cushing's disease*, causes a raised plasma cortisol, with a moon-shaped face, hirsutism, increased blood pressure and retention of sodium, causing oedema.

Underactivity, occurring in *Addison's disease*, causes a low plasma cortisol, with a low blood pressure, muscular weakness, pigmentation of the skin, low serum sodium with excessive loss of sodium chloride in the urine.

Blood tests for steroids

Plasma cortisol (II-hydroxycorticosteroids, II-OHCS)

The average normal cortisol level is 150–600 nmol/litre (6–22 µg/100 ml) in adults and 370–680 nmol/litre (15–25 µg/100 ml) in children. It is a very good indicator of adrenal cortical activity and it varies considerably during the day, with a minimum just after midnight (50–250 nmol/litre) and a maximum at about 08.00 hours (200–700 nmol/litre). It is secreted by the adrenal cortex in response to stimulation by adrenocorticotrophic hormone (ACTH) secreted by the pituitary gland; it opposes the effect of insulin in the control of carbohydrate metabolism. Plasma cortisol is raised in adrenal cortex overactivity, whether primary (*Cushing's syndrome*) due to *hyperplasia, adenoma or carcinoma of the adrenal cortex*; or *secondary to pituitary overactivity* (*Cushing's disease*; see ACTH, p. 57). Other causes of raised cortisol include *pregnancy, contraceptive steroids* and *oestrogen treatment of prostatic carcinoma*. Certain drugs, e.g. mepacrine and spironolactone, give false high levels. For patients on drugs see other specific steroids (p. 52). Reduced plasma cortisol occurs in *Addison's disease, hypothyroidism* and *hypopituitarism*. The Synacthen test (see pp. 53–54) assists in elucidating the cause.

The patient need not be fasted, but all forms of stress must be avoided before collection of 5 ml of blood into a heparin tube between 08.00 and 10.00 hours (or when investigating circadian rhythm, between 22.00 and 24.00 hours), the time of collection being stated on the request form.

Aldosterone

Aldosterone promotes potassium excretion and sodium retention. It is estimated in patients with hypertension who have a low plasma potassium. The aldosterone level is affected by diuretics, such as thiazides, frusemide and spironolactone, purgatives, liquorice derivatives, e.g. carbenoxolone, and oral contraceptives. All such drugs should be stopped for at least 3 weeks before aldosterone assay. The patient must also receive adequate sodium (<100 mmol/24 hours) and potassium (50–70 mmol/24 hours) as an inpatient for at least 3 days. Aldosterone assay should only be done if the plasma potassium is less than 3.7 mmol/litre; 10 ml of blood is collected into a heparin tube early in the morning before the patient has even raised his head off the pillow. Special arrangements must be made with the laboratory for the collection of blood, so that it can be transported without delay to a specialized laboratory for aldosterone and renin estimations. Urine aldosterone levels may also be estimated.

In aldosteronism the plasma aldosterone exceeds 300 mmol/litre. Urine aldosterone levels are also raised (normal 14–53 nmol/litre). In primary aldosteronism due to a tumour (*Conn's syndrome*) the plasma renin is low. In aldosteronism which is secondary, e.g. to a *renal lesion*, the plasma renin is high. Renin estimation can be performed on the same sample of blood when indicated by a high aldosterone level.

Other specific steroids

Other individual steroids may be measured by special techniques (radioimmunoassay or competitive protein binding). These enable cortisol to be measured in patients on drugs such as mepacrine or spironolactone which interfere with the simpler fluorimetric method. **NB**: *Any drugs taken by the patient must be noted on the request form.* Other steroids measured in this way include:

17-hydroxyprogesterone: the normal serum level is 1–10 nmol/litre in males, and in females during the follicular phase of the menstrual cycle, rising to 10–20 nmol/litre during the luteal phase. It is raised in *adult-onset congenital adrenal hyperplasia* (see also urine pregnanetriol, below).

11-deoxycortisol: (normal serum level 24–46 nmol/litre), raised in *adrenocortical insufficiency*.

Urine tests for steroids

Free cortisol

Most of the plasma cortisol is bound to protein but only the free cortisol is physiologically active. This is also the only part of the cortisol which is filtered out into the urine. So if properly collected, with complete absence of stress on the day preceding and on the day of the test, it provides a good assessment of active cortisol. The normal 24 hour excretion is <400 nmol (180 µg). Increased levels have the same significance as raised plasma cortisol but provide a more sensitive index of *adrenocortical overactivity*. They are suggestive but not diagnostic of *Cushing's disease*.

Total 17-oxogenic steroids (T-17OGS, also called 17-hydroxycorticosteroids or 17-OHCS, previously known as 17-ketogenic steroids)

This group includes cortisol and closely related compounds. The normal 24-hour excretion is 17–70 µmol (5–23 mg). Raised levels have the same significance as for free cortisol (above) and plasma cortisol (p. 51).

17-oxosteroids (17-OS, previously 17 ketosteroids)

These measure the products of androgens and closely related substances. The 24-hour excretion in females is 10–70 µmol (5–18 mg) and is almost entirely from the adrenal cortex. In males it is 20–100 µmol (8–25 mg) of which 10–20% is derived from the testis as products of testosterone. There is a non-specific reduction of 17-OS excretion in many illnesses. High levels occur in some forms of *virilism*.

Pregnanetriol

Estimations are of value in the investigation of *congenital adrenal hyperplasia* (see also, 11-oxygenation index p. 53) and disorders of ovulation, and in monitoring therapy. Table 4.1 gives normal excretion levels.

For initial investigation the patient must not be on cortisol or any synthetic analogue. No special preparation is required. Send complete 24-hour urine to laboratory for addition of 10 ml of 2% boric before onward transmission of 25 ml aliquot to SAS.

ll-oxygenation index

This relatively simple test is of great value in diagnosing *congenital adrenal hyperplasia*. It can be performed on any sample of urine. A 24-hour collection is unnecessary unless pregnanetriol (see p. 52) is being assayed at the same time. Normally the index is less than 0.5. This value is exceeded in various forms of *congenital adrenal hyperplasia*. The test is unreliable during the first week of life and in severe diarrhoea. Treatment with cortisol or cortisone gives a normal index but prednisone or prednisolone can elevate it.

Steroid excretion test

This is no longer considered a sufficiently sensitive test of adrenal cortical function. It has been replaced by the stimulation and suppression tests (see below).

Stimulation and suppression tests

The Synacthen or ACTH (stimulation) test detects *adrenal cortical insufficiency* (*Addison's disease*). Overactivity of the adrenal cortex is detected by the dexamethasone suppression test.

Synacthen (ACTH) test

This assesses the ability of the adrenal cortex to secrete cortisol in response to ACTH stimulation.

Screening (short Synacthen) test

At 09.00 hours 2 ml of blood are collected into a heparin tube and sent immediately to the laboratory for cortisol estimation (see p. 51). An intramuscular injection of 250 µg Synacthen in 1–2 ml of normal saline is then given. At 09.30 hours a further 2 ml sample of blood is collected into a heparin tube and again sent immediately to the laboratory. The plasma cortisol in the 09.00 hours specimen should be 0.2–0.7 µmol/litre (8–26 µg/100 ml). At 09.30 hours the plasma cortisol should be increased by at least 0.2 µmol/litre (7 µg/100 ml) to reach a minimum level of 0.5 µmol/litre (18 g/100 ml). Lesser values suggest *Addison's disease* (primary adrenocortical insufficiency due to atrophy, tuberculosis or carcinomatous deposits). A normal response excludes primary insufficiency but may not exclude secondary insufficiency due to reduced ACTH secretion by the pituitary gland (see combined test of anterior pituitary secretion, p. 58). An indeterminate result may be clarified by the definitive test, but if there is a strong clinical suspicion of *Addison's disease*, treatment with dexamethasone should be given immediately to avoid an adrenal crisis. Such treatment will not vitiate the results of a more prolonged ACTH stimulation (definitive) test if undertaken within a short time. **NB:** The alternative intravenous short Synacthen test (p. 54) is now preferred as a screening test.

Table 4.1 Pregnanetriol: normal excretion	
	µmol/24 hours
Children	0–4.8
Women: follicular phase	0.3–5.3
luteal phase	2.7–6.5
Men	1.2–7.5

Intravenous short Synacthen (tetracosactrin) test

This is an alternative screening test for adrenocortical insufficiency, including ACTH deficiency.[4] With the patient in a relaxed, unstressed state, 2 ml of blood is collected into a heparin tube and sent to the laboratory for cortisol estimation (see p. 51). Synacthen (tetracosactrin) 250 μg is then injected intravenously. After 30 minutes a second 2 ml sample of heparinized blood is collected and sent to the laboratory. With a normally responsive adrenal cortex, the plasma cortisol at 30 minutes is 550 nmol/litre or above, and this correlates with a normal pituitary–adrenal axis. A 30 minute level of 400–550 nmol/litre is equivocal and a definitive (long Synacthen) test should be undertaken (if not contraindicated by a strong clinical suspicion of *Addison's disease*, when treatment with dexamethasone should be given immediately to avoid an adrenal crisis).

Definitive (long Synacthen) test

At 09.00 hours 2 ml of heparinized blood are collected as before. Over the next 5 hours an intravenous infusion of 0.5 mg Synacthen in 500 ml of normal saline or 5% dextrose is given at the rate of approximately 0.1 mg Synacthen per hour. During the procedure a 2 ml heparinized sample is collected every hour. Each sample is sent immediately to the laboratory for separation of the plasma. The plasma cortisol should reach 0.8–1.4 μmol/litre (30–50 μg/100 ml) in at least one sample. Failure to reach this level indicates *Addison's disease*.

Dexamethasone suppression test (DST)

The DST is used to demonstrate overactivity of the adrenal cortex and to determine its cause. Dexamethasone is a synthetic steroid, given by mouth, which enters the bloodstream and suppresses the secretion of ACTH by the pituitary gland. In normal people, the reduction of the ACTH causes reduction in the steroids secreted by the adrenal cortex.

Overnight suppression test

Oral dexamethasone 1 mg is given at midnight, and at 09.00 hours the following morning 5 ml of blood is collected into a heparin tube for cortisol estimation. Suppression of the plasma cortisol below 100 nmol/litre excludes a diagnosis of *Cushing's syndrome*. If no suppression occurs, further investigation is needed.

Low dose dexamethasone suppression

On day 0, heparinized blood 5 ml is collected at 09.00 hours, after which dexamethasone 0.5 mg is given 6-hourly for 48 hours (including 03.00 hours). On day 2 (i.e. 48 hours after the first blood collection) a second 5 ml sample of heparinized blood is collected. A plasma cortisol below 50 nmol/litre indicates suppression.

High dose dexamethasone suppression

The procedure follows that of the low dose test except that the dose is quadrupled, i.e. 2 mg every 6 hours for 48 hours, giving a total of 8 mg/day. This test is only used in the differential diagnosis of *Cushing's syndrome*.[3]

Alternative DST, assessed by urinary excretion of 17- hydroxycorticosteroid

A complete 24-hour urine collection is made on five successive days. That from day 1 is the control. On days 2 and 3, dexamethasone 0.5 mg is given orally every 6 hours (i.e. eight doses). On days 4 and 5, dexamethasone 2.0 mg is given orally every 6 hours (i.e. another eight doses).

The substance measured in this test is the urinary 17-hydroxycorticosteroid. Normally the level on the control day is 8–33 µmol/day (3–12 mg/day). After the 0.5 mg doses the level falls to less than 7 µmol/day (2.5 mg/day) and after the 2 mg doses none can be detected.

In *Cushing's syndrome* due to *overactivity of the adrenal cortex* from hyperplasia the 17-hydroxycorticosteroid excretion is increased to 33–100 µmol/day (12–36 mg/day). Oral dexamethasone produces a reduction in the amount excreted, indicating that the overactive cortex can still respond in the same way as a normal gland.

In *Cushing's syndrome* due to *tumour of the adrenal cortex* the urinary excretion is increased to 50–160 µmol/day (19–60 mg/day) and there is no reduction following oral dexamethasone.

Other tests for diseases of the adrenal cortex

Blood pressure (see pp. 77–78).

Electrolytes in blood (see pp. 113–116), and urine (see sodium and potassium, p. 172).

Adrenal medulla

The adrenal medulla secretes catecholamines, 80% of which is epinephrine (adrenaline). It also secretes norepinephrine (noradrenaline) but most of this is produced by the sympathetic nervous system.[4] *To obtain blood for the estimation of plasma catecholamines it is necessary to have a venous catheter in place for 30 minutes before collecting a sample.*

Epinephrine (adrenaline)

The normal plasma level is 0.03–1.31 nmol/litre in resting conditions. It is raised in *phaeochromocytoma*. This is a very rare tumour and often as a screening test a 24-hour urine metanephrine screening test is used[4] *with the patient on a vanilla-free diet* (see catecholamines in urine, below).

Norepinephrine (noradrenaline)

The normal plasma level is 0.47–4.14 nmol/litre in resting conditions. It is raised in *phaeochromocytoma* and may exceed 10 nmol/litre.[4] See epinephrine above for screening test.

Catecholamines in urine

Some cases of high blood pressure are due to an adrenal medullary tumour (*phaeochromocytoma*) which secretes excessive epinephrine or norepinephrine into the blood. There is consequently an excess of epinephrine breakdown products in the urine, in the form of catecholamines, including VMA (vanillylmandelic acid). Excess catecholamine excretion also occurs with a *neuroblastoma*, a childhood tumour of the sympathetic nervous system. Normally less than 150 µg are excreted per day, of which VMA constitutes 5–35 µmol/24 hour, epinephrine <144 nmol/24 hour and norepinephrine <570 nmol/24 hour. For their estimation a complete 24-hour specimen of urine must be collected in a clean Winchester bottle containing 2 ml of concentrated hydrochloric acid. The bottle must be well sealed and sent to chemical pathology.

NB: For at least 48 hours prior to the test the patient must not eat food containing vanilla, e.g. tomatoes, bananas, cakes, sweets, coffee or tea. Aldomet should not be given for at least a week before the test. Any drugs taken should be noted on the request form.

Pituitary gland investigation

The pituitary gland has an anterior lobe and a posterior lobe (with small pars intermedia).

Perimeter or field analyser tests

These tests (p. 28) may show evidence of pressure on the optic nerve by a *tumour arising* from the *pituitary gland*.

X-Ray, CT scan and MRI

X-ray of the pituitary fossa may show enlargement by a tumour. X-ray may also show bone changes in acromegaly. A more accurate picture of the pituitary gland is provided by CT scanning (p. 21), with high dose intravenous contrast. An even better picture, which avoids the use and possible hazards of X- rays and contrast medium, is MRI (p. 21), with or without gadolinium enhancement.[5] So MRI is now the best method of imaging the pituitary gland.

Anterior pituitary hormones

The anterior pituitary produces a number of trophic hormones which control the function of other glands. A pituitary tumour may secrete hormone, e.g. prolactin produced by a *prolactinoma*. A pituitary tumour is also one of the causes of damage to the pituitary gland, resulting in a reduction in the blood level of other pituitary hormones, generally in the following order: MSH (melanocyte stimulating hormone), the gonadotrophins FSH (follicle stimulating hormone) and LH (luteinizing hormone), GH (growth hormone), TSH (thyroid stimulating hormone) and finally ACTH (adrenocorticotrophic hormone). It is now possible to measure the blood levels of these hormones, usually by radioimmunoassay. *The laboratory should be consulted if an assay is required.*

Assessment of anterior pituitary function

Basal anterior pituitary function may be assessed on 09.00 hours blood sample, collected under resting, unstressed conditions, for the measurement of the following[5]:

1. cortisol (p. 51)
2. total (or free) T_4 (p. 45)
3. TSH (p. 46)
4. testosterone (male, p. 188) or oestradiol (female, p. 187)
5. LH, FSH (p. 57)
6. prolactin (p. 57).

The ability to respond to stimuli is provided by dynamic tests such as the insulin tolerance test (ITT), the glucagon test, the clomiphene and gonadotrophin releasing hormone tests and the combined test of anterior pituitary function.

Luteinizing hormone (LH)

In males LH stimulates testosterone production in the testis;[5] the normal serum level is 1–7 U/L. In females LH stimulates ovulation;[5] the normal pre-ovulatory level is 2.5–10 U/L, rising at midcycle to 25–70 U/L and then falling to 1–10 U/L during the post-ovulatory phase. After the menopause the level is less than 30 U/L. Its assessment is of value in determining the cause of amenorrhoea in a nonpregnant woman. A normal menstrual cycle excludes LH deficiency in the female. Normal plasma testosterone (p. 188) excludes LH deficiency in the male.

Follicle stimulating hormone (FSH)

In males FSH controls spermatogenesis; in females FSH controls the development of ovarian follicles and consequently oestrogen secretion; in both sexes it stimulates the gonads to secrete inhibin,[5] which tends to inhibit the pituitary from overstimulating the gonads.

Prolactin

Prolactin stimulates the breast to produce milk. Serum prolactin assay is of value in the investigation of pituitary/hypothalamic disease, *galactorrhoea* (excessive production of milk), *infertility* and *gonadal disorders*. In this test 5 ml clotted blood is collected between 09.00 and 11.00 hours, early in the week, avoiding any stress which causes prolactin levels to rise. Most disorders of its secretion result in raised serum prolactin levels (>360 U/L), including *prolactinoma*, the commonest hormone-secreting pituitary tumour. Low serum prolactin is rare but can occur after *severe postpartum haemorrhage* from pituitary infarction, preventing breast feeding. Prolactin levels tend to vary from day to day; so with borderline results repeat samples should be collected.[5]

Adrenocorticotrophic hormone (ACTH)

ACTH stimulates the adrenal cortex to produce cortisol. The normal plasma ACTH level varies from 8 to 50 ng/litre at 09.00 hours to 1–17 ng/litre at 20.00 hours. Usually blood is collected between 09.00 and 10.00 hours. It is essential to use a plastic (not glass) syringe; 15 ml is taken into an ice-cooled heparin tube and sent immediately to the forewarned laboratory. Its assay distinguishes between *primary* and *secondary adrenal insufficiency*, plasma ACTH being raised in the former and reduced in the latter. It also assists in determining the cause of *Cushing's syndrome* once this has been diagnosed. In *adrenal adenoma* and *carcinoma* ACTH is undetectable. High normal or slightly raised levels suggest *adrenal hyperplasia* due to excess pituitary ACTH (*Cushing's disease*). Values above 200 ng/litre suggest ectopic ACTH from a *hormone-secreting tumour* of lung or other site.

(Human) growth hormone (HGH or GH)

Growth hormone is also known as diabetogenic hormone: a large baby may be the first sign that a mother has *diabetes mellitus*. Secretion of growth hormone is very irregular. The normal serum level is 0–50 mU/litre (0.7–7 ng/ml), usually below 4 mU/litre, but can vary greatly over a few minutes. So results can be misleading unless there is a gross increase as in *acromegaly* and *gigantism*. The CSF level is always below 5 mU/litre (2 ng/ml) even with an *HGH-secreting tumour*, unless it has extended outside the sella turcica when higher values occur. *HGH deficiency* is demonstrated by the insulin tolerance test or the glucagon test.

NB: *Growth hormone deficiency* in children may not persist into adult life, and so repeat testing is mandatory.[6]

Insulin tolerance test (ITT)
This is also called the insulin stress test or insulin-induced hypoglycaemia stimulation test. It is used in the investigation of *hypopituitarism* and provides information about the secretion of human growth hormone (HGH) and adrenocorticotrophin (ACTH) assessed from cortisol levels. Informed written consent is required (see p. 2). The ITT is safe provided it is performed under constant medical supervision with 40–50% glucose solution ready for intravenous injection in case of *severe hypoglycaemia*. The patient has to fast overnight, and details of the test are available from the laboratory (insulin injection is as for 'combined test of anterior pituitary function', below). It is contraindicated in heart disease and epilepsy, and instead the glucagon test (below) should be used. Most normal subjects reach an HGH level of at least 40 mU/litre during the test, with an increase in HGH level of more than 25 mU/litre over the basal figure. Undetectable HGH indicates total HGH deficiency, and below 15 mU/litre partial HGH deficiency. With such low figures blood glucose levels must be checked to ensure that hypoglycaemia actually occurred.

Glucagon test
This test can be used for the detection of *hypopituitarism in children or in patients with heart disease or epilepsy*. Glucagon (see p. 149) is given as a single dose of 0.5 mg in children, 1.0 mg in adults under 90 kg and 1.5 for those over 90 kg. Blood samples are taken for growth hormone (HGH) and cortisol at 0, 60, 90, 120, 150, 180, 210 and 240 minutes. In normal subjects serum HGH levels usually start to increase at 90 minutes and rise to above 20 mU/litre. In *hypopituitarism* there is a diminished response.

Clomiphene and gonadotrophin releasing hormone (LH/FSH-RH) tests
These tests for pituitary gonadotrophin secretion are of limited diagnostic value. They are of no value if serum LH and/or FSH values are high, indicating *primary gonadal failure*. They can be of assistance in assessing the amount of pituitary tissue present after attempted pituitary ablation. Details are available from the laboratory.

Combined test of anterior pituitary function
This test provides an assessment of ACTH, HGH, TSH, prolactin and gonadotrophin secretion. The patient fasts overnight. An intravenous cannula or butterfly needle is inserted into an antecubital or forearm vein. By injecting 2 ml of saline–heparin (20 ml saline with 1000 units heparin) from time to time the system is kept patent. After allowing 45 minutes for the patient to relax, basal samples of blood are collected for glucose, HGH, TSH, prolactin, FSH and LH. At zero time soluble insulin (measured in a tuberculin syringe) is injected followed by 200 µg TRH (see p. 47) and 100 µg LH/FSH-RH in 5 ml sterile water intravenously and washed in with 2 ml of saline–heparin. The amount of insulin injected depends on the clinical state. If *hypopituitarism* is definitely suspected, 0.1 units per kg body weight is given. If suspicion is less certain, as with delayed puberty, the standard dose of 0.15 units/kg is given. Where insulin resistance is suspected, as in *acromegaly* or *Cushing's syndrome*, 0.2–0.3 units/kg is used. To be effective blood glucose should fall to 2.2 mmol/litre (40 mg/dl) or less and be at least half the basal level. Slight sweating and faintness should occur but 40–50% glucose solution should be ready for injection in case of severe hypoglycaemia, with constant medical supervision.

Normally the basal cortisol is at least 140–170 nmol/litre (5–6 μg/100 ml) and rises to 500 nmol/litre (18 μg/100 ml). The increase above basal level should be at least 195 nmol/litre (7 μg/100 ml). Deficient rise in cortisol indicates deficient ACTH secretion provided the adrenal glands are responsive, demonstrable by the Synacthen test. HGH response is as described under the insulin tolerance test and TSH response as for the TRH (thyrotropin releasing hormone) test.

Effects of the anterior pituitary on other endocrine glands

In *Simmond's disease (hypopituitarism)* there is often insufficient thyrotropic hormone to stimulate the thyroid adequately. So thyroid function tests may show the changes of *hypothyroidism*, but serum TSH is reduced, whereas in *primary hypothyroidism* it is increased (see TSH, p. 46). Similarly there may be insufficient ACTH to stimulate the adrenal cortex adequately. So tests for adrenal cortical activity often show similar results to *Addison's disease*. However, the Synacthen test (p. 53) differentiates them, giving a normal response in *Simmond's disease*, unlike *Addison's disease*.

In *Cushing's disease* due to basophil adenoma of the pituitary, too much ACTH is produced, stimulating the adrenal cortex excessively. So the tests will show evidence of excessive adrenal cortical function. The dexamethasone suppression test (p. 54) distinguishes this from *primary adrenal overactivity (Cushing's syndrome)*. In addition plasma ACTH can now be estimated, after consulting with the laboratory.

Assessment of posterior pituitary function

The posterior pituitary secretes vasopressin (antidiuretic hormone, ADH) and oxytocin. Vasopressin (ADH) acts on the kidney tubules, causing them to reabsorb more water, thus restricting the volume of urine.[5] Oxytocin stimulates uterine contraction during childbirth. The main effect of damage to the posterior pituitary is a reduced secretion of vasopressin (ADH) and so the patient tends to develop *diabetes insipidus*, characterized by the passage of a large volume of dilute urine. Direct measurement of plasma vasopressin greatly assists in the diagnosis of posterior pituitary damage, which previously could only be assessed by the water deprivation and ADH stimulation tests.

Vasopressin (antidiuretic hormone, ADH)

The normal plasma vasopressin (ADH) is 0.9–4.6 pmol/L. Its secretion is stimulated by hypotension, low blood volume and increased plasma osmotic pressure. A *tumour* encroaching on the posterior pituitary tissue causes reduced vasopressin secretion with resultant *diabetes insipidus*. The laboratory should be consulted if an assay is required.

Water deprivation test

The patient is totally deprived of fluid for several hours so that his body weight falls by about 3%. Urine is collected at about hourly intervals. Normally the urine specific gravity increases to well above 1020. If ADH is deficient it does not rise above 1010. For the small volumes of urine involved it is more practicable to have the osmolality measured by the laboratory. Normally this rises to 800 mosmol/kg or more but in *diabetes insipidus* it fails to do so. Conversely the plasma osmolality, measured from blood taken into a heparin tube, normally does not rise above 300 mosmol/kg. In *diabetes insipidus* it exceeds this figure, the blood becoming more concentrated as a result of dehydration.

ADH stimulation test

This is only necessary if the water deprivation test results indicate *diabetes insipidus* and ADH estimation (p.59) is not available. The patient is given as much fluid as he wishes; 20 μg des-amino d-arginine vasopressin (DDAVP) is instilled intranasally. Over the next 4 hours urine is collected hourly. In patients with *cranial diabetes insipidus* the urine osmolality rises to 600 mosmol/kg or more. Failure to respond suggests that the dilute urine is due to kidney disease, i.e. *nephrogenic diabetes insipidus* (see also osmolality, p. 116).

Gonadal endocrine function investigations

See p. 187.

Pancreatic secretion of insulin

See p. 144.

Reference

1. Butler, J and Pope, R. Thyroid dysfunction. In: Marshall, W J and Bangert, S K, (eds). *Clinical Biochemistry; Metabolic and Clinical Aspects*. New York. Churchill Livingstone. 1995: 331–354.

2. Kelman, G R *Physiology: A Clinical Approach*. Edinburgh. Churchill Livingstone. 1980: 123.

3. Kelman, G R. *Physiology: a Clinical Approach*. Edinburgh. Churchill Livingstone. 1980: 124.

4. Drury, P L. Adrenal disorders. In: Marshall, W J and Bangert, S K, (eds). *Clinical Biochemistry: Metabolic and Clinical Aspects*. New York. Churchill Livingstone. 1995: 315–329.

5. Howlett, A H. Hypothalamic and pituitary disorders. In: Marshall, W J and Bangert, S K, (eds). *Clinical Biochemistry: Metabolic and Clinical Aspects*. New York. Churchill Livingstone. 1995: 295–313.

6. Monson, J P. Adult growth hormone deficiency. Journal of the Royal College of Physicians of London. 1998: 32(1): 19–22.

CHAPTER FIVE

Tests related to breathing

Respiratory system

Index of tests	Page		
Blood gases and pH	73	Nasal sinus X-rays	62
Bronchography	63	Nose	61
Bronchoscopy	74	Peak flow rate (PFR)	67
Chest X-rays	63	Pernasal swab	62
Diphtheria bacilli	62	Pleural fluid	66
Diphtheria carriers	62	Pleural needle biopsy	75
Dynamic lung volumes	68	Postbasic tests	72
Fine needle aspiration (FNA) of lung	75	Pulmonary angiography	64
Flow volume curve or loop	68	Rhinoscopy	61
Gastric washings	66	Static lung volumes	71
Laboratory examination of sputum	65	Streptococci	63
Larynx	63	Thoracoscopy	74
Laryngeal swab	66	Throat	62
Lung function tests	67	Throat swab	62
Lung scan	63	Transfer factor	71
Mediastinoscopy	74	Tubercle bacilli	66
Mediastinotomy	74	Vincent's angina	63
Nasal swab	62		

Introduction

The function of breathing is to provide a change of air in the lung alveoli. As air enters through the nose, throat and larynx it is warmed and moistened before reaching the delicate lining epithelium of the alveoli. Here, oxygen diffuses through the thin alveolar lining to reach the haemoglobin in the red blood cells, and carbon dioxide diffuses out into the alveoli to be expelled in the expired air. Many of the tests on the upper respiratory tract are performed by the otorhinologist and those on the lung by the chest physician or surgeon, the radiologist and the lung function technician.

Upper respiratory tract investigations

Nose
Rhinoscopy
This is the examination of the interior of the nose.

1. Anterior rhinoscopy is carried out through the nostrils with the aid of a nasal speculum and good illumination.

2. Posterior rhinoscopy is the examination of the nasopharynx, which is carried out through the mouth with the aid of a reflecting mirror (warmed, e.g. with a spirit lamp) or else with a pharyngoscope. The patient's pharynx is sprayed with local anaesthetic to permit vision behind the soft palate. No food is permitted until recovery from the local anaesthesia. Swabs may be taken for bacteriology or tissue for histology (taken into fixative, e.g. formol saline).

Nasal swab

One of the following techniques is normally used:

1. Swab from anterior nares (nostrils). Using a sterile bacteriological swab, material is collected from just within the anterior nares. This is the method of choice for the detection of *Staphylococcus* carriers, when swabs should also be taken from wrists, perineum and groin.

2. Pernasal swab (see below).

Pernasal swab

This swab is supplied by the laboratory. It is supported on a thin flexible metal wire. It is introduced through the anterior nares and passed directly posteriorly along the floor of the nose, until the posterior nasopharynx is reached. Care must be taken to choose the side of the nose which is free from any obstruction, e.g. by septal deflection. This method is used in suspected infections by *Meningococcus*, whooping cough (*Bordetella pertussis*) and nasal diphtheria (*Corynebacterium diphtheriae*). The swab should be sent to the laboratory, without delay, or in a transport medium e.g. Stuart's medium (p. 12).

X-ray of nasal sinuses

Disease of sinuses renders them radioopaque, demonstrable by taking appropriate skull X-rays.

Throat

Throat swab

Sterile swabs are supplied by the laboratory. The patient is placed so that the pharynx is well illuminated. If necessary the tongue may be depressed by a spatula. The specimen should be collected by rubbing the swab firmly over the tonsillar area. If a membrane is present this should be lifted gently and the swab taken from the deeper layers. Gargling with antiseptics, or drinking hot fluids, should be avoided for an hour or so prior to taking the swab.

Diphtheria bacilli

In all cases of throat infection a swab should be sent to the laboratory. If the case is *diphtheria* the result will be 'C. diphtheriae present' or '+ve for KLB' (KLB=Klebs Löffler bacillus – the cause of diphtheria). A repeated negative result usually means the case is not one of diphtheria.

Swab results are also useful in assessing when a convalescent case of diphtheria is clear of infection.

'Carriers'

Some persons, whether convalescent from diphtheria or not, carry diphtheria bacilli in their throats when perfectly well, and they may be a source of infection to others. In such cases a 'virulence' test is done to decide whether the bacteria present are capable of causing diphtheria or not. If 'virulent' the patient must be isolated until clear of infection. If 'non-virulent' they may be disregarded.

Both nasal and aural swabs may also be taken from patients who have a chronic discharge, and who may be potential carriers of diphtheria.

Streptococci

Many persons harbour streptococci in the throat which may or may not be harmful to others. The ones most liable to cause trouble are 'haemolytic streptococci', i.e. those capable of haemolysing blood. These are especially dangerous to maternity cases, and may cause *puerperal sepsis*.

Anyone working in a maternity ward who has a sore throat should have a throat swab and a nasal swab taken. Clinical staff with a throat swab 'positive for haemolytic streptococci' must be excluded until three negative results have been obtained. It may be necessary for carriers of streptococci to have the tonsils removed.

Vincent's angina

In cases of this disease a throat or gum swab will reveal the presence of the causal organisms: spirochaetes and fusiform bacilli.

Larynx

See Laryngoscopy, p. 27 and Laryngeal swab, p. 66.

Lower respiratory tract investigations

Chest X-rays

X-ray examinations include:

1. *Straight radiographs* of chest (posteroanterior and lateral) and of sinuses.
2. *Tomography.* This is a technique for obtaining a radiographic 'section' (usually coronal) of the chest at a given depth. It is of value in investigating a small tumour or cavity.
3. *Computerized tomography* (CT) scans (see pp. 38, 84).
4. *Screening.* The lungs and their movements are observed by a fluoroscopic screen placed in front of the patient via an image intensifier and television link.
5. *Bronchography.* The bronchial tree may be clearly outlined by the introduction of contrast medium. It is used for the diagnosis of bronchiectasis and other bronchial abnormalities, e.g. tumours. A laryngeal catheter is passed through the nose to the larynx and radioopaque medium injected through this. About 10 ml of medium is injected, the patient meanwhile lying on the side which it is desired to show, so that the medium will run by gravity into the lung concerned. It runs into the lower bronchioles, rendering them opaque to X-rays. This shows up dilatation from *bronchiectasis* or constriction from a *tumour.*
6. *Lung scans,* using radioisotopes (see p. 22). These provide evidence of the blood flow through the lungs. No preparation is required, but the patient must give informed consent (p. 2) after being reassured that only tracer doses of radioisotope are used. The latter is usually technetium attached to small aggregates of albumin. This is injected intravenously at the beginning of the test. With the patient lying in appropriate positions, a gamma camera is passed over the patient's body. Normally

this shows evenly distributed blood perfusion over the whole lung. This finding excludes *pulmonary embolism*.[1] When a blood vessel is obstructed, as in a *pulmonary embolism*, there is an absence of perfusion over the affected zone. If the straight X-ray film shows no lesion in this zone, a *pulmonary embolus* is likely, but if the X-ray shows evidence of a lung lesion in the unperfused zone, this lesion is likely to be the cause of the perfusion abnormality. If there is concern that *pulmonary embolism* or other vascular abnormality may coexist with the lung lesion seen on straight X-ray, this may be resolved by pulmonary angiography (see below).

7. *Pulmonary angiography* involves injecting the pulmonary arteries with radioopaque material in order to visualize the blood vessels in the lung. It may be used when *pulmonary embolism* can be neither excluded nor confirmed by a lung scan (see p. 63). This is particularly relevant in older patients with peptic ulcers, where the use of anticoagulants could precipitate bleeding and/or where embolectomy is contemplated. Pulmonary angiography is also used to demonstrate blood vessel abnormalities and occasionally in the investigation of tumours. The patient should be tested for iodine sensitivity and the radiologist notified if sensitivity is suspected. Nothing should be taken by mouth after midnight preceding the test. The patient should be told that ECG leads would be attached for monitoring the heart (p. 79), that a catheter would be inserted into the leg vein for introducing the dye, that the injection of the dye would cause a warm flush to be felt, also that coughing might occur and that bed rest would be necessary for 12–24 hours after the test. The patient should give written permission for the test (see p. 2). Following the test the patient's TPR (temperature, pulse and respiration) should be recorded at regular intervals and the catheter site checked for bleeding or inflammation. Evidence of hypersensitivity to the dye, usually within 2–6 hours of the test, should be reported (treatable with antihistamines or steroids).[2]

8. *Miniature mass radiography* (MMR). By using miniature films, population surveys may be carried out at a relatively low cost. Suspect cases are then examined using full-size films.

The following are examples of conditions which may be demonstrated by X-rays:

- *Abscess of the lung*. A cavity, perhaps with a fluid level, is seen.
- *Bronchiectasis*. Certain changes are visible on a straight X-ray, but the bronchial dilatations are better demonstrated by bronchography (see p. 63).
- *Pleural effusion and empyema*. An opacity is seen, perhaps with a fluid level, which can be seen to move with respiration and posture on screen examination.
- *Fibroid lung*. The collapsed lung is visible, and possibly some displacement of the heart which is pulled over by the contraction of the lung.
- *Growths*. These are visible and may be primary or secondary. Primary growths include *carcinoma of the lung* and *mediastinal tumours*. Secondary growths may be deposits of *sarcoma* or *carcinoma* from primary growths in other parts of the body. Enlarged mediastinal glands in *Hodgkin's disease* may be seen.
- *Hydatid cysts*. These have a typical circular appearance with clear-cut edges and possibly a fluid level.

Malignant cells

Malignant cells may be seen in effusions accompanying *growths of the lung*.

Purulent fluid

In *pneumococcal empyema* the pus is thick, creamy yellow, and contains numerous pneumococci. In *streptococcal empyema*, the pus is thinner and contains streptococci. In *tuberculous* cases the pus is greenish-yellow in colour, and tubercle bacilli may be demonstrable. See also infected fluids, p. 11.

Guinea pig test

In a doubtful case of tuberculosis with a clear effusion where culture for tubercle is negative, some of the fluid can be sent for injection into a guinea-pig (susceptible to even a small number of tubercle bacilli).

Lung function tests

Lung function tests provide a measure of the efficiency of the respiratory system. They are used in the diagnosis of chest diseases, in monitoring the response to treatment and in the assessment of risk prior to anaesthesia and surgery. The simpler tests such as measurement of the peak flow rate and dynamic lung volumes are sometimes performed by nurses and doctors on the ward. More complex procedures such as measurement of static lung volumes, transfer factor and postbasic tests are performed by physiological measurement technicians in a lung function laboratory.

Bronchodilators should not be taken for 4 hours before the test (provided there is no medical contraindication); smoking and alcohol should be avoided for 12 hours or more and the patient should not wear restrictive clothing.

There are five main types of test:

1. Peak flow rate
2. Dynamic lung volumes and flow volume curve or loop
3. Static lung volumes
4. Transfer factor
5. Postbasic tests.

Peak flow rate (PFR)

This is the maximum expiratory flow rate that can be sustained for 10 milliseconds following a full inspiration. It is very effort-dependent and the patient is usually given two practice runs with encouragement to make the maximum possible inspiration, sealing the lips tightly round the mouthpiece and then giving a short, sharp very fast blow into the instrument. The average of the next three attempts is then recorded with a rest period of at least 1 minute between attempts to avoid broncho-constriction. Instruments used for this test include the Wright peak flow meter (**Fig. 5.1a**) and the mini-Wright peak flow meter (**Fig. 5.1b**), the latter being cheap enough for home use by appropriate outpatients. The method of using both instruments is as outlined above. The normal PFR is related to age, height and sex (**Fig. 5.2**, adults, and **Fig. 5.3**, children 5–18 years). The figure is reduced if there is airways obstruction from any

Fig. 5.1 (a) Wright peak flow meter (Airmed); (b) Mini-Wright peak flow meter (Airmed)

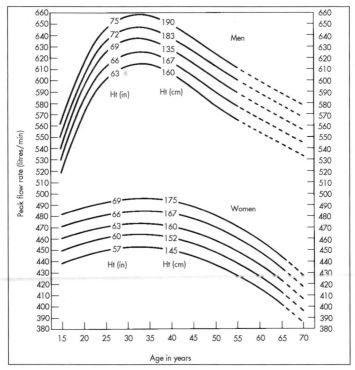

Fig. 5.2 Peak flow rate in normal adults. In men values up to 100 litres/minute less than predicted, and in women up to 85 litres/minute less than predicted, are within normal limits (Gregg and Nunn, *British Medical Journal*. 1973: 3: 282)

cause, e.g. *chronic bronchitis or asthma*. In the latter condition the peak flow rate can be greatly improved by treatment which relieves the broncho-constriction.

Dynamic lung volumes and flow volume curve or loop

1. Forced vital capacity (FVC). This is the maximum volume of air that can be forcibly exhaled following a full inspiration.

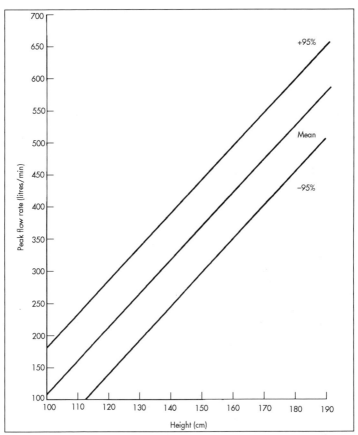

Fig. 5.3 Peak flow rate in normal boys and girls aged 5–18 years, 95% of results falling within the outer lines (Godfrey et al. *British Journal of Diseases of the Chest.* 1970: 64: 15)

2. Forced expiratory volume in 1 second (FEV$_1$). This is the maximum volume of air that can be forcibly exhaled in one second following a full inspiration. Normally the FEV$_1$ is about 80% of the FVC (**Fig. 5.4a**). This ratio is reduced in *obstructive airways disease*, viz. *asthma, chronic bronchitis* and *emphysema* (**Fig. 5.4b**). However, in restrictive conditions such as *fibrosis of the lung* and *deformities of the chest wall* there is a reduction in the FVC which may be proportionately greater than the reduction in the FEV$_1$. So the expiration ratio may be normal or higher than normal (**Fig. 5.4c**).

The instrument used for measuring dynamic lung volumes is a spirometer, an example of which is shown in **Fig. 5.5**. A clip on the nose ensures that all the air is exhaled and inhaled through the mouth. As with the peak flow rate the patient needs encouragement and practice in making maximal respiratory efforts before averaging the results of three tests. The patient should sit in a chair, in case of syncope, with arms about 25 cm (10 inches) above seat level.

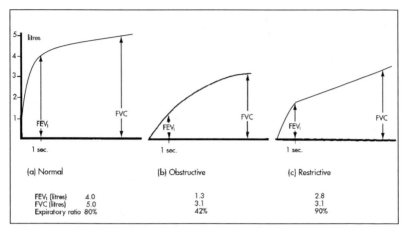

Fig. 5.4 Forced expiratory volume in 1 second (FEV₁), forced vital capacity (FVC) and expiratory ratio (FEV₁ / FVC 100): (a) normal, (b) obstructive, e.g. asthma or chronic bronchitis and emphysema, (c) restrictive, e.g. lung fibrosis or chest wall deformity

The results are plotted graphically as in **Fig. 5.4** for FEV₁ and FVC, and **Fig. 5.6** for flow volume loops. The latter represents the rates of flow recorded during maximum forced expiration, 'ABC', and inspiration, 'CDA'. A normal flow volume loop is shown in **Fig. 5.6a**, and by dotted lines in **Fig. 5.6b**, **c** and **d**. In the record of an *asthmatic* (**Fig. 5.6b**), 'A' is slightly to the left of the normal, indicating that the lungs are slightly

Fig. 5.5 Spirometer (Vitalograph Ltd.). Expiration via the elephant tubing expands the bellows inside the spirometer, causing the recording pen to move down the chart. At the same time the record chart moves from left to right and so a curved line is recorded

overinflated on full inspiration; the maximum rate of expiration 'B' is reduced and the rate of flow approaches nil more gradually than normal, indicated by BC being less steep and slightly 'scalloped'. After bronchodilators the asthmatic record reverts towards normality.

In *emphysema* (**Fig. 5.6c**) the lungs are even more overdistended so 'A' is shifted further to the left of normal; the 'scalloped' appearance of 'BC' is more evident and there is no improvement after bronchodilators; in both **Fig. 5.6b** and **c** the lungs contain more air than normal after full expiration so 'C' is shifted to the left. With restricted chest movement (*restriction*, **Fig. 5.6d**), the filling of the lungs at maximum inspiration is greatly limited and so 'A' is shifted to the right; reduction in the height of 'B' reflects the diminished flow.

Static lung volumes

The static lung volumes are shown diagrammatically in **Fig. 5.7**. They are usually measured in one of two ways:

1. The closed circuit helium rebreathing method. By measuring the dilution of the helium in the circuit, the lung volumes can be calculated.

2. Body plethysmograph. The patient sits in an airtight chamber and breathes normally while connected to a volume measuring system, usually a pneumotachygraph. By varying the type of breathing and monitoring the pressure changes in both the lung and the cabinet, the various lung volumes can be calculated on the basis of Boyle's law. The normal values for male and female adults are shown in **Table 5.1**.

Transfer factor

The transfer factor (or diffusing capacity) of the lung for carbon monoxide is the rate of uptake of the gas per minute for a pressure gradient of 1 mm of mercury (mmHg) across the alveolar capillary membrane. Carbon monoxide is used as the tracer gas because it behaves similarly to oxygen and has a high affinity for haemoglobin. Normal values are dependent on age, sex and body size.

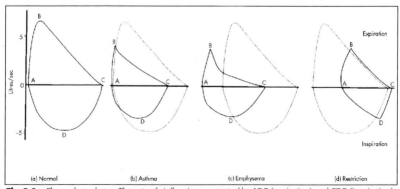

Fig. 5.6 Flow volume loops. The rate of air flow is represented by ABC (expiration) and CDE (inspiration), the volume of air in the lung being represented by the corresponding point on the line AC, in: (a) a normal subject, (b) asthma, (c) emphysema, (d) restriction, e.g. lung fibrosis or chest wall deformity

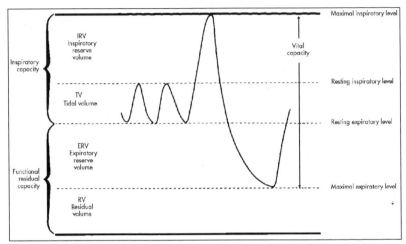

Fig. 5.7 Static lung volumes. Tidal volume represents the volume of air inspired and expired during normal quiet respiration. The other volumes are self-explanatory.

Postbasic tests

1. *Ear lobe capillary blood pH and gas analysis.* This is used in diagnosis to assess the oxygen requirement and the effectiveness of oxygen therapy in addition to the routine monitoring of blood gas levels. See pp. 73–74.

2. *Exercise-induced asthma test.* This involves monitoring spirometry tests before and after exercising for 6 minutes on a treadmill at 85% of predicted maximum cardiac efficiency. It is used in the diagnosis of bronchial reactivity, such as *asthma*.

3. *The 6 minute walking test.* This is performed in the hospital corridor. The total distance walked is measured, and rests are allowed as necessary. It is used to assess disability and effect of treatment such as rehabilitation programmes.

4. *Progressive multistage exercise test.* This involves exercise to exhaustion on a treadmill. Ear lobe blood is taken at rest and at the end of the exercise for the pH and blood gas analysis. Pulse rate, cardiac output and oxygen consumption are monitored. The results indicate whether dyspnoea is due to heart or lung disease. It detects early lung disease with great precision. It is used in the assessment of training and rehabilitation programmes, drug treatment and for diagnosis. This test is

Table 5.1   Average normal values for static lung volumes (Litres). More accurate figures are provided by a nomogram with corrections for age, height and sex.

		Men	Women	
Vital capacity	IRV	3.3	1.9	Inspiratory capacity
	TV	0.5	0.5	
	ERV	1.0	0.7	Functional residual capacity
	RV	1.2	1.1	
Total lung capacity		6.0	4.2	

IRV = Inspiratory reserve volume; TV = tidal volume; ERV = Expiratory reserve volume;
RV = residual volume

not usually used for diagnosis when routine tests have resolved the cause of breathlessness.

5. *Portable oxygen assessment.* The effect of breathing oxygen on the measured distance achieved in the 6 minute walking test is assessed, and used to determine whether portable oxygen therapy is indicated.

6. *Long-term oxygen therapy assessment.* The oxygen concentration needed to raise the arterial oxygen above a defined level is measured. Care is taken to ensure that there is not a dangerous rise in the carbon dioxide concentration. It is used to assess the need for prescription of 'oxygen concentrators'.

7. *Airways resistance and conductance.* This test provides additional information about any narrowing of the airways and 'stiffness' of the lungs. It evaluates the mechanical properties of the lungs.

Blood gases and pH

The pH of the blood is the degree of acidity or alkalinity. This can be measured by means of an instrument called a pH meter. A pH of 7 is neutral. Increase in the pH above 7 corresponds to an increase in alkalinity. Decrease below 7 corresponds to an increase in acidity.

For this test 2–5 ml of very fresh heparinized blood are usually needed, collected with a heparinized syringe. With the newer pH meters a finger-prick sample will suffice. Normal blood is slightly alkaline, having a pH of 7.36–7.44 (corresponding to a hydrogen ion concentration of 35–45 nmol/L). The body maintains this pH at the stable level necessary for life by means of buffer systems; one of the most important is the bicarbonate/CO_2 system. Bicarbonate is controlled by the kidneys (metabolic) and CO_2 by the lungs (respiratory). Only when the buffer systems break down does the pH fall outside the normal range. In *acidosis*, e.g. diabetic coma or respiratory distress, the pH may fall below 7.35; below 7.2 is critical. In *alkalosis*, e.g. from severe vomiting or excessive alkali therapy, the pH may be increased above 7.42; above 7.6 is critical.

The pH meter may also be used to measure the carbon dioxide pressure (pCO_2) and oxygen pressure (pO_2) in blood, also the standard bicarbonate and the base excess. The normal values are as follows:

Carbon dioxide pressure (pCO_2)	34–45 mmHg (4.8–5.9 kpa)
Oxygen pressure (pO_2)	90–1000 mmHg (12.0–13.3 kpa)
Standard bicarbonate	21.3–24.8 mmol/litre
Base excess	−2.3 to +2.3 mmol/litre

Measurements are usually performed on arterial blood ($paCO_2$, paO_2), often on capillary blood, but rarely on venous blood. A non-invasive technique for obtaining a close approximation to blood oxygen saturation is *pulse oximetry* (see p. 81).

In respiratory distress the pCO_2 is increased [over 70 mmHg (9.8 kpa) is critical], and the pO_2 reduced [under 50 mmHg (6.7 kPa) is critical]; the standard bicarbonate, the base excess and the pH are also all reduced. This is an example of severe respiratory acidosis. Other combinations of these findings give a measure of the severity of respiratory or metabolic acidosis or alkalosis. Blood gas estimations are used when testing for brain death (see p. 210).

For these estimations anaerobically collected fresh heparinized arterial blood is required, normally collected by the medical officer using a heparinized syringe. The laboratory will collect arterialized capillary blood in noncyanotic cases. In adults, the hand is placed in water at 45°C (just above body temperature) for about 5 minutes immediately before the blood is collected. The sample must be analysed within half an hour of collection.

Blood gas analysers are sometimes used on a ward or special care unit, under the supervision of the laboratory.

Tests undertaken by the thoracic surgeon or physician

Before any of the following tests are performed the surgeon or physician must first explain the nature of the test to the patient and obtain written consent (see pp. 2–3).

Bronchoscopy

By means of a bronchoscope the main bronchi and their branches can be inspected. Instead of a rigid bronchoscope, a flexible fibreoptic instrument is often used. No food is taken for several hours before this procedure is carried out. A sedative is given, and the patient prepared for the theatre. Its chief value is in the diagnosis of growths, when small portions of tissue are biopsied for histological examination. Bronchial brushings (spray-fixed) and washings (fresh) are sent for cytological examination. Bronchoscopy is also used for removing foreign bodies from the air passages. See also Other alternatives to sputum (p. 66).

Thoracoscopy

After artificial pneumothorax has been induced and the skin at the site of inspection sterilized and anaesthetized, the pleura may be inspected with the aid of a thoraco-scope. This is an endoscope which is introduced through the chest wall into the pleural cavity. It is of value in the diagnosis of disease involving the pleura and is occasionally used for cutting adhesions which prevent the full collapse of the lung. It is also used for endoscopic cervical sympathectomy.

Mediastinoscopy

This is the direct inspection of mediastinal structures with a special viewing instrument, the mediastinoscope. It is performed in the operating theatre under general anaesthesia through a small incision in the suprasternal fossa. Preparation of the patient is as for any such procedure. It is of value in the diagnosis of mediastinal lymph node enlargement, e.g. from *lymphoma*, *sarcoidosis* or *tumour* deposits. Morbidity and mortality from this procedure are less than 2%. Superior vena caval obstruction is a contraindication.

Mediastinotomy

This is an alternative procedure to mediastinoscopy, preferred by many surgeons and offering similar information. It also is performed in the operating theatre under general anaesthesia. A small incision is made in the second intercostal space. In addition it permits examination of the anterior mediastinum and is not contraindicated by obstruction of the superior vena cava.

Pleural needle biopsy
Needle biopsy can provide the diagnosis of lesions such as *tuberculosis* and *mesothelioma*. It is often performed when a pleural effusion is present but may be done in its absence. The skin over the suspected lesion is cleaned and then infiltrated with local anaesthetic. Abram's needle is the type most frequently used. The tissue specimens it provides are small, and so several samples are collected. Most of the material is placed in formol saline for histology but some unfixed material is also sent to the microbiology department for culture. Contraindications and complications, which are the same as for fine needle aspiration of the lung (below), are rare. Repeat biopsy may be indicated if the first is inconclusive; alternatively thoracoscopy or open pleural biopsy may be required.

Fine needle aspiration (FNA) of lung
This technique is used to determine the nature of any discrete mass seen in the lung on X-ray which remains undiagnosed after sputum cytology, serological tests and sometimes bronchoscopy. It is being used with increasing frequency following improvements in radiological control, fine needles and cytological methods.

For an afternoon test the patient may eat a normal breakfast and have coffee at 11.00 hours but no lunch. Premedication is advisable, such as valium 10 mg orally, codeine phosphate 30 mg intramuscularly and hyoscine hydrobromide 0.4 mg intramuscularly, together given 30 minutes before examination. The patient lies on the X-ray table with the affected area closest to the radiologist. The skin overlying the lesion is marked, cleaned and infiltrated with local anaesthetic. The needle is introduced vertically, held in special forceps. The patient must then hold his breath as the needle is advanced into the lesion under radiological control and a small amount of tissue aspirated. The needle is then removed and the aspirated material immediately spread on glass slides, put into 95% alcohol and taken to the laboratory for staining and interpretation. If no tumour cells are found in the first aspirate the procedure is repeated twice more with additional alcohol fixed specimens for special stains and unfixed material for culture.
Contraindications to this test are:

- An uncooperative patient with an uncontrollable cough or unable to lie flat for 10 minutes or so

- Suspected hydatid cyst or arteriovenous malformation

- A significant bleeding diathesis

- Poor respiratory reserve such that the patient could not withstand a large *pneumothorax*.

It is not uncommon for a small pneumothorax to occur, but one large enough to require treatment (intubation) occurs in less than 5% of cases. There is sometimes slight haemorrhage which may produce a haemoptysis, but this should not cause concern; severe haemorrhage is rare. Lung FNA has proved extremely valuable for diagnosis of *focal lung lesions*, mainly *tumours*, and for planning appropriate treatment.

References

1. Pagana, K D and Pagana, T J. Lung scan. In: Pagana, K D and Pagana, T J, (eds). *Mosby's Diagnostic and Laboratory Test Reference*. St Louis. Mosby Year Book. 1992: 488–490.

2. Pagana, K D and Pagana, T J. Pulmonary angiography. In: Pagana, K D and Pagana, T J, (eds). *Mosby's Diagnostic and Laboratory Test Reference*. St. Louis. Mosby Year Book. 1992: 604–606.

CHAPTER SIX

Tests related to circulation

Cardiovascular system

Index of tests	Page
Aneurysms	83
Angiocardiography	84
Angiography	83
Apical heart rate	79
Arterial disease test	85
Blood pressure measurement	77
Cardiac catheterization	83
Cardiac function	79
Cardiac monitoring	80
Central venous pressure (CVP)	85
Computerized tomography (CT) scan	84
Coronary angiography	84
Doppler ultrasound	85
Echocardiography	85
Electrocardiogram (ECG)	79
Exercise tolerance tests	79
Lymphangiography	83
Heart X-ray	83
Renin–angiotensin system	78

Introduction

The main functions of the circulation are to carry oxygenated blood and dissolved food material to the tissues, and remove waste products from the tissues to the lungs and kidneys. The circulation also provides transport for phagocytes, hormones and many other substances. Most of the tests on the cardiovascular system are undertaken by the cardiac physician, the radiologist and the ECG technician. Blood pressure measurement and cardiac monitoring are often undertaken by the nurse.

Blood pressure

Blood pressure (BP) measurement

The BP is the pressure the blood exerts on the wall of a blood vessel. The arterial BP is the one commonly recorded. It is expressed as a figure which indicates the height in millimetres of a column of mercury (mmHg) that would be supported by the pressure in question. For many years it has been estimated by means of a sphygmomanometer containing a column of mercury with an attached millimetre scale. However, mercury is a poison and, just as with barometers, the use of a mercury column has been almost entirely replaced by an aneroid system, with a manometer dial calibrated in mmHg, having the same significance as before. A cuff is placed around the upper arm which can be inflated by means of a rubber bulb, and it is attached to the manometer by a length of rubber tubing.

There are two readings to be taken in measuring the blood pressure:

1. *Systolic*. The pressure corresponding to systole, or contraction of the ventricle of the heart.

2. *Diastolic*. The pressure corresponding to diastole, or relaxation of the ventricle.

The simplest way to take the systolic pressure is to feel the pulse at the wrist, inflate the armband, and note the figure reading (in mmHg) at which the pulse disappears.

It is, however, desirable to record both systolic and diastolic pressures, and for this purpose a stethoscope is placed over the brachial artery in the region of the elbow. Air is pumped into the armlet till no sounds are audible. The pressure is then allowed to fall slowly by opening the valve. At the point when regular sounds become audible, a reading is taken: this is the systolic pressure. The pressure is still allowed to fall, and the sounds change in character, ultimately becoming practically inaudible, at which point another reading is taken: this is the diastolic pressure (many sphygmomanometers give an automatic readout of the systolic and diastolic pressures).

The difference between the two readings is termed the pulse pressure. Normal systolic blood pressure may vary from 100 to 140 mmHg. It tends to increase with age. Normal diastolic pressure varies from 60 to 90 mmHg. A blood pressure reading is usually expressed thus: 120/80, 210/140, etc. This indicates that the systolic pressure is 120 and the diastolic 80, and so on.

A high blood pressure is found in cases of *essential hypertension, chronic renal disease, cerebral compression, toxaemias of pregnancy*, etc. A low blood pressure (hypotension) is found in cases of *haemorrhage, shock, severe acute infections, Addison's disease,* excess hypotensive drug etc., when the systolic blood pressure may fall below 90 mmHg.

Estimation of the blood pressure is one of the commonest of all tests, and is carried out on the majority of patients.

Renin–angiotensin system

In cases of hypertension where there is evidence of possible unilateral kidney disease, revealed for example by intravenous urography (IVU, p. 168), it is feasible to collect blood for renin–angiotensin estimation from each renal vein to see whether excess is being produced by one kidney compared to the other. This assists in deciding whether surgical removal of a damaged kidney may relieve hypertension. For this test 5–20 ml of blood are collected into a universal container to which a special enzyme inhibitor has been added. The collection is usually carried out by a radiologist after he has introduced a catheter from the femoral vein into the inferior vena cava. Prior to the test all drugs are stopped, particularly hypotensive drugs. Sometimes a diuretic is given on the morning of the test to exaggerate any renin–angiotensin difference between the two kidneys. The patient must give informed written permission for this test (see p. 2).

Cardiac function
Exercise tolerance tests
These are methods of estimating the reserve power of the heart in cases of *cardiac disease.*

The patient is given some definite amount of physical effort to carry out, e.g. walking a certain distance, climbing a certain number of steps, stepping on and off a stool several times, etc., and the effect on the heart is noted. The pulse rate is taken before the test, immediately following exercise and again after a rest of 2 minutes. If the reserve power of the heart is sufficient for the task in question, the pulse rate should not be unduly increased by the exercise, and should have returned to its original rate after the 2 minutes' rest.

Another method of estimating the reserve power of the heart is to see how much physical effort the patient can carry out without developing any signs of cardiac distress, e.g. severe palpitation, shortness of breath, faintness or pain.

Apical heart rate
With a stethoscope over the apex of the heart two heart sounds – 'lub-dup' – are normally heard for each heart beat. It is advisable to count the heart rate in this way in heart conditions such as *atrial fibrillation* where some heart impulses fail to reach the radial pulse.

Electrocardiogram (ECG)
Electrical impulses are set up by cardiac contractions, and these may be recorded in the form of a graphic chart, an electrocardiogram, or displayed on an ECG monitor. After consultation with the physician in charge it is usual for a patient on beta-blockers to stop taking the tablets the day before the test. Most inpatients are tested on the ward using a portable ECG machine. Electrodes are attached to the chest and limbs after the chosen sites (from which hair has been shaved if necessary) have been cleaned with spirit swabs and electrode gel applied to provide electrical conductivity between skin and electrode. It is quite painless, but informed written consent should be obtained (see p. 2). Outpatients attend the ECG department and females should be advised to wear separate top and trousers or skirt to facilitate access to the chest. Often the effect of exercise on the ECG is tested.

The ECG records the electrical changes associated with atrial contraction (P wave), passage of the impulse from atria to ventricles (PR interval), ventricular contraction (QRS complex) and ventricular repolarization (T wave) (**Fig. 6.1**). If there is atrial fibrillation the P wave is replaced by multiple waves (**Fig. 6.2**). If conduction from atria to ventricles is slowed by partial heart block, the length of the PR interval is prolonged (**Fig. 6.3**). If the ventricular muscle is damaged, as in *myocardial infarction* due to *coronary thrombosis,* the pattern of the ST segment and/or T wave is altered (**Fig. 6.4**).

Now that cardiac monitoring is a routine on intensive care wards, it is necessary to become familiar with the normal ECG and to distinguish between a trivial abnormality, such as atrial ectopic beat, and a major disaster, such as a *ventricular fibrillation* (**Fig. 6.5**)

Fig. 6.1 Normal ECG

Fig. 6.2 Atrial fibrillation

Fig. 6.3 Partial heart block (prolonged PR interval)

Cardiac monitoring

Practically every bed in units for the intensive care of cardiac patients now has a cardiac monitor (**Fig. 6.6**). This is an electronic apparatus with electrodes which are attached to the patient. The instrument can then monitor the heart rate and ECG. It detects any change in the heart rhythm, recording it automatically and warning the staff so that appropriate treatment can be given at an early stage, e.g. by a defibrillator.

Ambulatory monitoring enables a continuous record, of up to 48 hours' duration, to be made of the electrical impulses emitted by the heart during unrestricted activity, rest and sleep. A small portable ECG monitor (**Fig. 6.7**), which includes a clock, is carried by the patient together with the electrodes and gel securely attached to the patient's

Fig. 6.4 Myocardial infarction (raised ST segment)

Fig. 6.5   Venticular fibrillation

body, as shown. The patient carries a diary to record the time and nature of all activities undertaken. There is also a marker with a button which the patient presses if chest pain, faintness or other symptoms occur. After completion of the test, the monitor is carefully removed, together with the strapping, electrodes, gel, etc. The magnetic tape is extracted and rapidly played back, using a computer to detect any abnormalities. Apart from being a diagnostic tool, it is also used to check artificial pacemaker function and the effectiveness of drugs used to control *arrhythmia*.[1]

Pulse oximetry

When a patient is in intensive care, and particularly if on a ventilator, or undergoing major surgery, it is important to keep a constant check on the oxygen saturation (SaO_2) in the arterial blood, without having to take blood samples, i.e. by a non-invasive technique. This is provided by oximetry. A sensor is clipped to the ear or finger. It warms the tissues to increase the blood flow, so that the oxygen saturation is almost equal to that of arterial blood, and it measures the oxygen saturation by passing a beam of light through the tissues and measuring the light absorption. If the haemoglobin is 90% saturated with oxygen, this is expressed as an SaO_2 of 90%. Oximetry is also used for testing the response to bronchodilators in an *asthmatic attack,* in sleep laboratories and for other studies where blood oxygenation may be affected.[2]

Chemical markers for myocardial ischaemia

Myocardial ischaemia occurs when the blood supply to any part of the heart is insufficient to supply its oxygen needs. *Angina* is the pain caused by this deficiency. If it is sufficiently severe or prolonged the heart muscle is damaged *(myocardial infarction)* and chemical substances are released from the damaged heart muscle cells. These

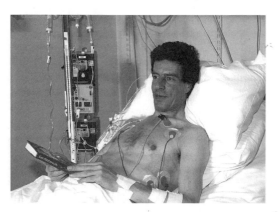

Fig. 6.6   Cardiac monitor

Thor : the Dark World 3D

Fig. 6.7 Portable cardiac monitor

include myoglobin, troponin T, troponin I, creatinine kinase (CK or CPK) and other enzymes.

Myoglobin

This is one of the earliest substances to be released into the blood after *myocardial infarction*, a raised level being detectable after 2 hours, reaching its peak at 6–9 hours and returning to normal by 24–36 hours.[3] It is a protein which is present in both cardiac and skeletal muscle, so that damage to either causes a rise in the serum level. It is measured by radioimmune assay and the laboratory should be consulted concerning its estimation.

Troponin T

This is another protein released from heart muscle following *infarction*. It can be measured by immunoassay, the normal serum level being 0–0.1 µg/L. A level of 0.2 µg/L or more is 98% diagnostic of *myocardial infarction* at 12–24 hours after the event.[3] It is also being used to determine which patients with *unstable angina (severe transient myocardial ischaemia)* are likely to progress to *myocardial infarction*.[3] **Troponin** I is similar and may be more specific for heart (as opposed to skeletal) muscle.[3] The normal serum level is 0–0.4 µg/L. The laboratory should be consulted concerning troponin estimation.

Other chemical markers

Other enzymes of value in the diagnosis and assessment of myocardial infarction are *creatine kinase (CK), phosphokinase (CPK, p. 117)*, *lactic dehydrogenase (LDH)* and, more specifically, *alpha hydroxybutyrate dehydrogenase* (αHBD, p. 117).

Imaging examination of the cardiovascular system

Heart

The heart is clearly visible on X-ray examination, enabling the heart size to be assessed. In certain types of heart disease the heart assumes a distinctive shape, e.g. boot-shape in *hypertension*. Calcification is sometimes seen in *valvular disease* and *pericarditis*. A *pericardial effusion* can also be demonstrated.

Aneurysms

Aneurysms (dilatations) of large vessels are sometimes visible on straight X-ray but are better shown on angiogram (see below). Ultrasound (p. 20) is also useful for demonstrating *abdominal aneurysms*. See also CT scan, p. 84.

Angiography

Injection of radioopaque dye into a vessel and rapid filming provides an angiogram. This outlines the vessel showing any *obstruction, aneurysm,* or *abnormal course*. The patient should give informed written consent (see p. 2). An angiogram of the aorta is called an aortogram, of arteries an arteriogram, and of veins a venogram or phlebogram. A number of specialized investigations may be undertaken, e.g. splenic venogram, hepatic arteriogram or renal arteriogram, which outline the vasculature in the respective organs. Abnormal vessels may be demonstrated in *tumours of the viscera* and *obstruction of the arteries* seen, e.g. in the legs in *intermittent claudication* (see also angiogram of cerebral vessels, p. 39).

Lymphangiography

Certain lymph nodes and vessels can be demonstrated by injection of ultrafluid Lipiodol through a tiny cannula into a lymph vessel in the dorsum of the foot (occasionally between the fingers) to produce a lymphangiogram. This is of value in showing lymph node involvement in *pelvic carcinoma* and *Hodgkin's disease*.

To locate the fine lymphatics in the feet a blue dye is injected between the toes. For a few hours after the procedure the patient may appear blue and the urine become green. The examination takes at least 3 hours and is tedious for both patient and radiologist. The injected oil eventually enters the neck veins and reaches the lungs, where it temporarily impairs function. It requires informed written consent (p. 2) and is contraindicated in patients with severe *lung disease*.

Cardiac catheterization (including angiocardiography)

This test enables the heart, coronary arteries and great vessels to be scrutinized. It is carried out with full aseptic precautions and is performed in the X-ray department. It involves passing a fine flexible catheter into a vein or artery in order to reach the heart. It is usually undertaken to determine the nature and degree of cardiac abnormality when surgery is contemplated.

Before the test the patient is usually admitted to the ward, where pulse, temperature and respiration are recorded, together with blood pressure, weight and urinalysis (see pp. 160–163). Preliminary tests include ECG, chest X-ray, full blood count, urea and electrolytes, hepatitis screening, blood group and the cross-match of two units of blood.

The procedure must be explained to and discussed with the patient before obtaining signed consent. The night before the test the right femoral and brachial areas are shaved. A little iodine is applied to the skin to exclude sensitivity to iodine in the contrast medium. A night sedative may be needed. No food or drink should be taken for 4–6 hours before the test.

Premedication and also prophylactic antibiotic are given 1 hour before. The latter is continued for a further 2 days.

A cardiac catheter, usually made of polythene tubing, is introduced into the relevant vessel, generally in the cubital fossa or the femoral region. Its progress is watched under X-rays until it is seen to enter the heart. Blood is then withdrawn, e.g. from the pulmonary artery, right ventricle, right atrium and superior vena cava. Blood pressures may also be measured at these sites. The samples of blood removed are examined for their oxygen and carbon dioxide content. Normally these remain practically the same in all the samples. Where there is a short circuit between the left and right sides of the heart, a marked rise in the oxygen content will be found to occur when the catheter has reached the site of the defect, e.g. right atrium in *atrial septal defect*.

Angiocardiography

This involves the injection of radioopaque dye through the catheter, so that by means of X-rays many abnormalities of the heart structure can be demonstrated. A cine film is often taken (cineradiography).

Coronary angiography

This is a similar technique for outlining the coronary arteries. It may be used in conjunction with the exercise tolerance test (p. 79) to assess coronary artery sufficiency before undertaking a cardiac bypass or a coronary angioplasty (the introduction of a balloon into the coronary artery to dilate any sites of narrowing).

After completion of the catheterization, the patient is returned to the ward and kept in bed under observation for 6–8 hours. Temperature, pulse, respiration and blood pressure are recorded regularly and a close watch kept on the site of introduction of the catheter, where a pressure pad is used to discourage haematoma formation.

Computerized tomography (CT) scan

A CT scan (p. 21) can provide an accurate, sometimes three-dimensional image of an intrathoracic lesion such as a *tumour* or *aneurysm*. The patient should fast overnight for a morning scan or following a light (08:00 hours) breakfast for an afternoon scan. This is to ensure that the stomach is empty at the time of the scan, minimizing any danger of aspirating gastric contents if a contrast medium is injected, which sometimes causes nausea. Informed written consent should be obtained (see p. 2).

Heart scan

Using radioisotopes (see p. 22) it is possible to study cardiac function, the blood flow through the heart and coronary arteries, and the extent of a *myocardial infarction*.

Being a non-invasive technique it is safer than cardiac catheterization but can provide comparable information.[4] Informed written consent is required (see p. 2).

Where available, *positron emission tomography* (p. 23) and another test with comparable precision, *single-photon emission computerized tomography* (*SPECT*), can be used to provide three-dimensional images of the functioning heart. Zones of *infarction* of the heart muscle can be accurately delineated.[4]

Doppler ultrasound

The sound of a car horn changes to a lower note as the car passes by. This alteration in sound frequency is known as the Doppler effect, a principle used to measure changes in velocity of a moving object. A Doppler probe generates its own inaudible sound beam. If the beam reflects off a moving object, such as a fetal heart valve or a moving column of blood, the Doppler effect causes a slight frequency change which the instrument presents as an audible sound in the loudspeaker.

Echocardiography

An ultrasound beam is directed at the heart. Movement of the heart walls and of individual valves is detected by the Doppler principle. The record may be displayed on a screen or on paper. It is used in the diagnosis of valvular disease and pericardial effusion.

Testing for arterial disease

The brachial systolic blood pressure is measured using a sphygmomanometer cuff on the upper arm and the Doppler probe placed over the brachial artery (instead of a stethoscope, as described on pp. 77–78). The cuff is then applied to the lower leg and the blood pressure measured at the dorsalis pedis or tibial arteries. The two pressures are compared. If the pressure at the ankle is less than 60% of the brachial pressure this indicates significant *occlusive arterial disease*. A practical consequence of a pressure less than 60% is that firm support bandaging of the type used to treat *venous ulceration* could occlude the arterial blood supply and cause *gangrene*.

Phonocardiography

The heart sounds may be recorded graphically. This is carried out by means of a special instrument called a phonocardiograph. By this means it is possible to detect and record heart sounds which are inaudible or difficult to distinguish by the ear. By means of an electrocardiogram (p. 79) recorded simultaneously it is possible to correlate the heart sounds with the heart action. It is of value in the interpretation of heart murmurs.

Central venous pressure (CVP)

This is the pressure in the large veins returning blood to the heart. It is normally between -20 mm (- 2 cm) and +80 mm (+8 cm) of water. It is raised in *heart failure* or following *excessive intravenous infusion*. It is low in *dehydration* and following *haemorrhage*. There are also fluctuations with respiration and pulsations with the heart beat.

The pressure is measured by a CVP line. This is a fine plastic catheter inserted aseptically, usually via the arm, and long enough to place the tip in the superior vena cava close to the heart. The other end is connected via a three-way tap to a sterile manometer set and a standard 'drip' set with a suitable infusion fluid. When taking a measurement a spirit level is used to align the sternal notch of the patient with the zero point on the manometer. The CVP line is of particular value when the intravenous fluid requirements are uncertain. Informed written consent must be obtained (see p. 2).

Reference

1. Pagana, K D and Pagana, T J. Holter monitoring (ambulatory monitoring, ambulatory electrocardiography). In: Pagana K D and Pagana T J, (eds). *Mosby's Diagnostic and Laboratory Test Reference*. St Louis. Mosby Year Book. 1992: 414–415.

2. Pagana, K D and Pagana, T J. Oximetry (pulse oximetry, ear oximetry, oxygen saturation). In: Pagana, K D and Pagana, T J, (eds). *Mosby's Diagnostic and Laboratory Test Reference*. St. Louis. Mosby Year Book. 1992: 537–538.

3. Hooper, J and Bangert S K. Clinical biochemistry in the investigation of acute chest pain and the acute abdomen. In: Marshall, W J and Bangert, S K, (eds). *Clinical Biochemistry; Metabolic and Clinical Aspects*. New York. Churchill Livingstone. 1955: 779–787.

4. Pagana, K D and Pagana, T J. Cardiac nuclear scanning. In: Pagana, K D and Pagana, T J, (eds). *Mosby's Diagnostic and Laboratory Test Reference*. St Louis. Mosby Year Book. 1992: 160–163.

CHAPTER SEVEN

Tests related to blood (1)

Haematology | **blood transfusion**

Index of tests	Page		Page
Abnormal haemoglobins	100	Haemoglobin	88
'Absolute values'	89	Haemoglobin S	98
Activated partial thromboplastin time (APTT)	96	Haemoglobins, abnormal	100
Antenatal blood tests	104	Haemolytic anaemias	98
Antibodies	99	Haemorrhagic disorders	93
Antiglobulin (Coomb's) test	107	Haptoglobin	98
Autohaemolysis	99	Heinz body test	100
Bacterial activity	103	Hess's test	94
Bleeding time	94	International normalized ratio (INR)	95
Blood group tests	103	Iron	91
Blood transfusion essentials	105	Iron-binding capacity	91
Blood transfusion reaction investigation	107	Iron saturation	91
Blood counts	88	Kaolin–cephalin time	96
Bone marrow puncture	93	Kleihauer test for fetal cells in maternal blood	105
Capillary microscopy	94	Lymph node biopsy	93
Capillary resistance test	94	Packed cell volume (PCV)	90
Clot retraction	94	Parasites in blood	92
Clotting time	94	Plasma fibrinogen	96
Coomb's test	107	Platelet count	93
Differential white cell count	92	Prothrombin and proconvertin test	95
Disseminated lupus erythematosus (DLE) tests	103	Prothrombin consumption test	96
Erythrocyte sedimentation rate (ESR)	89	Prothrombin ratio	95
Euglobin lysis time (ELT)	97	Recalcification time	94
Factor assays	96	Red cell appearance	91
Ferritin	91	Red cell count	89
Fetal cells in maternal blood	105	Red cell mass	90
Fibrindex (fibrinogen index)	96	Red cell osmotic fragility	99
Fibrinolysin	97	Red cell survival	100
Fluorescent antibody technique	103	Reticulocyte count	90
Gammaglobulin neutralization test	108	Rhesus type	104
Glandular fever tests	101	Rheumatoid arthritis tests	101
Glucose-6-phosphate dehydrogenase		Schumm's test	101
(G6PD) deficiency	100	Serum iron	91
Haematocrit	90	Sickle cell anaemia	98
Haemolysins	99	Streptokinase resistance test	98
Haemolytic disease of the newborn	105	Thrombin clotting time	98

Index of tests	Page		
Thrombotest	95	Viscometry	88
Transfusion reaction investigation	107	Wet film	98
Two-stage prothrombin test	95	White cell count	92

Introduction

Blood consists of plasma in which cells and platelets are suspended. The most numerous cells are the red blood cells (erythrocytes) which contain haemoglobin for carrying oxygen. In anaemia the amount of circulating haemoglobin is reduced, often due to blood loss; in haemolytic anaemia red cells are destroyed more rapidly than they can be replaced. About a tenth of the cells are white cells (leucocytes) whose main function is to combat any infection occurring in the body. The platelets and clotting factors in the plasma enable blood to clot, a mechanism for controlling blood loss from injury. Replacement of lost blood by transfusion is safe provided the donor blood is infection-free and compatible. Incompatible blood contains red cells which react with antibodies in the recipient's plasma, causing a blood transfusion reaction. Tests on all the above are performed in the haematology department which may also undertake some immunological tests, e.g. for glandular fever and rheumatoid disease, unless there is a separate department of immunology.

Haematology

This section deals with the tests concerning blood cells, bleeding and clotting and other investigations performed in the haematology department.

Blood counts and related investigations
Blood counts
The tests most commonly needed are the haemoglobin (below), red cell appearance (p. 73) and white cell count (p. 92). These can all be undertaken on one 4 ml sequestrenated sample of blood and are usually performed on automated equipment which provides seven separate results: haemoglobin, red cell count, white cell count, haematocrit (p. 90) and also the three main absolute values: mean cell volume (MCV), mean cell haemoglobin (MCH) and mean cell haemoglobin concentration (MCHC) (p. 90). Platelet counts (p. 93) are also frequently required, especially to monitor drug toxicity. The other common investigation is the differential white cell count (p. 92).

Haemoglobin
Haemoglobin is a pigment in the red blood cells, which combines with oxygen to form a reversible compound (oxyhaemoglobin).

Estimation of the haemoglobin content of the blood is thus a measure of its oxygen-carrying capacity. It is undertaken on finger-prick blood sample or alternatively on a venepuncture sample taken into a sequestrene (EDTA) tube. Estimation is usually done in the hospital laboratory but can be done in the clinic or sideroom with an instrument such as Reflotron (Boehringer–Mannheim).

The average adult level is about 14.5 g/dl (14.5 g/100ml) or 100%. It is higher in men (13.0–18.0 g/dl), and lower in women (11.5–16.5 g/dl). At birth the cord blood haemoglobin is about 13.6–19.6 g/dl, falling to about 12–15 g/dl in the first few weeks of life. In *anaemia* this figure is reduced below 11.5 g/dl. If it drops below 8 g/dl cardiac failure may develop. In *polycythaemia* it is increased to over 18 g/dl. It is also increased following *fluid loss*, e.g. from *burns, vomiting, diarrhoea, diuresis* or *excessive sweating.*

Red cell count

The red cell count is normally about 5.00×10^{12}/litre (5 000 000 red cells per mm^3), being slightly higher in males (4.5–6.5×10^{12}/litre) than females (3.8–5.8×10^{12}/litre). The figure is decreased in *anaemia* and increased in *polycythaemia*. The latter may be primary (*polycythaemia rubra vera*) or secondary, for example to altitude, *renal disease* or *chronic obstructive airways disease*. Dehydration from any cause, e.g. *shock, vomiting, diarrhoea, excessive sweating* or *diuresis*, also causes a rise in the red cell count.

After haemorrhage it is about 24 hours before the full reduction of the red cell count and haemoglobin can be demonstrated.

Erythrocyte sedimentation rate (ESR)

If blood which has been treated with anticoagulant is left to stand, the red cells start to sediment under the influence of gravity. Normally the red blood cells do not show much tendency to aggregate on standing, with the result that sedimentation is slow. In certain diseases they run together very readily to form rouleaux which sediment more rapidly.

The Westergren method is the one most commonly used. For the rarely used Wintrobe method, blood is collected into a sequestrene bottle and sent to the laboratory without delay. The Westergren method is often performed in the ward and will therefore be described in more detail.

For the test 0.5 ml of 3.8% sodium citrate is placed in a test tube; to this is added 2 ml of freshly taken blood and the sample is mixed. This mixture is then introduced into a graduated Westergren tube to the zero mark and the tube fixed into position on a special rack.

The distance fallen by the red blood cells is read at the end of 1 hour and sometimes after 2 hours. Normally it is 0–15 mm/1st hour for men and 0–20 mm/1st hour for women and children; over the age of 50 years it is 0–20 mm/1st hour for men and 0–30 mm/1st hour for women. It is of great value in estimating the progress in cases of *tuberculosis, rheumatic fever* and *vasculitis*.

It is raised in many other diseases, e.g. *infections, infarctions* and *cancer*, particularly in *multiple myeloma. Anaemias* generally cause a rise in the sedimentation rate, for which allowance must be made. With the Wintrobe method a correction factor may be applied and a result corrected for *anaemia* included in the report.

Viscometry

This is the measurement of the viscosity of whole blood or plasma and is performed on sequestrenated blood. Blood viscosity is increased when there is increase in the PCV (see p. 90). Plasma viscosity is increased when there is a raised ESR (see above). The increase is due to raised protein concentration, particularly fibrinogen. Some workers claim that plasma viscometry is a better test than the ESR, being quicker to perform.

It is also more reliable for a stored specimen, for up to 3 days, and so can be used for postal samples (for which the ESR is unreliable). The normal plasma viscosity is 1.50–1.72 mPa/S for both males and females.

Haematocrit (packed cell volume or PCV)

As soon as possible after applying the tourniquet the appropriate volume of venous blood is collected into a container with anticoagulant (e.g. sequestrene), mixed and sent to the laboratory. A representative portion is placed in a haematocrit tube and spun on a centrifuge until all the red cells are tightly packed at the bottom of the tube. Using automated equipment the haematocrit is a computed result based on the MCV (see below) and red cell count. The normal haematocrit is 0.40–0.52 (40–52%) in men and 0.36–0.47 (36–47%) in women. In *anaemia* it is reduced below these figures. It is increased in *polycythaemia* and *dehydration*. In the newborn the normal cord blood haematocrit is 0.44–0.62 (44–62%).

It may be used to screen for anaemia, to indicate the degree of fluid loss, to correct the sedimentation rate for *anaemia* and to calculate certain absolute values (see below). With a micro-haematocrit the test may be performed on a finger-prick sample.

'Absolute values'

Mean cell haemoglobin concentration (MCHC) indicates the degree to which cells are packed with haemoglobin. It is normally 32–35 g/dl and is reduced in *iron deficiency*. It is about the most reliable of the 'absolute values'.

Mean cell diameter (MCD) is the average diameter of the red cell, expressed in micrometres (μm). The average normal MCD is 7.2 μm (normal range 6.7–7.7 μm).

Mean cell volume (MCV) is the average volume of a single red cell, expressed in femtolitres (fL). Normally it is 80–96 fL. In *pernicious anaemia* it is usually above 104 fL.

Mean cell haemoglobin (MCH) is the average amount of haemoglobin in each red cell, normally 28–32 pg.

Interpretation

In *microcytic hypochromic anaemia*, e.g. *iron deficiency*, all the absolute values are diminished.

In *macrocytic anaemias*, e.g. *pernicious anaemia* (PA), the absolute values are usually all raised with the exception of the MCHC, which is either normal or reduced (if iron deficiency is also present).

Red cell mass

This test measures the total volume of all the circulating red cells. Blood is collected by the laboratory staff. The red cells are tagged with radioactive chromium, washed and reinjected into the patient. After 10–20 minutes blood is again collected. The haematocrit and radioactivity are measured. The red cell mass can then be calculated. Normally this is 30 ml/kg for males and 27 ml/kg for females. It is increased in *polycythaemia*, sometimes to more than twice the normal figure.

Reticulocyte count

Very young red blood cells may be recognized by the fact that they take up a special stain that does not affect the mature red blood cells.

These young cells are called reticulocytes, because the stain demonstrates a network inside the cell (*reticulum* is Latin for a little net). The normal reticulocyte count is $25-85 \times 10^9/L$ (or 0.5–2.4%). A rise in the reticulocyte count is called a reticulocytosis and occurs as a *response to* satisfactory *treatment* in cases of *anaemia*. It also occurs following *haemorrhage* or *haemolysis*, due to the body's own power of regeneration.

On the routine blood film (e.g. stained with Leishman's stain) these young red cells have a bluish tinge described as polychromatic; so an increased number of polychromatic cells (called polychromasia) implies a *reticulocytosis*.

The 'stippling' of the red blood cells in *lead poisoning* and in *haemolytic anaemias* is also associated with a *reticulocytosis*.

Red cell appearance

On some haematological reports the appearance of the red cells, as seen on the stained film, is described. A cell of normal size is described as normocytic and one of normal colour as normochromic. Large cells, as seen for instance in *pernicious anaemia*, are called macrocytic, and small ones, as in *iron deficiency*, microcytic. Also in *iron deficiency anaemia* the cells are incompletely filled with haemoglobin, giving them a pale appearance, described as hypochromic. Cells resembling targets (target cells) are seen in *Mediterranean anaemia* and in liver disease. *Anisocytosis* means excessive variation in size. *Poikilocytosis* means irregularity in shape (see also blood film, p. 98).

Iron

For the following tests 5–20 ml of clotted blood are required. It must be collected with an iron-free syringe (a plastic disposable syringe is satisfactory) into a specially prepared iron-free container.

Serum iron

The normal value is 1–3 mmol/litre (60–180 µg/ml). Low figures are found in the *iron deficiency anaemias*, *scurvy* and *polycythaemia*. Raised levels occur in *infective hepatitis* (see p. 139) and in *haemochromatosis*.

Iron-binding capacity

The iron in serum is bound to a protein. This measures the maximum amount of iron with which the protein can combine. Normally it is 4.5–8 mmol/litre (250–450 µg/ml). It is increased in *iron deficiency* (more empty spaces left to bind with iron).

Iron saturation

This is calculated from the above results. It is the proportion of iron actually present compared to the total iron-binding capacity, expressed as a percentage. Normally it is 15–50%. In *iron deficiency* it is usually less than 10%. In *pernicious anaemia* and *haemochromatosis* it is usually nearly 100%.

Ferritin

Ferritin is a protein containing iron. The normal serum level is 20–450 ng/ml (µg/L) in males and 10–200 ng/ml (µg/L) in females. It is reduced in *iron deficiency* and increased when there is iron overload, as in *haemochromatosis* or in patients who have had *multiple transfusions*, e.g. for *Mediterranean anaemia*. For its estimation 10 ml of clotted blood is required. It provides a means of assessing the total iron storage in the body, 1 ng/ml of serum ferritin being approximately equivalent to 8 mg of storage iron in the body. False high values can occur in liver diseases.

Parasites in blood

If a blood film is taken during an attack of *malaria* the parasites can be seen in the red blood cells. The best time for blood to be collected is about 2 hours after the temperature peak. The disease may recur several years after the original infection, especially with *benign tertian malaria*. If a fever occurs in a person who has been in districts where the anopheline mosquito breeds, a blood film should be taken. *Latent malaria* may be activated by some other disease, e.g. *pneumonia*, in which case there is a double diagnosis.

Blood parasites are found in other tropical diseases, e.g. trypanosomes in *sleeping sickness*, and spirochaetes in *relapsing fever*.

White cell count

The normal range of the white cell count is $4.0–11.0 \times 10^9$/litre ($4000–11\ 000$/mm^3). An increase above 11.0×10^9/litre is known as a leucocytosis. This occurs in *infections* such as *pneumonia*, *appendicitis*, etc. A low figure in such conditions indicates a poor resistance on the part of the patient.

A great increase occurs in most types of *leukaemia*, especially in chronic myeloid leukaemia, sometimes up to 50.0×10^9/litre or more.

A decrease in the number below 4.0×10^9/litre is known as a *leucopenia*. It occurs in *typhoid* fever and *aplastic anaemia*; *drugs*, *poisons* and *irradiation* are important causes of *leucopenia*. An occasional cause is a leucocyte antibody. To detect this, a special blood sample is collected by the laboratory.

Persons exposed continuously to *X-rays*, *radium* or other forms of radioactivity, and certain industrial workers, should have regular blood counts. Most people, if exposed excessively, first show an increase in the red cell count, followed later by a fall in the white cell count, and still later by an *anaemia*.

Differential white cell count

There are several different types of white cells, and the proportion of each type differs in various diseases. The differential count, previously carried out by microscopical examination of a stained film of blood on a glass slide, is now usually done by automation. Normal figures are:

Polymorphs	$1.5–7.5 \times 10^9$/litre ($1500–7500$/mm^3)
Lymphocytes	$1.0–4.5 \times 10^9$/litre ($1000–4500$/mm^3)
Monocytes	up to 0.8×10^9/litre (800/mm^3)
Eosinophils	up to 0.4×10^9/litre (400/mm^3)
Basophils	up to 0.2×10^9/litre (200/mm^3)

To convert the percentage to the absolute figures as given above, the percentage figure for each type of cell is multiplied by the total cell count, e.g.

Total white blood cells 10.0×10^9/litre
Polymorphs 60%
$\therefore 60/100 \times 10.0 \times 10^9$/litre $= 6.0 \times 10^9$/litre

In most *acute infections* and in *sepsis* the polymorphs are increased. In *glandular fever* the lymphocytes and monocytes are increased. The eosinophils are increased in *allergic conditions*, e.g. *asthma*. In *leukaemia*, abnormal cells of a primitive type are seen in the differential count.

A reduced polymorph (neutrophil) count is called a neutropenia. If polymorphs are less than 1.0×10^9/litre (1000/mm³) it is often called an agranulocytosis, most cases being the result of drugs or X-rays damaging the bone marrow.

Bone marrow puncture

Examination of the bone marrow is an important part of the investigation of obscure anaemias. Informed written consent must be obtained (see. p. 2)

The sites in which this is usually performed are the iliac crests and the sternum. In the obese the vertebral spines may be used.

A sterile trolley is required providing: dressing towels, skin antiseptic, swabs, 2% procaine hydrochloride with syringe and needles, and a tenotomy knife or small scalpel. The special marrow puncture needle, together with syringe to fit, are usually provided by the laboratory.

Marrow is aspirated from the bone cavity (sternum or iliac crest) with full aseptic precautions, and spread on slides, for later microscopic examination.

This procedure confirms the diagnosis in *leukaemia, multiple myeloma* and other blood disorders.

Lymph node biopsy

This procedure is often used to determine the cause of an enlarged lymph node. Informed written consent must be obtained (see p. 2). The equipment required is similar to that for elliptical surgical skin biopsy (see p. 8), with similar antiseptic preparation of the skin. Local anaesthetic is injected round the lymph nodes as well as into the skin. Through a skin incision, e.g. of the axilla (groin nodes may be difficult to interpret histologically), one or two enlarged nodes are removed. If infection is a possibility, part of the material should be placed in a dry container for microbiology, the remainder being put into fixative for histology, usually 10% formol saline, often buffered. Causes of enlargement include *primary tumours (lymphoma,* e.g. *Hodgkin's disease)* and secondary *lymph node tumour deposits, leukaemia, tuberculosis* and *cat-scratch fever* (the microscopic appearance in these conditions is often diagnostic).

Investigations for haemorrhagic disorders

Haemorrhagic disorders can be due to deficiency (reduction or absence) of one or more clotting factors, circulating anticoagulants, fragility of the blood vessel walls or excess of fibrinolytic (clot-destroying) activity. Commonly-used screening tests are the activated partial thromboplastin time (p. 96), or the kaolin cephalin time (p. 96).

Routine blood examination (haemoglobin, white cell count and blood film)

This may reveal that a bleeding disorder is due to a blood disease such as *leukaemia* or a *platelet abnormality*. The findings may indicate the need for a bone marrow puncture (above).

Platelet count

Blood platelets are normally present in the blood to the number of $150–400 \times 10^9$/litre (150 000–400 000/mm³). They are an essential component of the process of blood clotting and haemorrhage control. Reduction of the platelets below a level of 40×10^9/litre (40 000/mm³) is liable to be followed by a haemorrhage. Blood for this test is usually collected by the laboratory, but a sequestrene sample is very satisfactory. Platelets are diminished in *thrombocytopenic purpura, pernicious anaemia (PA), aplastic anaemia, acute leukaemia* and other conditions, including *autoimmune disease* with platelet antibody formation. For detection of the latter, blood is collected by the laboratory staff. Platelets are increased following operation, especially splenectomy. If the count exceeds 1000×10^9/litre (1 000 000/mm^3) thrombosis may occur. The platelet count is not altered in *haemophilia*.

Capillary resistance test (Hess's test)
A circle 6 cm in diameter is marked out on the antecubital fossa. It is carefully examined under a bright light for any skin blemishes. A sphygmomanometer cuff is placed round the arm at least 3 cm above the circle. A pressure of 50 mmHg is maintained accurately for 15 minutes. After release the number of small haemorrhages (petechiae) appearing in the circle is counted. Up to eight is normal. It is increased when there is increased capillary fragility, e.g. in *thrombocytopenic purpura*.

Capillary microscopy
The capillaries at the base of the fingernails may be examined under the microscope, using an Anglepoise lamp and a drop of immersion oil on the nail bed. Vascular abnormality such as increased capillary tortuosity may be demonstrated, usually associated with a prolonged bleeding time.

Bleeding time (Ivy's method)
Three small puncture wounds are made on the anterior aspect of the forearm, after a sphygmomanometer cuff has been applied and the pressure set at 40 mmHg. The bleeding points are blotted at half-minute intervals, and the average time taken for two of the punctures to stop bleeding is taken. Normal bleeding time is 3–8 minutes. It is prolonged in *purpura, acute leukaemia, severe pernicious anaemia*, and certain abnormalities of the blood vessels. It is normal in *haemophilia*.

Clotting time (method of Lee and White)
One millilitre of freshly collected blood is placed in each of four dry tubes, 0.6 cm in diameter, placed in a water bath at 37°C. The clotting time is estimated as the average time taken for the first three tubes to clot. The normal time is 4–7 minutes. It is prolonged in *haemophilia, Christmas disease, obstructive jaundice* and during *heparin treatment*.

Recalcification time
This is the time for a fibrin clot to appear after the addition of calcium to plasma. It is more sensitive to slight disorders than the clotting time (above). Normally it is 90–125 seconds. It is increased in most coagulation disorders, e.g. *haemophilia, Christmas disease*, etc. Blood is collected by the laboratory staff.

Clot retraction
When blood has clotted the clot retracts, so that after 1 hour at 37°C normally 42–62% of the original blood volume is serum. If platelets or fibrinogen are deficient it may fail to retract normally and show increased friability. Blood is collected by the laboratory staff.

Prothrombin ratio (Quick's one-stage test)
International normalized ratio (INR) or British ratio (BR)

Prothrombin is essential for blood clotting, when it is converted into thrombin. This in turn converts fibrinogen into fibrin. Prothrombin cannot yet be estimated chemically. It is measured indirectly by the time taken for citrated plasma to clot after it has been activated. This is called the prothrombin time. Normally it is 11.5–15.5 seconds. If the prothrombin time of a patient's plasma is twice as long as that of normal plasma, this is expressed as a prothrombin ratio of 2.0. The prothrombin index in this example would be 50% but this term is being abandoned in favour of prothrombin ratio, now usually known as the INR (internationally normalized ratio, to avoid confusion with prothrombin activity which is also expressed as a percentage).

The normal INR is <1.4. In the postoperative management of *heart valve replacement* and in the treatment of *deep vein thrombosis (DVT)*, *pulmonary embolism* and *transient ischaemic attacks* by anticoagulants, the drugs should be adjusted to maintain the INR at 1.9–2.3. For *recurrent DVT* and *pulmonary embolism, arterial disease,* including *myocardial infarction, arterial grafts* and *cardiac prosthetic valves*, a ratio of 3.0–4.5 is required. If the ratio increases above this level there is a danger of haemorrhage.

The estimation is done by the laboratory on blood collected in a fresh citrate tube, usually specially provided for the purpose, particular care being taken to add the right amount of blood and mix well. It is also of value in investigating *haemorrhagic disorders* and *liver disease.*

There used to be considerable variations in the prothrombin ratio results between one hospital and another. By using a standardized reagent (Manchester Reagent) comparable results are produced at most hospitals, the standardized ratio being expressed as the British ratio (BR), which is almost identical with the international normalized ratio (INR).

Two-stage prothrombin test

This is designed to estimate prothrombin more specifically than the preceding test. Normally prothrombin is 100%. The figure is reduced in prothrombin deficiency and also by prothrombin inhibitor occurring in some cases of *disseminated lupus erythematosus (DLE).*

Prothrombin and proconvertin test

This differs from the Quick's one-stage prothrombin test in that fibrinogen and factor V are added, making it more sensitive to changes in factor VII, factor X and prothrombin (all of which depend on vitamin K for their formation). The specimen is collected by the laboratory staff. It can be performed on capillary plasma, a great advantage in small children. The normal range is 70–130%. It forms the basis of the Thrombotest (see below).

Thrombotest

This may be used instead of the prothrombin ratio to control anticoagulant therapy. The test may be carried out directly on finger-prick blood, thus avoiding venepuncture. The therapeutic level is 10–20%, normal being taken as 100% (see prothrombin and proconvertin test, above).

Plasma fibrinogen
Fibrinogen is necessary for blood clotting, being converted by thrombin into fibrin which is the essential constituent of blood clot. For its estimation blood is collected in a sequestrene or heparin bottle. Normal plasma fibrinogen is 1.8–5.4 g/litre (180–540 mg/100 ml). This level increases during pregnancy. An abrupt fall in the fibrinogen to levels below 1 g/litre (100 mg/100 ml) may occur in a pregnant woman when there is *intrauterine death* of the fetus. This can lead to dangerous haemorrhage. A rapid method of estimating fibrinogen is therefore of great value (Fibrindex, below). Low plasma fibrinogen also occurs in severe *liver disease* and as a *congenital abnormality*.

Fibrindex (fibrinogen index)
This test gives a quick estimate of the patient's fibrinogen level; 2 ml of blood in a prothrombin bottle is required. The result is reported as the time taken for the patient's plasma to clot after it is added to thrombin. Normally it clots in 5–12 seconds; in moderate fibrinogen deficiency the time is 12–30 seconds, and in severe deficiency it is over 30 seconds. It is chiefly used in obstetrical emergencies and following thoracic operations. The thrombin clotting time (p. 98) is equally informative.

Prothrombin consumption test
When healthy blood clots, most of the prothrombin is used up. In clotting defects much prothrombin may still remain in the serum. This test measures how much of the original plasma prothrombin remains in the serum. This is the prothrombin consumption index (PCI), normally 0–30%, usually below 10%. A raised result indicates a clotting defect, requiring further tests to be described.

Activated partial thromboplastin time (APTT)
This is the most commonly used screening test for clotting disorders prior to undertaking coagulation factor assays (see below). It is used in the detection of *Factor VIII deficiency* (*haemophilia*) and *Factor IX deficiency* (*Christmas disease*) when the APTT is prolonged. It is also used in the control of *heparin therapy*. The normal APTT is generally in the range 30–40 seconds but the local laboratory guide should be followed. Blood for the test is a venous sample taken into a citrate container (to the mark indicated).

Kaolin cephalin time
This is sometimes used as an alternative to the activated partial thromboplastin time (above) in the preliminary investigations of a suspected coagulation defect. It is the time taken for plasma to clot when incubated in the presence of calcium, kaolin and cephalin (a platelet substitute made from the brain). Normally the kaolin cephalin time is 45–60 seconds, but the figure varies in different laboratories. It is prolonged in all coagulation defects except those due to defects or diminution of platelets or fibrinogen. Blood for this test is collected by laboratory staff.

Coagulation factor assays
In cases of *haemorrhagic* and *coagulation disorder* it is possible to identify exactly which factor(s) are abnormal by means of factor assays.
The normal levels for these coagulation factors are as follows:

Factors II, V, VII, VIII, IX, X, XI, XII	50–150 IU/dL
Factor V Leiden	50–150 IU/dL

Von Willebrand factor	45–150 IU/dL
Protein C	80–135 IU/dL
Protein S	80–120 IU/dL
Antithrombin III	80–120 IU/dL
Activated protein C resistance	2.12–4.0
Fibrin degradation products	<100 mg/L
D-Dimer screen	<0.5 mg/L

Disseminated intravascular coagulation (DIC) screening

In DIC, multiple fibrin clots occur in blood vessels throughout the body. The normal coagulation factors (see above) become used up and there is a life-threatening bleeding tendency which may be associated with a *haemolytic anaemia*. Causes of DIC include *amniotic fluid embolism* complicating delivery, a *retained dead fetus*, and *bacterial septicaemia*. Screening for DIC is an investigation involving a number of tests, characteristic findings being as follows:[1]

Bleeding time (p. 94)	prolonged
Prothrombin ratio (p. 95)	prolonged
Activated partial thromboplastin time (p. 96)	prolonged
Euglobin lysis time (below)	normal or prolonged
Platelet count (p. 93)	reduced
Plasma fibrinogen (p. 96)	reduced

Thromboplastin generation test (TGT)

Factor assays (see above) have largely replaced the TGT. It is however occasionally used, e.g. for demonstrating circulating anticoagulants (*pseudohaemophilia*).

Fibrinolysin

Fibrinolysin is a substance causing lysis and breakdown of blood clot (fibrin), excess leading to a haemorrhagic tendency. If the clot remains solid after 24 hours incubation, the test is regarded as negative (normal). Increased fibrinolysin is sometimes found after *massive blood loss*, after treatment with the *heart–lung machine* and occasionally in *liver disease, heart failure* and *certain obstetric emergencies*. Blood is collected by the laboratory staff.

Euglobin lysis time (ELT)

This is a test for measuring fibrinolytic activity. For this test a citrated blood sample (to the volume indicated) is required. In the laboratory, the euglobin fraction of the plasma is precipitated, redissolved and allowed to clot. The time taken for the clot to undergo lysis is the euglobin lysis time, normally 150–300 minutes. In primary fibrinolysis (too much fibrinolysin), as can occur with *carcinoma of the prostate, shock* or streptokinase administration,[2] this time is reduced, to 30 minutes or less, with an associated haemorrhagic tendency. The test is used to differentiate primary fibrinolysis from DIC (above) in which the ELT is normal or prolonged.[2]

Thrombin clotting time

This detects inhibitors to the normal clotting process. About 2 ml of blood is taken into a tube containing 0.2 ml of 3.13% sodium citrate. The normal range is 10–15 seconds. It is prolonged in *disseminated intravascular coagulation (DIC), liver disease* and *heparin therapy*. The test is used to monitor *streptokinase treatment of thromboembolic disorders*.

Streptokinase resistance test

The use of streptokinase in the treatment of *thromboembolic disorders* is sometimes monitored by this test but usually by the thrombin clotting time (see above).

Investigations for the haemolytic anaemias

The *haemolytic anaemias* are those due to destruction of the circulating red cells.

Haemoglobin estimation

An unexplained fall in the haemoglobin level (see p. 88) may be the presenting feature of a *haemolytic anaemia*.

Blood film

Certain features may suggest a *haemolytic anaemia*, e.g. small densely-staining red cells (apparent microspherocytes); considerable polychromasia or reticulocytosis (see pp. 90–91); nucleated red cells ('normoblastic showers'); elliptical red cells (elliptocytes); red cell fragments; target cells, poikilocytes and iron deficiency changes (see red cell appearance, p. 91) may also be present.

Haptoglobin

Serum haptoglobin estimation is used as a test for intravascular haemolysis. Haptoglobins are glycoproteins which combine readily with any free haemoglobin released from haemolysed red cells to form compounds which are rapidly catabolized.[3] As a result the serum haptoglobin level falls. The normal range is 0.3–2.0 g/litre (30–200 mg/100 ml). The level is greatly reduced in *haemolytic anaemia*, but the reduction is transient as the liver generates more haptoglobin. It is estimated either chemically or by electrophoresis, 5 ml of clotted blood being required. The haptoglobin level is also reduced in *glandular fever, liver diseases* and the rare congenital deficiency of *ahaptoglobinaemia*. The haptoglobin level is increased *in infections, malignancy including Hodgkin's disease, tissue damage, systemic lupus erythematosus (SLE)* and in *steroid therapy*. It can be used as a guide to progress in these conditions, comparable to sedimentation rate.

Wet film

A drop of blood diluted with normal saline is examined microscopically. Small spherical red cells (microspherocytes) or elliptical red cells (elliptocytes) may be seen.

Tests for sickling and haemoglobin S

In the test for sickling the amount of oxygen in a drop of diluted blood is lowered artificially, which in *sickle cell anaemia (SCA)* produces sickle-shaped (crescent-shaped) cells. SCA is the most severe of the *haemolytic anaemias*. It is a hereditary condition, characteristically affecting people of African origin, due to the presence of abnormal haemoglobin S in the red cells. Tests are based on the fact that haemoglobin S is converted into crystals by reducing agents (see also abnormal haemoglobins, p. 100).

Direct antiglobulin test

This is a test for antibody coating the red blood cells (see p. 107).

Blood group

Haemolytic disease of the newborn results from a difference in blood group between mother and fetus, usually of the Rhesus type, as described on p. 104.

Serum bilirubin

This is only raised if there is much haemolysis (see p.138).

Red cell osmotic fragility

Red blood cells are stable in normal saline because its osmotic pressure is equal to that inside the cells. If the saline is progressively diluted, osmotic pressure draws fluid into the cells until a point is reached when the cells burst. This is known as *haemolysis*.

In certain *haemolytic anaemias*, e.g. *acholuric jaundice* and the *acquired haemolytic anaemias*, the red cells are more fragile, and haemolysis occurs with less dilute solutions of saline than normally; 10 ml of heparinized blood is required for the fragility test.

The result, usually accompanied by a graph, is given thus:

> **Normal control:**
> Haemolysis commences at 0.45%.
> Haemolysis is complete at 0.35%.
> **Acholuric jaundice:**
> Haemolysis commences at 0.6%.
> Haemolysis is complete at 0.45%.

In certain *haemolytic anaemias* the red cells are more resistant than normal against low osmotic pressures, e.g. *Mediterranean anaemia* and *sickle cell anaemia*.

Antibodies

In *haemolytic anaemia* with a positive direct antiglobulin test (p. 107), e.g. the *acquired haemolytic anaemias*, antibody can be obtained (eluted) from the surface of the patient's red cells and then tested against various known red cells. See antibody testing, p. 105.

Haemolysins

These are antibodies which cause the red cells to rupture. They are demonstrated by incubating the patient's serum with suitable suspensions of red cells under certain conditions, such as warmth, cold and acidity. An example is Ham's test for a haemolysin active in acidified serum: it is positive in *paroxysmal nocturnal haemoglobinuria*. Fresh specimens are essential, preferably collected by the laboratory staff. Sometimes two specimens are required, one being placed immediately in a water bath at 37°C to clot and the other in an ice bath at 0°C. The latter is necessary to detect the cold antibody causing paroxysmal cold haemoglobinuria by the Donath–Landsteiner test.

Autohaemolysis

This test is performed to help diagnose *hereditary spherocytosis* and, to a lesser extent, other types of *haemolytic anaemia*. From a fresh sample of clotted blood the red cells are incubated at 37°C in their own serum with and without added glucose. Normal values after 48 hours incubation are:

Without added glucose	0.2–2% haemolysis
With added glucose	0.01–0.9%.

Haemolytic red cells show increased *haemolysis* without added glucose, which is corrected to some degree by added glucose.

Abnormal haemoglobins

Some forms of *haemolytic anaemia* are due to the red cells containing abnormal haemoglobin as a congenital anomaly. *Mediterranean anaemia* (*thalassaemia*) is a typical example, in which a certain proportion of the haemoglobin is of the type normally found in the fetus, known as fetal haemoglobin (haemoglobin F). This may be detected by the alkali resistance test, fetal haemoglobin being abnormally resistant to alkali; 10 ml of heparinized blood is sufficient for both this and the following tests.

Other types of haemoglobin, such as the haemoglobin S found in *sickle cell anaemia* and similar congenital abnormalities, may be detected by electrophoresis. Sufficient for this test may be obtained by finger-prick (see also tests for sickling and haemoglobin S, p. 98). Normal levels for the different types of haemoglobin are as follows:

Haemoglobin A	>95%
Haemoglobin A_2	2–3%
Haemoglobin A_1C	3.8–6.4%
Haemoglobin F	<2%

Abnormal haemoglobin may also result from certain drugs and poisons such as chlorates and carbon monoxide (p. 207), also following incompatible blood transfusion. These may be detected by spectroscopy. For this test about 2 ml of sequestrenated, heparinized or oxalated blood should be sent to the laboratory.

Glucose-6-phosphate dehydrogenase (G6PD) deficiency

Some people are born with red cells lacking an enzyme called glucose-6-phosphate dehydrogenase. This inherited defect only becomes evident on exposure to certain drugs or chemicals such as sulphones or naphthalene (mothballs) which cause the red cells to break down, resulting in *haemolytic anaemia*. The haemolytic process stops when exposure to the offending substance ceases. The following tests are of value.

Heinz body test

Incubation of the defective cells with a reducing agent, e.g. acetyl phenylhydrazine, causes more Heinz bodies to develop than in normal blood.

Glutathione stability test

Defective cells incubated as above contain less reduced glutathione than normal cells.

Methaemoglobin reduction test

Defective cells accelerate the reduction of methaemoglobin under appropriate conditions.

Assay of glucose-6-phosphate dehydrogenase activity

This is the most reliable test and is available in most laboratories.

Blood for all the above tests is collected by the laboratory staff.

Red cell survival

The shortened length of life of the red cells in *haemolytic anaemias* can be demonstrated by the radioisotope method. Ashby's method is now seldom used.

Radioisotope method
Red cells, preferably from the patient himself, are tagged with radioactive chromium and reinjected into the patient's bloodstream. By measuring the radioactivity with an instrument like a Geiger counter the lifespan of the red cells can be estimated.

Ashby's method
Blood of a compatible but slightly different blood group is transfused into the patient. Samples of blood are then collected, daily for the first week and then at longer intervals, usually by finger-prick. The transfused cells can be recognized by their blood group, and their time of survival measured.

Schumm's test
When haemolysis occurs in the bloodstream, e.g. following incompatible blood transfusion and in certain *haemolytic anaemias*, methaemalbumin is released from the haemolysed cells. This is detected in the plasma or serum by Schumm's test, using spectroscopy. About 5 ml of either anticoagulated or clotted blood may be used for the test.

Urine tests
Urobilin (see pp. 138, 163) is increased in *haemolytic anaemias*, especially during an active phase. Haemoglobin appears in the urine in certain severe *haemolytic anaemias*, e.g. *paroxysmal nocturnal haemoglobinuria*.

Other tests in haematology
Tests for glandular fever
Paul–Bunnell test
This test is positive in many cases of *glandular fever*. The patient's serum, after absorption with ox cells, is found to agglutinate the red cells from a sheep, even after considerable dilution of the serum. A finger-prick sample is sufficient for a preliminary screening test. If this is positive a full test may be done, requiring 5 ml of clotted blood (but see monospot, etc., below).

Monospot and monosticon
These are proprietary tests for glandular fever similar in principle to the Paul–Bunnell but more rapid. A positive monospot or monosticon with a positive Paul–Bunnell screening test may be considered diagnostic of *glandular fever.*

Tests for rheumatoid arthritis
Differential agglutination test (DAT, Rose's test, Rose–Waaler test)
This is also called sheep cell agglutination test (SCAT). Serum from many patients with *rheumatoid arthritis* agglutinates sheep red cells which have been specially sensitized. A DAT of 1 in 16 or more is regarded as positive. Positive results are found most frequently in *adult rheumatoid arthritis* and in *systemic lupus erythematosus*, less frequently in *childhood rheumatoid arthritis* (*Still's disease*) and in *hepatitis*. For this test 5–10 ml of clotted blood is required.

Hyland RA test
A drop of diluted patient's serum is tested on a slide against latex particles coated with gammaglobulin. Agglutination of the particles is reported as a positive test. The results usually correspond to those with the DAT.

It is best to use both tests in each case, the results being most reliable when the two tests agree.

Autoantibody tests for rheumatic diseases
Antibodies against the patient's own cell components occur in the different types of *rheumatic disease*. Those with high specificity are known as 'disease markers'. These diagnostic markers are present in 80% of cases of *Sjögren's syndrome* and *Wegener's disease* and in a smaller proportion of *polymyositis* and *scleroderma*. Their detection is undertaken in special laboratories for *rheumatic diseases,* using serum from clotted blood samples. The autoantibody findings in normal people are as follows:

Adrenal antibody	Negative at 1:10 dilution
Anticentromere antibody	Negative at 1:40 dilution
Anticardiolipin antibody	
. IgG	0–23 U/ml
IgM	0–11 U/ml
Anti double-stranded DNA (ELISA)	0–73 U/ml
Antineutrophil cytoplasmic antibodies	Negative
Anti-proteinase 3	Negative
Anti-MPO	Negative
Antinuclear antibodies	Negative at 1:20 dilution
Gastric parietal cell antibodies	Negative at 1:20 dilution
Testicular interstitial cells	Negative at 1:10 dilution
La antibodies	Negative
Mitochondrial antibodies	Negative at 1:20 dilution
RNP antibodies	Negative
Ro antibodies	Negative
Skeletal muscle antibodies	Negative at 1:60 dilution
Sm antibodies	Negative
Smooth muscle antibodies	Negative at 1:20 dilution
Antibodies to thyroid colloid and microsomal antigen	Negative at 1:20 dilution
Rheumatoid factor	<30 k IU/L

Test for HLA-B27 antigen
Histocompatibility (HLA) antigens identify the tissue type of an individual and are of great importance in ensuring that a donor organ such as kidney or heart used for transplant is compatible with the recipient. Only 5–7% of normal people have the histocompatibility antigen HLA-B27, but 80–90% of patients with *ankylosing spondylitis* and/or *Reiter's disease* have this antigen, making its detection a helpful indicator in these conditions. The laboratory should be consulted to confirm its feasibility before collecting the 10 ml of heparinized blood required for this test.[4]

Tests for systemic (disseminated) lupus erythematosus (SLE, DLE)

LE (lupus erythematosus) 'cell preparation' test
For this test 5 ml of heparinized blood is required. In the laboratory it is appropriately incubated and smears of the white cells examined. Cells, usually polymorphs, containing large round masses of structureless material are reported as LE cells. Their finding strongly suggests *systemic (disseminated) lupus erythematosus.*

Hyland LE test
A drop of the patient's serum is tested on a slide against latex particles coated with gammaglobulin. Agglutination of the particles is reported as a positive test. The results usually correspond to the 'cell preparation' test for *lupus erythematosus* and are most reliable when the two tests agree.

Antinuclear factor (ANF)
Serum from patients with *systemic lupus erythematosus* may contain a factor which reacts with the nuclei of normal human cells. This can be demonstrated on a slide using the fluorescent antibody technique (see below). A positive result strongly supports the diagnosis of *SLE.*

Fluorescent antibody technique

This technique can be used to detect the presence of antibody in the patient's blood against various tissue elements, e.g. thyroid in *autoimmune thyroid disease* (p. 48), stomach in *pernicious anaemia*, or nuclei of any tissue in *DLE* (see antinuclear factor above).

The patient's serum is layered over a section or smear of fresh tissue. Any antibody present will then combine with the corresponding tissue element. All the uncombined serum is washed off. Antibody, being a globulin, can be demonstrated by adding a fluorescent antiglobulin and examining microscopically.

Bactericidal activity

For this test (also called nitroblue tetrazolium, NBT) 20 ml of venous blood is collected into a mixture of heparin and dextran. The dextran causes the red cells to form rouleaux and sediment rapidly, leaving the leucocytes in suspension. After treatment with tetrazolium, the actively bactericidal cells show a deep blue precipitate when examined under the microscope. During infections more than 50% of the cells show this change in normal people. In patients with granulomatous disease less than 10% of the cells show evidence of bactericidal activity.

Blood transfusion

Blood group tests

There are four main blood groups: A   B   AB   O
Of the population of the United Kingdom:

46% are group O

42% are group A

9% are group B

3% are group AB

Russians, Arabs, and Turks show a higher percentage of group B.

To ascertain a person's blood group, his cells are placed against known sera; thus A cells are agglutinated by anti-A serum but not by anti-B serum.

B cells are agglutinated by anti-B serum and not by anti-A serum. AB cells are agglutinated by both sera and O cells are not agglutinated by either.

A person's blood group is named after the antigens in his red cells. In practice it is checked by also testing for the antibodies in his serum. Thus group A blood contains anti-B antibody in the serum; group B blood contains anti-A antibody; group O blood contains both antibodies; and group AB blood contains neither.

It is the presence of these antibodies that makes it vital that blood of the right group is selected for blood transfusion. In addition to ABO there are other blood group systems, the most important being the rhesus (Rh) type described below. Less commonly investigated blood groups include MNS, P, Kell, Duffy, Kidd, Lewis, etc. More are being discovered.

The fact that blood groups are inherited is of legal importance in cases of disputed paternity of a child, but genetic fingerprinting is more reliable (see p. 184).

Rhesus type

Of the population 85% are rhesus positive. This means that their cells are agglutinated by a serum which also agglutinates the cells of a rhesus monkey. People whose cells are not agglutinated by the serum are rhesus negative.

This is of importance in haemolytic disease of the newborn as well as in blood transfusion.

A rhesus-negative mother and a rhesus-positive father may have a rhesus-positive child, and in a small percentage of cases the mother produces antibodies which pass through the placenta and damage the red cells of the fetus. As a result, the baby may be stillborn, or else develop severe jaundice and anaemia shortly after birth. This condition, *haemolytic disease of the newborn*, does not occur in the first pregnancy, unless the mother had previously been stimulated to produce antibodies, e.g. by transfusion with rhesus-positive blood.

Haemolytic disease of the newborn (p. 105) may also be due to other types of incompatibility, in the rhesus, ABO or other blood group systems.

Antenatal blood tests

All pregnant women should have an antenatal blood test during the third or fourth month. A venepuncture sample is taken into three containers: 2 ml sequestrenated blood for haemoglobin estimation, 5 ml clotted blood for rubella and syphilis antibodies (see pp. 18, 200–201), and 5 ml clotted blood for grouping. The latter is rhesus typed and the serum screened for antibodies (see antibody testing, p. 105). All rhesus-negative women are ABO grouped and if they have no living children they are booked for hospital delivery (see Kleihauer test, p. 105). If an antibody is detected it is identified and the husband's blood group investigated (genotyped) to assess the probable outcome in this and future pregnancies. Women with antibodies have a blood sample taken each month for the antibody level (titre) to be measured. If a sharp rise in titre is found, measures may be instituted to monitor and protect the baby, e.g. amniocentesis (see p. 191), early induction of labour, exchange transfusion of baby, or in severe cases intrauterine transfusion.

Haemolytic disease of the newborn

This condition is the result of a pregnant woman producing antibodies against the red cells of the fetus. It is usually due to red cells of a previous fetus escaping into the mother's bloodstream during delivery. Such antibodies can also be the result of a transfusion, e.g. of rhesus-positive blood into a rhesus-negative woman (see Rhesus type, p. 104 and HPL, p. 190).

Kleihauer test for fetal cells in maternal blood

This test is of value in the *prevention of haemolytic disease of the newborn*. A sequestrenated sample of blood is collected from the mother at exactly 10 minutes after delivery. When treated with acid and stained film examined microscopically, the fetal cells stand out quite clearly and can be counted. If fetal cells are detected in the mother's blood and the baby is rhesus-positive with the same ABO group as the mother, she is in danger of being stimulated to produce rhesus antibody. This can be prevented by injecting the mother with rhesus antibody within 72 hours of delivery, destroying the fetal cells before they have time to sensitize her. This procedure is being adopted for all rhesus-negative women.

Routine tests for haemolytic disease of the newborn

As soon as a baby with suspected haemolytic disease is born, the following samples should be sent to the laboratory:

1. From the mother – two 5 ml samples of clotted blood; one 2 ml sample of sequestrenated blood.
2. From the baby (cord blood) – 10 ml of clotted blood; 5 ml of clotted blood; 2 ml of sequestrenated blood.

A positive direct antiglobulin test (p. 107) indicates that the baby has haemolytic disease; its nature is revealed by the blood groups. The baby's haemoglobin and serum bilirubin levels give guidance on the severity of the condition and indicate whether exchange transfusion is required.

Antibody testing

The patient's serum is tested against cells having known antigens, including the patient's own cells. By finding which antigen is common to all the cells that are agglutinated by the serum, the antibody can be named. More than one antibody may be present (see also antenatal blood tests, p. 104).

Essentials of blood transfusion

The chief importance of blood groups is in blood transfusion. For example, if group A blood is transfused into a patient who is group O, the transfused cells will be agglutinated and haemolysed by the antibodies present in the patient. The patient will suffer a severe reaction, with jaundice and kidney failure, which may result in death. It is therefore essential that blood used for transfusion is compatible with the patient's blood, wherever possible of the same group and rhesus type. *All patients likely to require blood transfusion should therefore be grouped and rhesus typed at the earliest opportunity. Where transfusion is certain, the blood must also be crossmatched.* This entails placing the red cells of the donor with serum of the patient and then examining for agglutination. Grouping and crossmatching normally takes a minimum of 1–2 hours. For this purpose, about 5 ml of blood are collected in a dry sterile tube and sent to the laboratory. It must be fully labelled with forenames, surname, age, address and ward and accompanied by a fully completed request form. If there is a history of previous transfusions, or if the patient is a woman whose children have had haemolytic disease at birth or who has a history of miscarriage, these facts must be stated on the request form.

The regional blood transfusion centres play an important part by collecting the blood from the donors, ensuring as far as possible that it is free from infection, such as hepatitis and AIDS, grouping it and distributing it to all the hospitals. The blood group labels on blood containers were previously colour coded. This has been discontinued since the Gulf War, when the colours gave rise to problems. By international agreement black and white labels are now used (**Fig. 7.1**).

It is vital that the units of blood are stored in a refrigerator with a rigidly controlled temperature of 4°C and an alarm system to warn if temperature varies. Blood must not be stored in an ordinary ward or domestic refrigerator (unless specially modified) and must not be warmed or frozen. It may be kept for up to 3 hours in an insulated transporting box freshly issued from the blood bank.

Fig. 7.1 Blood group labels

The investigation of transfusion reactions

Transfusion reactions may be either non-haemolytic or haemolytic.

Non-haemolytic reactions include pyrexial and allergic reactions to the transfusion fluid, circulatory overloading, air embolism (more likely if positive pressure is used) and septicaemia from infected transfusion fluid. The latter can be proved only by isolating the same organism from the patient and from the transfusion fluid. This is one reason for not destroying or washing out the packs or bottles after transfusion.

Haemolytic reactions result from the destruction of either donor or recipient red cells following transfusion. The following must be available for investigation:

1. The remains of all transfused fluids (blood, plasma, saline, etc)

2. Two post-transfusion samples of blood from the recipient: 10 ml of clotted blood, 10 ml of citrated blood, collected from a vein well away from the transfusion site

3. All urine passed after the transfusion reaction

4. A pre-transfusion blood sample should be available in the blood bank.

Typical findings following a haemolytic transfusion reaction are set out in Table 7–1.

Antiglobulin (Coombs') test

The presence of antibodies coating the red cells, e.g. of a newborn baby with *haemolytic disease*, may be detected by antiglobulin which causes the cells to agglutinate. Antiglobulin is also known as antihuman globulin since it contains antibodies active against human globulins. Rhesus antibody and all other antibodies are globulin. Antiglobulin will thus detect the presence of any antibody coating the red cells.

Coated red cells which agglutinate with antiglobulin are said to give a positive antiglobulin test. If washed cells direct from the patient are found to be so agglutinated it is reported as a positive direct antiglobulin test. In addition to haemolytic disease of the newborn, a positive direct antiglobulin test may be found in *acquired haemolytic anaemia*. This indicates that the patient has produced antibodies against his own red cells (an example of autoimmunity). Following mismatched blood transfusion, blood from the patient often (but not always) gives a positive direct antiglobulin test, the donor cells being coated with antibody from the patient.

Antiglobulin may also be used to detect antibodies in the serum. After appropriate cells have been placed in contact with the serum they are washed and then tested for antibody coating, using antiglobulin. This is known as the indirect antiglobulin test, the donor cells being incubated in patient's serum, washed, and then tested for coating.

Table 7. 1 Haemolytic transfusion reaction: typical findings		
	Pre-transfusion	*Post-transfusion*
Serum bilirubin. (p. 138)	normal	raised
Serum haptoglobin (p. 98)	normal	reduced
Direct antiglobulin test (above)	negative	variable
Schumm's test (p. 101)	negative	positive
Free haemoglobin in plasma (p. 100)	absent	present

Gammaglobulin neutralization test

This distinguishes between antibody of gammaglobulin type and that of non-gammaglobulin type. Gammaglobulin antibody is likely to be of importance in causing *haemolytic disease of the newborn* whereas non-gammaglobulin is unlikely to. About 5 ml of clotted blood is required. Antiglobulin neutralized with gammaglobulin no longer reacts with cells coated by antibody which is gammaglobulin. It continues to react with cells coated by antibody which is non-gammaglobulin.

References

1. Pagana, K D and Pagana, T J. Disseminated intravascular coagulation. In: Pagana, K D and Pagana, T J, (eds). *Mosby's Diagnostic and Laboratory Test Reference*. St. Louis. Mosby Year Book. 1992: 275–277.

2. Pagana, K D and Pagana, T J. Euglobin lysis time. In: Pagana, K D and Pagana, T J, (eds). *Mosby's Diagnostic and Laboratory Test Reference*. St. Louis. Mosby Year Book. 1992: 328–329.

3. Pagana, K D and Pagana, T J. Haptoglobin. In: Pagana, K D and Pagana, T J, (eds). *Mosby's Diagnostic and Laboratory Test Reference*. St. Louis. Mosby Year Book. 1992: 398–399.

4. Pagana, K D and Pagana, T J. HLA-B27. In: Pagana, K D and Pagana, T J, (eds). *Mosby's Diagnostic and Laboratory Test Reference*. St. Louis. Mosby Year Book. 1992: 412–413.

CHAPTER EIGHT

Tests related to blood (2)

Chemistry (chemical pathology)

Index of tests	Page		
Alcohol	117	Hyperlipoproteinaemia	119
Aldolase	116	Hypernatraemia	115
Alkaline phosphatase	111	Hypokalaemia	115
Alpha$_1$ (a_1) antitrypsin	110	Hyponatraemia	114
Alpha-fetoprotein (AFP)	119	IgA, IgD, IgE, IgG, IgM	118
Alpha hydroxybutyrate dehydrogenase (aHBD)	117	Immune paresis studies	118
Amino acids	110	Immunoglobulins	118
Aminotransferases	116	Inorganic phosphate	111
Ammonia	139	Insulin	148
Anion gap	115	Iron	91
Bilirubin	138	Lactic dehydrogenase (LDH)	117
Caeruloplasmin	112	Magnesium	110
Calcitonin	111	5-nucleotidase	117
Calcium	110	Osmolality	115
Carcinoembryonic antigen (CEA)	120	Oxygen saturation (pulse oximetry)	81
Cholesterol	111	pH	73
Cholinesterase	116	Phenylalanine	193
Complement components C_3 and C_4	112	Phosphatases	111
(Complement) C_1 esterase inhibitor	112	Phosphorus	111
Copper	112	Potassium	115
Cortisol	51	Progesterone	187
C-reactive protein (CRP)	112	Prostate specific antigen	185
Creatinine	112	Protein electrophoresis	118
Creatine phosphokinase (CPK)	117	Proteins	118
Cyclic AMP (adenosine monophosphate)	113	Pseudocholinesterase	116
Drugs	203	Reaction (pH)	73
Electrolytes	113	Sugar (glucose)	145
Enzymes	116	Sodium	114
Ferritin	91	Tonicity	115
Fibrinogen	118	Transaminases	116
Fluid volumes	115	Transpeptidase	117
Gammaglutamyl transferase (gGT)	117	Triglycerides	119
Gases	73	Tumour markers	119
Glucose	145	Urea	165
Gases	73	Uric acid	120
Glucose	145	Water and electrolyte balance	114
Hyperkalaemia	115	Zinc	120

Introduction

In addition to the cells, clotting factors, etc., described in the last chapter, blood contains many other chemical substances. These include sugar (glucose), cholesterol, triglycerides, salts (electrolytes), vitamins, hormones, drugs, proteins (including enzymes), amino acids and breakdown products such as urea. Tests for all these substances are undertaken by the department of *chemical pathology* (biochemistry). With automation, less blood is required for multiple tests than is specified for the individual tests described.

Chemical analysis of blood

Alpha, (a,) antitrypsin
This is a glycoprotein involved in the response to acute infections and tissue damage. These conditions cause a raised serum level unless there is a congenital deficiency of a_1 antitrypsin. Deficiency is associated with *neonatal cholestasis, juvenile cirrhosis* and *emphysema*, with a lowered resistance to lung infections and a great susceptibility to the effects of smoking. About 5 ml of clotted blood are required for the test. It must be collected *without a tourniquet* and sent immediately to the laboratory. The request form should summarize the results of liver or lung function tests, liver biopsy or chest X-ray findings, family history of lung disease and urine findings. Family studies on close relatives of an affected individual provide a basis for genetic counselling.

Alpha-fetoprotein (AFP)
see p. 119.

Amino acids
- Blood or urine amino acids may be measured in specialized laboratories, thus enabling inherited metabolic disorders to be investigated. Arrangements must be made with the local laboratory for collection and transport of specimens.
- Phenylalanine, see phenylketonuria p. 193.

Ammonia
See p. 139.

Bilirubin
See pp. 138, 140.

Calcium and magnesium
Some 5 ml of blood are collected without a tourniquet into a dry tube and sent to the laboratory without delay. The normal calcium is 2.1–2.6 mmol/litre (8.5–105 mg/100 ml), slightly higher in young children. (Since half the calcium is bound to albumin the above values depend on a normal albumin level.) Symptoms of tetany (see p. 50) occur when the figure is as low as 1.5 mmol/litre (6 mg/100 ml). Low readings are found in *hypoparathyroidism, renal dwarfism, osteomalacia, coeliac disease*, in some cases of *rickets*, and in *chronic nephritis*. High readings occur in *parathyroid hyperplasia and tumour* (causing generalized *osteitis fibrosa*, see also p. 50), *sarcoidosis* and *vitamin D excess*.

Serum magnesium, normally 0.6–1 mmol/litre (1.5–2.6 mg/100 ml), may be estimated on the same specimen as for calcium above. Low levels may occur in *tetany* and *renal failure*.

Inorganic phosphate (phosphorus)

This may be estimated on the same specimen as for calcium above. The normal phosphate is 0.8–1.45 mmol/litre (2.5–4.5 mgP/100 ml) for adults and 1.3–1.9 mmol/litre for children. It is raised in *chronic nephritis, prolonged diabetic coma, hyperparathyroidism, rickets* and *osteomalacia*.

NB: Misleading high levels occur artefactually from blood samples which are haemolysed or which are not separated on the day of collection.

Alkaline phosphatase

About 5 ml of blood is sent to the laboratory in a dry tube. The normal serum level is 45–105 U/L (over 21 years). There is a significant increase in the serum level during infancy, childhood, adolescence (up to 21 years) and pregnancy. This reflects the increased osteoblastic activity associated with bone growth, maximal during puberty and adolescence. Abnormal increase occurs in *cirrhosis of the liver, obstructive jaundice* and many bone diseases including *rickets* and *hyperparathyroidism*. To determine whether a raised serum alkaline phosphatase is of liver or bone origin, isoenzyme studies may be performed; alternatively 5-nucleotidase (p. 118) or γGT estimation (p.117) may be undertaken.

NB: Calcium, phosphorus and alkaline phosphatase are frequently estimated on the same specimen. A single 5 ml sample of clotted blood suffices.

Calcitonin

This hormone, produced by the thyroid, inhibits the resorption of calcium from bone. The normal serum level is 20–40 pg/ml. It is raised in *medullary carcinoma of thyroid*, also in *pseudohypoparathyroidism*, some renal diseases and occasionally in malignant *tumours of the breast, lung* and *other organs*. The laboratory should be contacted before collecting 10 ml blood into an ice-cooled heparin tube.

A reduced level, occurring in *hypoparathyroidism*, is not demonstrable by routine assay.

Cholesterol

About 10 ml of blood are collected (clotted or in EDTA). Provided the patient is fasting, triglycerides and other lipids (see p. 119) may be estimated on the same sample. These are usually estimated in the hospital laboratory. Cholesterol and triglycerides may also be estimated in the clinic or sideroom with an instrument such as Reflotron (Boehringer–Mannheim). The estimation is done on plasma in which the normal cholesterol level is 3.6–5.7 mmol/litre (140–220 mg/100 ml) at 20 years of age. It increases gradually with age.

The figure is raised in long-continued *biliary obstruction* and in some cases of *chronic nephritis* (with proteinuria), *diabetes, myxoedema* and *pregnancy*.

The figure may be decreased in *thyrotoxicosis, liver disease* and *chronic wasting diseases*.

Elevated serum cholesterol levels increase the risk of ischaemic heart disease. The WHO recommended upper limit of normal for total cholesterol in serum is 5.2 mmol/litre. The levels at which a raised cholesterol is considered to increase risk are:

5.7 mmol/litre (20–30 years)

6.2 mmol/litre (30–40 years)

6.7 mmol/litre (over 40 years).

Cholesterol is carried in the blood as lipoprotein, mainly LDL (low density lipoprotein) and HDL (high density lipoprotein). HDL is protective and should be more than 0.9 mmol/litre.

Complement components C_3 and C_4

The term 'complement' includes a number of enzymes in blood involved in immunity and activated by antigen–antibody complexes. Serum C_3 and C_4 levels are generally a guide to overall complement activity; the normal range for C_3 is 65–190 mg/dl and for C_4 is 15–50 mg/dl. They are raised in many conditions involving inflammation, e.g. *infections*, *injuries* and *infarction*. Reduced levels are of more diagnostic value and occur in *acute nephritis* and *disseminated lupus erythematosus* (*DLE*). About 5 ml freshly taken clotted blood is required.

(Complement) C_1 esterase inhibitor

This is a globulin which inhibits activated complement, limiting its possibly harmful effects. It is deficient in sufferers from *hereditary angioneurotic edema* (*HANE*) who develop episodic swelling of various parts of the body, sometimes with serious effects. If detected, family studies are indicated. In the active phase C_4 is also low but C_3 is usually normal (see preceding section). About 5 ml of freshly collected blood is required.

Copper and caeruloplasmin

The normal serum copper is 13–24 µmol/litre (70–150 µg/100 ml). Caeruloplasmin is the copper-binding protein with a serum level of 200–400 mg/litre in adults and children (1–10 years) and 120–300 mg/litre in infants and adolescents (10–15 years). Serum copper and caeruloplasmin are reduced in *Wilson's disease* (*hepatolenticular degeneration*), the copper usually being less than 2 µmol/litre. Low levels also occur when serum proteins are reduced, as in *starvation* and *nephrosis*. Increased levels are caused by *pregnancy, the pill, oestrogens, leukaemia* and *infections*. About 5 ml of clotted blood are required for the estimation of copper and caeruloplasmin.

C-reactive protein (CRP)

This is an abnormal protein which appears in the blood during the active phase of many diseases. The results are expressed as 0, 1+, 2+, 3+, 4+ and 5+. The normal is usually 0 or occasionally 1+. Quantitatively the normal serum level is <10 mg/L. Raised values occur in *bacterial infections, rheumatic fever, myocardial infarction* and widespread malignant disease, corresponding roughly to the ESR (see p. 89). About 5 ml of clotted blood are required for the test.

NyoCard is a near patient test for C-reactive protein assay.[1] It is of value in determining whether an inflammatory process is present and in monitoring its progress.

Creatinine

Creatinine is a waste product from creatine. Creatine is necessary for muscle contraction. Normally serum contains 50–100 µmol/litre (0.6–1.2 mg/100 ml) of creatinine in men and 50–80 µmol/litre (0.6–0.9 mg/100 ml) in women. It is excreted through the glomeruli of the kidney and the blood level is a useful index of their function. The blood creatinine rises in *kidney diseases* when a sufficient number of glomeruli are damaged, and is later to rise than the blood urea. A blood creatinine of over 420 μmol/litre (5 mg/100 ml) in *chronic nephritis* is of serious significance.

The test is usually carried out in the hospital laboratory on 2–5 ml of clotted blood. It may also be done in a clinic or sideroom using an instrument such as the Reflotron® (Boehringer–Mannheim).

Cyclic AMP (adenosine monophosphate)

The normal plasma level of cyclic AMP is 12–20 nmol/litre. The main clinical value of its estimation is in the diagnosis of *hypoparathyroidism*. In this condition the plasma level rises to peak values about 20 minutes after injection of parathormone. This does not occur in *pseudohypoparathyroidism*. The laboratory should be contacted for details of the test (see also p. 50).

Drugs

See p. 203.

Electrolytes

Electrolytes are the chemical substances called salts. For example, common salt is sodium chloride (NaCl). It consists of positively charged sodium ions and negatively charged chloride ions. When it is dissolved in water these ions dissociate and move about almost independently. In blood the two chief electrically positive ions (cations) are sodium and potassium; the two chief electrically negative ions (anions) are chloride and bicarbonate (measured as carbon dioxide or CO_2). These are the substances usually estimated when an electrolyte investigation is requested. Table 8.1 sets out normal values for blood electrolytes.

The result is given in millimoles per litre (mmol/l). This is a method of expressing the actual proportions of the different substances present. For sodium, potassium and chloride the figures are numerically the same as those for milli-equivalents per litre (mEq/l), the units previously used.

Electrolyte estimation is of great value in *dehydration* from *diarrhoea, vomiting, burns* or *excessive sweating; oedema* from *kidney failure, heart failure* or other causes; *diabetic ketosis, Addison's disease* and other endocrine disturbances; and also in the *control of steroid therapy*. Electrolyte estimation is not only a guide as to the treatment to be adopted but later estimations are also a check on the effectiveness of the treatment. It must be emphasized however that mere correction of the electrolyte disturbance in a condition such as intestinal obstruction is of little value unless the obstruction is also relieved by operation. But used in conjunction with treatment of the cause, correction of the electrolyte disturbance can be lifesaving.

Table 8.1 Blood electrolytes: normal values

	Normal average	Normal range
Sodium (Na)	140 mmol/litre	137–144 mmol/litre
Chloride (Cl)	100 mmol/litre	95–107 mmol/litre
Potassium (K)	4 mmol/litre	3.5–4.9 mmol/litre
Bicarbonate (CO_2)	25 mmol/litre (adults)	20–28 mmol/litre
	20 mmol/litre (children)	18–23 mmol/litre

For electrolyte estimation, 10 ml of blood should be placed in a heparin container and sent to the laboratory without delay. A wet syringe or container, or squirting the blood through a fine needle, can haemolyse the blood and make the potassium estimation unreliable. Delay in sending the specimen to the laboratory also leads to erroneous results.

Water and electrolyte balance

Water forms 70–90% of our diet, even apparently solid foods consisting largely of water. The normal daily intake for an adult is about 2.5 litres of water, with a minimum total requirement of 1.5 litres. We also eat daily about 5 grams (g) of sodium chloride, of which only half is salt added during cooking and flavouring, and 2–3 grams of potassium, which is found in meat, tea and fruit.

Approximately 70% of the body, by weight, consists of water (75% in children). In a man of 70 kg this represents about 50 litres. Water within the cells forms half the body weight (about 35 litres). Water in the plasma is about 3.5 litres and the remainder is in the tissue spaces surrounding the cells. The tissue space fluid and the plasma together are known as extracellular fluid, which measures about 15 litres (20% of the body weight). The electrolyte level in the serum or plasma is the same as that in the tissue space fluid.

Dehydration results when 5% of the body weight is lost as water, i.e. about 3 litres for an adult. Twice this loss may be fatal. The fluid loss is mainly from the tissue spaces, with some loss from the plasma which causes haemoconcentration, reflected by raised haemoglobin (p. 88) and haematocrit (p. 90) readings.

When the water content of the body decreases the electrolyte levels tend to rise; when it increases they tend to fall and *oedema* tends to occur. Often, however, water loss is associated with electrolyte loss. Thus in severe sweating or vomiting there is much loss of chloride. If the fluid lost is replaced by water alone, the chloride level in serum and tissue fluid falls. The importance of maintaining the balance between water and electrolytes is thus clear.

In the management of patients with dehydration or oedema, *accurate measurement of all fluid intake and output is essential*. This is a duty which largely falls on the nurse. It is more important than frequent electrolyte estimations. Inaccurate charting is useless and may be dangerous. It may also be necessary to check salt intake and sometimes output as well. Investigations of value are the plasma or serum osmolality, electrolytes, blood urea, haematocrit and, possibly, measurement of extracellular fluid volume.

Which electrolytes?

The electrolyte estimations most frequently used in the management of patients with electrolyte imbalance are sodium and potassium, together with urea.

Sodium

A *low plasma sodium* (*hyponatraemia*), of 120 mmol/litre or less, causes headaches, confusion, fits and eventually death. Some *hyponatraemia* is very common postoperatively, particularly in patients receiving a low salt infusion such as dextrose–saline (which may be counteracted by alternating with 'normal saline'). Infusions of amino acids, mannitol, etc., which are deficient in sodium, have a similar effect. *Hyponatraemia* also occurs in *acute uraemia, hyperglycaemia* and the later stages of *Addison's disease*.

A *high plasma sodium* (*hypernatraemia*), of 160 mmol/litre or more, causes thirst, mental confusion and later coma. Almost always due to water depletion, it is most commonly found in unconscious or confused patients who are unable to drink, particularly if they suffer from a head injury causing *diabetes insipidus* or have *extensive burns*. It also occurs in *infants with gastro-enteritis* or *pneumonia*, and in cases of poisoning who have been given a strong salt solution as an emetic (a dangerous and possibly lethal practice). **NB**: *Hypernatraemia* often occurs before clinical signs of dehydration are evident. Accurate monitoring of fluid balance provides an early alert.

Potassium

A *low plasma potassium* (*hypokalaemia*), of 3 mmol/litre or less, causes muscle weakness and loss of tone, cardiac arrhythmias with characteristic ECG changes and occasionally muscle cramps or even *tetany* (see p. 50). If prolonged, it causes *kidney damage*, which in turn makes the *hypokalaemia* worse.

Hypokalaemia is usually due to loss of potassium from the body:

- from the gut, e.g. *prolonged vomiting or diarrhoea* (including excess laxatives), *intestinal fistulae, villous tumours of the colon*; or

- in the urine, e.g. *thiazide diuretics* (e.g. frusemide), *excess liquorice, tobacco-chewing, prolonged saline infusion, Cushing's syndrome, steroid therapy, synacthen or ACTH therapy*, and *stress*.

Other causes are chronic starvation, glucose and insulin therapy, alkalosis, and pyloric stenosis with alkalosis.

A *high plasma potassium* (*hyperkalaemia*), of 6 mmol/litre or more, causes characteristic ECG changes with the danger of cardiac arrest. **NB**: A false high result occurs if the blood sample is haemolysed or if there is delay in separating off the serum.

Hyperkalaemia may be due to excessive intake, e.g. from *failure to stop potassium therapy*, or else failure to excrete potassium, as in *Addison's disease* or as a result of certain diuretics, e.g. spironolactone. Other causes are *severe tissue damage* and *ketoacidosis* from badly controlled *diabetes mellitus*. The latter is reversed by treatment with insulin and fluids, which can then cause *hypokalaemia*. So it is very important to monitor the plasma potassium before the level falls too far.

Anion gap

This term is used to denote the anion difference between the sum of the two main cations, Na^+ and HCO_3^-. This gap is mainly accounted for by the anionic nature of most proteins in plasma.[2] Its normal value is 12–16 mmol/L (usually nearer 15 mmol/L). This test is only likely to be helpful in cases of acidosis where the cause is not obvious.[2]

Osmolality (tonicity)

This is the osmotic pressure produced by all the substances dissolved in the blood. The normal level is 285–295 milliosmol/kg (mosmol/kg). It is increased in *dehydration*, e.g. from *burns*, and decreased in *water retention*, e.g. in *pre-eclampsia*. By repeating the test after pitressin the distinction between *pituitary and renal diabetes insipidus* may be made (see also p. 59). Only a small sample of clotted blood is required, or alternatively the heparinized blood supplied for electrolytes.

Measurement of fluid volumes

The volume of plasma, extracellular water and total body water can be measured by dilution techniques, using suitable chemical or radioactive substances.

A measured dose of the chosen substance is administered, e.g. radioactive bromide (see radioisotopes, pp. 22–23) by mouth for extracellular fluid volume or Evans blue intravenously for plasma volume. After sufficient time for complete distribution, a blood sample is collected. The amount of substance present is estimated. From the degree of dilution, the extracellular fluid volume or the plasma volume can be calculated. These methods are used in certain centres for investigating *dehydration, oedema, malnutrition* and *obesity*.

Enzymes

Enzymes are substances which promote chemical reactions in the body. When cells are damaged, their enzymes escape into the body fluids and tend to raise the blood level above normal values. *It should be noted that the normal values tend to vary from one laboratory to another*, depending on the reagents and temperatures used. Where values are quoted below they are the accepted national figures but *the normal range should always be obtained from the local laboratory*. For each test about 5 ml of clotted blood is required.

Aldolase

Raised values occur in all types of tissue damage, e.g. muscle, heart and liver. It is non-specific and now little used. Haemolysis invalidates the result.

Alkaline phosphatase

See p. 111.

Aminotransferases (transaminases)

The type of aminotransferase usually estimated is aspartate transferase (AST) (glutamic oxalacetic transaminase, GOT). The normal blood level is 1–31 U/L. It is higher in children than adults. Alanine aminotransferase (ALT) (glutamic pyruvic transaminase, GPT) estimation (normal 5–35 U/L) is now considered less useful. Increase in the blood AST level occurs in *acute liver damage*, in *heart muscle damage* due to *coronary artery disease* and in *skeletal muscle damage* from injury and disease. In *acute liver disease* the level may be greatly increased (see Table 9.2, p. 140). In *heart muscle damage* the increase is considerably less and may only last a few days. However, this can be very helpful if the clinical and ECG changes are doubtful, when samples should be collected on three successive days.

The estimation of AS (AST) and AL (ALT) is usually carried out in the hospital laboratory on a sample of clotted blood (2–5 ml). They may also be estimated in the clinic or sideroom using an instrument such as Reflotron® (Boehringer–Mannheim).

Cholinesterase (pseudocholinesterase)

This enzyme is necessary for nervous tissue to return to normal after it has been stimulated. The normal level is slightly higher in males than in females. In some families this enzyme is present in smaller amounts and in unusual form (*familial cholinesterase deficiency*). This results in delayed recovery of normal respiration after anaesthesia in which a muscle relaxant (suxamethonium) has been used. Such delayed postoperative recovery is an indication for cholinesterase estimation in the patient and blood relatives. An acquired form of *cholinesterase deficiency* can occur after exposure to certain pesticides and phosphate-rich fertilizers, leading to general lethargy.

Creatine phosphokinase (CPK), creatine kinase (CK)

This enzyme occurs mainly in heart muscle, skeletal muscle and brain.[3] Estimation of this enzyme is used in the diagnosis of *myocardial infarction*, for which the MB isoenzyme (CK-MB) is even more specific. The normal serum level is 24–170 U/L in females and 24–195 U/L in males, with higher values in children. Normally less than 5% of the enzyme consists of the MB isoenzyme. Exercise increases the level of CPK, so the patient must be at rest for 2 hours before collection. Abnormal increase occurs 6–36 hours after *heart* or *skeletal muscle damage* and also with *muscular degeneration* and *dystrophy*.

Gammaglutamyl transferase (γGT, transpeptidase)

This enzyme provides a very sensitive indicator of all types of *liver disease*, the normal serum level of 4–35 U/L (<50 U/L in males). It is almost invariably raised when there is damage to liver cells. It is also raised in *pancreatic disease* and in 50% of patients with *cardiac infarction*. It is not raised in *bone disease* and so can assist in determining the cause for a raised serum alkaline phosphatase. **NB**: γGT is also increased by certain drugs, including alcohol and phenytoin. So the request form should state what drugs (including alcohol) the patient is receiving.

Estimation of gammaglutamyl transferase is usually carried out in the hospital laboratory on clotted blood (2–5 ml). It may also be undertaken in the clinic or sideroom using an instrument such as Reflotron® (Boehringer–Mannheim).

Lactic dehydrogenase (LDH)

Lactic dehydrogenase is an enzyme which occurs in many tissues, especially heart muscle, skeletal muscle, brain, liver, kidneys, red cells and lungs.[4] Normal serum levels are 10–250 U/L. Raised enzyme levels provide a measure of the extent of any tissue damage. Increased levels occur in *carcinoma with secondary deposits*, especially in the liver, and in *leukaemia*, *haemolytic anaemia* (including *sickle cell*), *pernicious anaemia*, *muscular dystrophy* and in some *chronic renal diseases*. The blood level also rises in *myocardial infarction*, of which it is more useful for retrospective diagnosis than for rapid diagnosis. Haemolysis of the specimen invalidates the result.

Alpha hydroxybutyrate dehydrogenase (aHBD)

This enzyme forms part of the LDH (lactic acid dehydrogenase) complex and its LDH-I-isoenzyme. The blood level is increased in *myocardial infarction* 36 hours to 6 days after the onset of pain. The increase is proportional to the extent of the infarction. It occurs chiefly in the heart, kidneys and red cells, so it is a more specific test for *myocardial infarction* than total LDH, but it is not very sensitive as an early marker.[5] Like LDH, haemolysis of the sample must be avoided.

5-nucleotidase

This enzyme is specific for liver.[6] Estimation of 5-nucleotidase is of value when there is a raised serum alkaline phosphatase (p. 111) for which the cause is uncertain. 5-nucleotidase serum level is raised in *liver disease*, but not in bone disease. If other enzymes are raised and the 5-nucleotidase is normal, liver disease may be excluded from the differential diagnosis.

Gases

See blood gases and pH, p. 73.

Oxygen saturation

See pulse oximetry, p. 81.

Phenylalanine

See phenylketonuria, p. 193.

Proteins

For the estimation of serum proteins about 5 ml of blood in a dry tube are required. The total proteins are 60–80 g/litre (6–8 g/100 ml) of which 35–55 g/litre (3.5–5.5 g/100 ml) is albumin and 15–33 g/litre (1.5–3.3 g/100 ml) is globulin.

Where the plasma proteins are requested the blood must be sent in a sequestrene or heparin container. The only difference from the serum proteins is the addition of fibrinogen, this being normally 2–4 g/litre (0.2–0.4 g/100 ml). Fibrinogen is usually estimated on its own (p. 96). The *albumin is diminished* in *liver* and *kidney diseases*; the *globulin is increased* in *liver diseases* and to a much greater extent in *multiple myeloma* and *kala-azar*. In starvation both albumin and globulin are diminished.

Protein electrophoresis

Separation of the serum protein into its various components may be carried out by electrophoresis. The passage of an electric current causes the different protein components to move at different speeds along a cellulose acetate strip, causing them to separate from each other. The globulin is separated into four parts called alpha$_1$ (a$_1$), alpha$_2$ (a$_2$), beta (β) and gamma (g) globulin. The abnormal gamma-globulin in multiple myeloma may be demonstrated by this method, also the deficiency of gamma-globulin in *agammaglobulinaemia*. Electrophoresis may also be performed using filter paper, starch gel or a starch block instead of cellulose acetate.

Immunoglobulins

These are globulins concerned with immunity, i.e. antibodies. Their estimation involves the use of a specific antibody against each immunoglobulin. That with the largest molecules is called macroglobulin or IgM (immunoglobulin M); its normal serum level is 0.5–2.0 g/litre (50–200 mg/100 ml). Gamma (g) globulin is IgG (immunoglobulin G); its normal serum level is 6–16 g/litre (0.6–1.6 g/100 ml). Other immunoglobulins are IgA, IgD and IgE. The blood IgM rises in the early stage of many infections. Then as the IgM falls the IgG rises, reflecting the molecular pattern of the antibodies being produced by lymphocytes. Excessive and abnormal (monoclonal) IgG is produced in *myelomatosis* and excessive IgM in *macroglobulinaemia*. IgE can now be estimated (after checking with the laboratory). The adult serum level is 0–840 (mean 95) U/ml, with lower levels in children. It is raised in many allergic conditions, particularly those with an immediate hypersensitivity reaction, e.g. *asthma*. The expensive RAST (radioallergosorbent test) which measures allergen-specific IgE is rarely positive if serum IgE is less than 300 U/ml.

Immune paresis studies

These are undertaken by the SAS when immune response is impaired, either as a congenital defect or secondary, e.g. to *lymphoma* or *nephrosis*. About 10 ml clotted blood and a 24-hour urine (p. 160) are required. Clinical history and details of vaccination, e.g. by tetanus toxoid, polio vaccine, BCG and Mantoux response, must be given.

Cryoglobulins

Cryoglobulins are abnormal globulins that precipitate at low temperatures and redissolve when warmed.[7] Normally none are present in blood. The highest serum levels occur in *myelomatosis*, *macroglobulinaemia* and *leukaemia*. *Cryoglobulinaemia* of lesser degree also occurs in *rheumatoid disease*, *lupus erythematosus* and several other conditions.[8] Symptoms of *cryoglobulinaemia* resemble *Raynaud's disease*, often with skin changes and occasionally with neurological symptoms. Before collecting blood for testing, the laboratory should be consulted and the patient should fast for 8 hours, to reduce serum turbidity. About 10 ml of blood is collected into a plain tube which has previously been warmed to 37°C, using a prewarmed syringe,[7,8] and then transferred to the laboratory in a warmed container.

Triglycerides

Triglycerides are the neutral fats, carried by the blood in the form of chylomicrons (microscopic fatty droplets) and lipoproteins. Their estimation is often carried out on the same 10 ml clotted or EDTA sample of blood that is used for cholesterol (p. 111) and HDL (high density lipid) cholesterol. This is usually done in the hospital laboratory. Cholesterol and triglycerides may also be estimated in the clinic or sideroom using an instrument such as Reflotron® (Boehringer–Mannheim). The normal fasting range for triglycerides is up to 2.1 mmol/litre in women. Raised values are found in some cases of *hyperlipoproteinaemia* which may be familial or due to a metabolic disorder, e.g. poorly controlled *diabetes mellitus*. Five basic types of *hyperlipoproteinaemia* have been distinguished by electrophoresis.

Tumour markers

Most of the tumour markers, including AFP, CEA, HPL and PSA, can be estimated on a 5–10 ml sample of clotted blood sent to the laboratory early in the day. The laboratory should be consulted about other tumour markers.

Alpha-fetoprotein (see also hCG, p.120)

This is a glycoprotein produced by the liver of the fetus and greatly reduced after birth. The normal adult serum level is 2–25 μg/litre (<10 kU/L). During pregnancy the maternal serum level is usually below 100 μg/litre between the 14th and 18th weeks; it reaches its maximum of 30–500 μg/litre between the 28th and 36th week, decreasing to the normal adult level by 5 weeks after delivery. In view of the wide range, units must be carefully checked (whether ng, μg, g, ml or litre). Estimation is of value in (1) tumour diagnosis and monitoring, (2) detection of fetal abnormalities and (3) other conditions:

- Serum AFP is raised in most (80–90%) *hepatocellular carcinomas* and *hepatoblastomas*, many *malignant teratomas* and *other germ cell tumours* (see also hCG, see below), some *alimentary tract carcinomas* and *secondary tumours of liver* and occasionally other tumours. Estimation before surgery (e.g. gonadectomy) and about 2 weeks afterwards provides a guide to the completeness of tumour removal. It can also be used to monitor radiotherapy.

- The pregnancy serum level is raised in *anencephaly, spinal tubal defects* and *fetal death* (see also amniocentesis, p. 191–192).

- Raised serum AFP occurs in *hepatitis*, especially in children. It is said to indicate a favourable prognosis in any *acute liver failure*. It is also raised in *cirrhosis, biliary atresia* and *ataxia telangiectasia*. No preparation of the patient is required. About 5 ml clotted blood should be sent to the laboratory early in the day.

Carcinoembryonic antigen (CEA)

This antigen was first demonstrated in carcinoma of the colon and in embryonic intestine. It is not specific for malignancy but can be used to *detect recurrence* of some cancers, e.g. *colonic carcinoma*, or to *monitor response to cancer therapy*. The normal serum level is less than 3 μg/litre, 3–10 μg/litre being borderline. It is raised in many conditions including *heavy smoking* (more than 15/day), *chronic lung disease, peptic ulcer, inflammatory bowel disease* and *cirrhosis*. Values above 20 μg/litre are suggestive of malignancy and above 50 μg/litre highly suggestive. In advanced malignancy the level may fall. About 5 ml clotted blood should be sent to the laboratory early in the day.

Human chorionic gonadotrophin (hCG)

The normal serum level of hCG is <5 U/L. It is raised in the presence of *choriocarcinoma* and *germ cell tumours*; it is of great value in their diagnosis and post-therapy monitoring. *Any female of child-bearing age with unidentified malignancy should have* serum levels of hCG and AFP measured, as should *all males under 45 with a suspicious lump in the testis or malignancy of unknown origin.*[9] **NB**: hCG is also raised during pregnancy.

Human placental lactogen (HPL)

See p. 190.

Prostate specific antigen (PSA)

See p. 185.

Ca 19-9

The normal serum level of Ca 19-9 is <33 U/mL. It is raised in a high proportion of *pancreatic carcinomas* and only a small proportion of patients with benign pancreatic disease;[10] and so it is very helpful in the often difficult diagnosis of *pancreatic carcinoma*. It is also raised in 65% of cases of *hepatobiliary cancer* and is of value in monitoring the response to therapy of both *pancreatic* and *hepatobiliary carcinoma*.

Ca-125

Ca-125 is a marker for *ovarian carcinoma*, for which it has a high sensitivity and specificity. The normal serum level is 0–35 kU/ml. It is of value as an adjunct to diagnosis[9] and post-therapy monitoring of epithelial cancers of the ovary[11] (comparable with AFP and hCG as markers for germ cell tumours of the ovary). **NB**: Although a raised serum level (>35 U/ml) reliably indicates active disease, a low serum level (<10 kU/ml) does not exclude active disease and so does not indicate a cure.[9]

Neurone-specific enolase (NSE)

Serum neurone specific enolase is normally <12 μg/L. It is raised in *lung cancer of small cell type* but is of limited specificity and sensitivity.[9]

Uric acid (urate)

The normal figure is 0.15–0.4 mmol/litre (2.5–7 mg/100 ml) for men and 0.1–0.35 mmol/litre (1.5–6 mg/100 ml) for women. About 5 ml of blood are sent to the laboratory in either a dry or a sequestrenated tube. The estimation may also be undertaken in a clinic or sideroom using an instrument such as Reflotron® (Boehringer– Mannheim).

In *gout* the figure may rise as high as 0.6 mmol/litre (10 mg/100 ml).

Zinc

Zinc is an essential part of many enzymes.[12] The normal serum level is 6–25 μmol/L. The effects of deficiency include *hair loss, dermatitis, growth retardation, poor wound healing, anorexia, lethargy* and *impaired sense of smell and taste*. Nuts, red meat and shellfish are sources, but processing of food tends to remove zinc from sources such as cereals (as in white flour). Deficiency can result from diminished intake, e.g. from parenteral feeding, impaired absorption, or increased loss, e.g. from a *gastro-intestinal fistula*. Excess intake interferes with copper metabolism and produces features of copper deficiency (*microcytic anaemia* and *neutropenia*).[12] Consult with the laboratory before sending a sample of about 5 ml of clotted blood.

References

1. Kenkre, J E, Hobbs, F D R, Carter, Y H. Evaluation of a C-reactive protein assay (Nyocard) as a near patient test in primary care. *Clinical Rheumatology*. 1994; 13: 359–360.

2. Marshall, W J. Hydrogen ion homeostasis, tissue oxygenation and their disorders. In: Marshall, W J and Bangert, S K, (eds). *Clinical Biochemistry: Metabolic and Clinical Aspects*. New York. Churchill Livingstone. 1995: 61–86.

3. Pagana, K D and Pagana, T J. Creatine phosphokinase. In: Pagana, K D and Pagana T J, (eds). *Mosby's Diagnostic and Laboratory Test Reference*. St Louis. Mosby Year Book. 1992: 248–250.

4. Pagana, K D and Pagana, T J. Lactic dehydrogenase. In: Pagana, K D and Pagana, T J, (eds). *Mosby's Diagnostic and Laboratory Test Reference*. St Louis. Mosby Year Book. 1992: 450–452.

5. Hooper, J and Bangert, S K. Clinical biochemistry in the investigation of acute chest pain and the acute abdomen. In: Marshall, W J and Bangert, S K, (eds). *Clinical Biochemistry: Metabolic and Clinical Aspects*. New York. Churchill Livingstone. 1995: 779–787.

6. Pagana, K D and Pagana, T J. 5-nucleotidase. In: Pagana, K D and Pagana T J, (eds). *Mosby's Diagnostic and Laboratory Test Reference*. St Louis. Mosby Year Book. 1992: 522–523.

7. Riches, P. Paraproteinaemias. In: Marshall, W J and Bangert, S K, (eds). *Clinical Biochemistry: Metabolic and Clinical Aspects*. New York. Churchill Livingstone. 1995: 493–506.

8. Pagana, K D and Pagana T J. Cryoglobulin. In: Pagana, K D and Pagana T J, (eds). *Mosby's Diagnostic and Laboratory Test Reference*. St Louis. Mosby Year Book. 1992: 251–252.

9. Beastall, G H and McAllister, E J. Tumour markers. In: Marshall, W J and Bangert, S K, (eds). *Clinical Biochemistry: Metabolic and Clinical Aspects*. New York. Churchill Livingstone. 1995: 705–716.

10. Pagana, K D and Pagana, T J. Ca 19.9 tumor marker. In: Pagana, K D and Pagana, T J, (eds). *Mosby's Diagnostic and Laboratory Test Reference*. St Louis. Mosby Year Book. 1992: 138–139.

11. Pagana, K D and Pagana, T J. Ca-125. In: Pagana, K D and Pagana, T J, (eds). *Mosby's Diagnostic and Laboratory Test Reference*. St Louis. Mosby Year Book. 1992: 134–135.

12. Bangert, S K. The clinical biochemistry of nutrition. In: Marshall, W J and Bangert, S K, (eds). *Clinical Biochemistry: Metabolic and Clinical Aspects*. New York. Churchill Livingstone. 1995: 173–198.

CHAPTER NINE

Tests related to eating and drinking

Nutrition and alimentary tract

Index of tests	Page		Page
Abdomen, radiograph of	137	Glucose tolerance tests	147
Abdomen, ultrasound of	137	Hippuric acid test	139
Ascitic fluid	150	Histamine test meal	135
Alcohol test meal	135	Ileal biopsy	149
Ascorbic acid	127	Intravenous cholangiogram	142
Barium meal	131	Intravenous glucose tolerance test	148
Barium swallow	130	Insulin secretion tests	144
Bile secretion	144	Insulin test meal	135
Bilirubin in urine	137	Intestinal absorption tests	149
Blood sugar (glucose)	145	Ketones in urine	145
Cholangiograms	142	Laparoscopy	150
Cholecystography	141	Laparotomy	151
Cobalamin	126	Liver radiology, ultrasound and MRI	137
Computerized tomography (CT)		Liver function tests	137
scan of abdomen	151	Liver function test interpretation	139
Dicopac test	136	Liver puncture biopsy	140
Double contrast radiography	131	Lundh test	144
Duodenal aspiration tests	143	Malabsorption of vitamin B_{12}	136
Duodenal biopsy	133	Milk	124
Duodenal X-ray	131	Mouth	128
D-xylose excretion test	150	Mucoviscidosis, sweat test for	143
Endoscopic retrograde		Oesophagitis	129
cholangiopancreatography (ERCP)	144	Oesophagoscopy	130
Extended glucose tolerance test	147	Oesophagus	129
Faecal fat	150	Oral cytology	128
Fine needle aspiration (FNA) of liver	141	Pancreatic biopsy and aspiration cytology	148
Folic acid	127	Pancreatic function tests	143
Food poisoning	128	Pancreatitis tests	142
Gall bladder and bile ducts	141	Pentagastrin test meal	134
Gastric secretion tests	134	Percutaneous cholangiogram	142
Gastrin	136	Plasma glucagon	149
Gastrocamera examination	134	Salivary gland aspiration cytology	129
Gastrointestinal bleeding scan	151	Salivary gland excision biopsy	129
Gastroscopy	132	Schilling test	136
Glucose (sugar) in urine	144	Secretin test	144
Glucose in blood	145	Serum alkaline phosphatase	138

Index of tests	Page		
Serum aminotransferases	139	Test meals	134
Serum amylase	142	Throat swab	129
Serum bilirubin	138	Transhepatic cholangiogram	142
Serum cholesterol	140	T-tube cholangiogram	142
Serum gammaglutamyl transferase	139	Urobilinogen and urobilin in urine	138
Serum iron	139	Vitamin A	125
Serum insulin	148	Vitamin B₁	125
Serum proteins	139	Vitamin B₁₂	126
Small intestinal biopsy	149	Vitamin B₁₂ malabsorption	136
Stomach and intestines	130	Vitamin C	127
Sugar in blood	145	Vitamin D	127
Sugar in urine	144	Vitamin deficiencies	125
Sweat test for fibrocystic disease	143	Vitamin K	128
Teeth	128	Xylose excretion test	150

Introduction

Adequate nutrition is essential for health. Tests on milk are performed in the Public Health Laboratory. Tests for vitamins A, B_1, C (ascorbic acid) and D are undertaken in chemical pathology; those for vitamin B_{12}, K and folic acid in haematology, and those for food poisoning in microbiology. The upper alimentary tract, liver and pancreas are mainly investigated by the gastroenterologist and radiologist. Tests for gastric secretion, gastrin, malabsorption of vitamin B_{12}, liver function, pancreatitis, pancreatic and bile secretion, and insulin secretion are mainly performed by chemical pathology. Urine tests for bile pigments, sugar and ketones are often performed by the nurse, using stick tests. The nurse may also use a more sophisticated 'near patient' test for blood sugar.

Nutrition

Milk

Milk has to be of a certain standard, and tests are carried out for the following purposes:

- To estimate the fat content and so detect any adulteration with water.
- To estimate the bacterial content and the possible presence of any bacteria which should not be present.

Several types of milk are marketed in England and Wales: pasteurized, sterilized and UHT (ultra high temperature-treated). Tuberculin-tested milk is not specially designated since the whole of England, Scotland and Wales is an attested area in which all cattle are tested to see that they are free from tuberculosis.

Pasteurized milk

This is milk which has been heated to a temperature of 62.8°C for half an hour (or using the high temperature short time method, 71.6°C for 15 seconds) and immediately cooled to 10°C or less. This destroys most of the bacteria. Pasteurized milk must give a 'negative' phosphatase test (2.3 Lovibond units or less). Phosphatase is an enzyme which occurs normally in milk but is practically destroyed by adequate pasteurization. In addition a sample of pasteurized milk which is taken on the day of delivery and kept below 18°C should, until 0900–10.00 hours of the day following delivery, fail to decolourize methylene blue in 30 minutes.

Sterilized milk

The milk is filtered, homogenized and heated to a temperature of at least 100°C for sufficient time (several minutes) to comply with the turbidity test. The bottles are sealed with airtight seals.

UHT (ultra high temperature-treated)

The milk is heated to a temperature of not less than 132.2°C for at least 1 second. UHT milk is tested by culture on a specialized medium for 48 hours at 37°C. The number of bacterial colonies is then counted and must be fewer than ten. Unopened cartons may be safely stored without refrigeration until the date of expiry. Once opened, the milk should be used at once or refrigerated.

Infection in milk

Certain diseases may be transmitted by milk, e.g. *tuberculosis, scarlet fever, epidemic diarrhoea, abortus fever, undulant fever, typhoid fever, diphtheria.* In some cases the milk is infected by 'carriers' who handle it.

Vitamin deficiencies
Vitamin A

Vitamin A precursors occur in the green and yellow parts of vegetables, including carrots. Deficiency can cause *'night blindness', xerophthalmia* and *keratomalacea*, one of the commoner causes of blindness in poor countries. The normal blood level of vitamin A is 0.7–7 µmol/litre (20–200 µg/100 ml). This can be estimated chemically, 10 ml of heparinized or clotted blood being required. Deficiency can also be detected by the dark adaptation test which shows impairment when the blood level falls below 0.35 µmol/litre (10 µg/100 ml). Deficiency occurs in *intestinal malabsorption*, excessive use of *liquid paraffin* and *dietary inadequacy*.

Vitamin B₁ (aneurine, thiamine)

Wheat germ, oatmeal and yeast are rich sources of vitamin B_1. Its deficiency is a causative factor in *beriberi, peripheral neuritis* and *Wernicke's encephalopathy*. The vitamin B_1 status of a patient was assessed, rather inaccurately, by measuring the blood pyruvic acid or more accurately by the pyruvic tolerance test, but is probably best estimated by erythrocyte transketolase activity[1].

Pyruvic acid

Normally the blood pyruvic acid is 0.045–0.110 mmol/litre (0.4–1.0 mg/100 ml). In *vitamin B₁ deficiency* it may be increased up to 0.22–0.33 mmol/litre (2–3 mg/100 ml) and is used as a test for this condition, although the pyruvic tolerance test (see below) is more sensitive. Some increase also occurs in *diabetes mellitus, congestive heart failure* and other conditions. The blood is usually collected by one of the laboratory staff.

Pyruvic tolerance test

This is a more sensitive test for vitamin B_1 deficiency than simple blood pyruvic acid level determination. The laboratory staff must be notified and may undertake the blood collection. The test is performed in the morning, the patient having fasted since 22.00 hours the previous evening (water may be drunk). A 2 ml fasting blood sample is collected as described below. Then 50 g of glucose is given orally in about 300 ml of water flavoured with diabetic squash. Further 2 ml blood samples are collected at 30 minutes, 1 and 2 hours after the glucose. Special care is required for blood collection. The syringe must not be warm. Either a 2 ml or 5 ml syringe is used, with a 21-gauge needle. The patient must not clench and unclench the hand. The tourniquet is kept on for the minimum of time, being removed immediately after the needle enters the vein. The 2 ml of blood is ejected into 8 ml of cold trichloracetic acid in a stoppered centrifuge tube. The blood pyruvic acid level should not exceed 0.132 mmol/litre (1.2 mg/100 ml) for any specimen. In vitamin B_1 deficiency this level is exceeded.

Erythrocyte transketolase activity

Assessment of the erythrocyte transketolase activity, with and without added thiamine pyrophosphate, is probably the most reliable test for vitamin B_1 deficiency.[1]

Vitamin B_{12} (cobalamin)

Vitamin B_{12} is essential for the normal production of red cells by the bone marrow. Normally blood serum contains 0.09–0.44 nmol/litre (120–600 ng/litre) of metabolically active vitamin B_{12} (cobalamin). In *pernicious anaemia* and *subacute combined degeneration of the cord* it is greatly reduced (due to failure of secretion of intrinsic factor by the stomach, essential for cobalamin absorption). It is also reduced in the *intestinal malabsorption syndrome* (together with folic acid, iron and vitamin D), in some cases of *carcinoma of stomach* and occasionally in *megaloblastic anaemias of pregnancy*. Often vitamin B_{12} deficiency can be inferred, as in typical *pernicious anaemia*, by the raised MCV, megaloblastic bone marrow, histamine-fast achlorhydria and slightly raised serum bilirubin. Confirmation should be obtained by laboratory estimation of vitamin B_{12} before starting therapy. Laboratories which use microbiological assay should be informed of any antibiotic (including antituberculous) or cytotoxic therapy, which can give false low results.

Laboratory assay of vitamin B_{12} (cobalamin)

About 10 ml of clotted blood is collected, using a new syringe, needle and universal container. Minute traces of contamination can vitiate the assay. The vitamin B_{12} is estimated in the laboratory either by radioisotope assay or by measuring the amount of growth of a specially chosen microorganism promoted by different dilutions of the patient's serum. The radioisotope method is more accurate and measures only the metabolically active cobalamin (see p. 136, Schilling and Dicopac tests).

Other tests for vitamin B_{12} deficiency

1. *Therapeutic response.* Administration of vitamin B_{12} to a patient with *pernicious anaemia* produces a reticulocytosis (see p. 90) on about the fifth day, detected by serial reticulocyte counts. This is followed by a steady rise in the haemoglobin level.

2. *Schilling* or *Dicopac* test (pp. 136). Using radioactive B_{12} it is possible to diagnose *pernicious anaemia* even in a patient who has been receiving treatment.

Malabsorption of vitamin B_{12}

See p. 136.

Folic acid

Folic acid is essential for the normal production of red blood cells by the bone marrow. Blood folic acid can be estimated by radioisotope or microbiological assay. The former can be performed on the same specimen as for vitamin B_{12} (see p. 126). Normally the blood level, reported as serum folate, is 3.6–13.7 µmol/litre (1.6–6.0 µg/litre). Laboratories which use microbiological assay must be informed of any recent antibiotic or cytotoxic therapy, since these can cause false low results. In deficiency, e.g. *megaloblastic anaemia of pregnancy* and the *malabsorption syndrome*, it disappears from the blood more rapidly than normal after intravenous administration. This is the basis of the *folic acid clearance test*. Absorption after oral administration may similarly be tested. However, during pregnancy folic acid is usually prescribed without laboratory testing.

Vitamin C (ascorbic acid)

Vitamin C occurs in fruit (especially citrus) and vegetables, including potatoes. Severe deficiency of vitamin C causes *scurvy*. Less severe deficiency leads to *impaired healing*. It may occur in some cases of gastric ulcer which have had prolonged medical treatment. Vitamin C deficiency can be detected either by the ascorbic acid saturation test or less reliably by blood ascorbic acid estimation. However, usually the deficiency is diagnosed clinically and vitamin C supplement is given without laboratory testing.

Ascorbic acid saturation test

After at least 3 hours fasting, the patient drinks an ascorbic acid solution. This contains 11 mg of ascorbic acid/kg body weight, i.e. a total of about 700 mg of ascorbic acid for an adult, dissolved in about 150 ml of water. The bladder is emptied at exactly 4 hours after the drink, and the urine discarded. The bladder is again emptied exactly 2 hours later and the 2-hour specimen of urine sent to the laboratory. Normally about 0.8 mg/kg is excreted, i.e. about 50 mg in adults. In *vitamin C deficiency* a total of about 3 mg or less is excreted. When excretion is found to be deficient the test is repeated on several consecutive days. Even normal people may not be fully saturated with vitamin C initially.

Blood ascorbic acid

About 5 ml of anticoagulated blood are required. Normally 10–100 µmol/litre (0.4–2.0 mg/100 ml) are present. Below 10 µmol/litre (0.2 mg/100 ml) suggests scurvy. The saturation test (see above) is more reliable than a blood estimation.

Radiological changes in scurvy

In scurvy, haemorrhage occurs under the periosteum of bones in the neighbourhood of joints, the changes being visible on X-ray which may also show that the epiphyseal lines are irregular.

Vitamin D

Fish liver oils are rich in vitamin D. The normal serum level of 25-hydroxycholecalciferol is 10–80 µg/litre in adults and children. In *rickets* and *osteomalacia* the level may be too low to be detectable. In intoxication from overdosage, *hypervitaminosis D*, serum levels exceed 400 μg/litre. For its estimation 10 ml of clotted blood are required.

Vitamin K

Intestinal bacteria normally synthesize much of the vitamin K, essential for the normal production of prothrombin and other blood clotting factors. Vitamin K deficiency is caused by inadequate synthesis and absorption, e.g. *obstructive jaundice*, the *malabsorption syndrome* and *haemorrhagic disease of the newborn*. As a result the prothrombin time is raised, i.e. the prothrombin ratio increased. The prothrombin ratio (p. 95) is also increased in patients treated by anticoagulants such as warfarin, phenindione (Dindevan), nicoumalone (Sinthrome) and ethylbiscoumacetate (Tromexan). The effect of these drugs is counteracted by vitamin K.

Food poisoning

This is almost always due to contamination of the food by organisms. The organisms most commonly found are those of the salmonella group, such as *S. typhimurium* and *S. enteritidis*. A notable outbreak was caused by *S. enteritidis* of phage type 4 infecting eggs. Severe outbreaks with fatalities, particularly in the very young, have been caused by pathogenic *E.coli (0157)*, originating from sheep or cattle, either directly from faecal contamination of playing fields or from infected private water supplies. Food poisoning is also caused by *Staphylococcus pyogenes* which produces an exotoxin (enterotoxin), often by viruses (see p. 157), occasionally by *Clostridium perfringens* and rarely by *Clostridium botulinum*. The latter organisms or their toxins may survive boiling for up to 20 minutes. The following should be sent to the laboratory in suspected cases of food poisoning (**NB**: the clinical history is of very great importance in establishing the diagnosis):

- Portion of food or water suspected
- Stools (as soon as passed)
- Vomited matter, or stomach contents from a gastric washout.

Upper alimentary tract

Tests related to the mouth
Teeth

X-ray examinations are frequently of value in dental conditions, and may show the following: apical abscess (an abscess at the root of a tooth); bone infection round teeth; dental cysts; unerupted teeth.

Oral cytology

By taking cytological smears from abnormal lesions in the mouth, particularly in older people, it is possible to detect cancer at the very early stage when it can be readily treated. The material may be collected either by touching or by scraping.

1. *Touch preparation*. Where the situation allows, a glass slide may be applied directly to the surface of the lesion. A gentle touch suffices, repeated at different sites on the slide, or on different slides, and immediately fixed.

2. *Scrape and smear.* The surface of the lesion is gently scraped with a spatula and the material spread evenly on a slide, avoiding a rotary motion. With either method the material must be fixed while still moist and the slide labelled immediately.

Aspiration cytology of salivary gland

Using a fine needle inserted through the skin or buccal mucosa it is possible to aspirate material from a salivary gland tumour for cytological diagnosis. No local anaesthetic is required. The technique is similar to that described for breast lumps (p. 195).

Excision biopsy of salivary gland

The definitive diagnosis of a salivary gland tumour is often made by histological examination after surgical excision of the lesion in theatre. Total excision minimizes the risk of recurrence. The specimen is placed in a labelled container with at least ten times its volume of fixative and sent to the histopathology laboratory. Preparation of the patient is as for any surgical operation.

X-ray examination of salivary gland

A straight X-ray of a salivary gland clearly reveals any foci of calcification, including the presence of a calculus in the salivary duct. It may also reveal evidence of a tumour or of inflammatory change. For more detailed information, a sialogram (below) may be needed. Dentures and any relevant jewelery should be removed before the examination.

Sialogram

The injection of contrast medium into a salivary duct enables a more clearly defined picture of the duct and related salivary tissue to be obtained. It is of particular value in demonstrating the exact site of a stricture or calculus. The procedure should be explained to the patient, who should give written informed consent (see p. 2). Some patients may find the idea of a substance being injected into the mouth disturbing and require moral support. The mouth should be rinsed with antiseptic mouthwash before the test to avoid introducing infection into the salivary gland from the mouth.[2]

Throat swab

See p. 62.

Tests related to the oesophagus (all requiring written informed consent, see p. 2)

Test for oesophagitis (Bernstein, Baker and Earlam test)

The patient swallows a pernasal catheter until its tip is 30–35 cm from the incisor teeth. Connected to the catheter by a Y-tube are two drip bottles with taps, one bottle containing normal saline (150 mmol/litre), the other containing hydrochloric acid (100 mmol/litre). Saline alone dripped into the oesophagus should cause no pain, and acts as a control. Switching to the acid (6–7 ml/min) causes pain if oesophagitis is present. Relief of the pain by sodium bicarbonate (100 mmol/litre) is characteristic. This test distinguishes the pain of oesophagitis from other causes of chest pain.

Oesophagoscopy

This is the examination of the inner lining of the oesophagus by means of a special instrument called an oesophagoscope. It is a tube with a light at one end, which is introduced into the oesophagus through the mouth. The patient must be told the nature of the test and written consent obtained by the oesophagoscopist. A flexible fibreoptic instrument is often used rather than a rigid one. It is of great value in the investigation of *growths* and *strictures* of the oesophagus, the removal of accessible *foreign bodies*, and the collection of small portions of tissue for histological examination and material for cytology, and also in the treatment of *oesophageal varices* by the injection of a sclerosant. The preparation and aftercare of the patient are as described below for gastroscopy. After dilation of an oesophageal stricture no food or drink should be taken until a post-investigational X-ray has been examined and perforation excluded. Pulse and temperature should be recorded 4-hourly.

Barium swallow

This is a modified barium meal (see p. 131), and is used when it is expected that a lesion of the oesophagus is present. The patient is prepared as for a barium meal but swallows a smaller amount of a more concentrated emulsion, and its course is watched under the fluoroscopic screen from the moment that the barium enters the mouth.

Obstruction of the flow may be due to a *stricture*, a *growth*, an *external mass* pressing on the oesophagus, such as an *aneurysm*, or failure of the gastro–oesophageal orifice to open, a condition known as *achalasia of the cardia* or *cardiospasm*.

A *diverticulum* of the oesophagus becomes visible as a barium-filled pouch. A *hiatus hernia* can also be demonstrated.

Examination of the oesophagus is usually carried out as the first part of routine barium meal.

CT scan and PET (positron emission tomography)

If oesophagoscopy or barium swallow show evidence of oesophageal cancer, a CT scan (p. 21) provides a guide as to the extent of the tumour and helps to determine whether it is operable. In a few centres PET (p. 23) is available, which can demonstrate small extensions of tumour which would otherwise be undetectable.

Tests related to stomach and intestines

Improved techniques have made it possible to examine the stomach with greater precision. These techniques include double-contrast radiography, gastroscopy using a flexible fibreoptic endoscope, multiple biopsies, brushing cytology and photography. By their use gastric cancer is being diagnosed at a curable stage with increasing frequency in Japan and more recently in Europe and America.

For testing gastric secretion, Pentagastrin has now become the method of choice (p. 134), apart from insulin stimulation (Hollander test, p. 135), which is used to check whether the operation of 'highly selective vagotomy' has been successful. Gruel, alcohol and histamine test meals are now little used. All tests, apart from the *H. pylori* antibody test, require written informed consent (see p. 2).

Double contrast radiography

A double contrast X-ray is obtained by introducing gas and barium into the stomach. It enables much smaller abnormalities to be demonstrated than with the ordinary barium meal.

Barium meal

The night prior to the examination the patient is given an aperient if constipation is present. Nothing is given by mouth, not even a cup of tea, for 8 hours before the barium meal.

In the X-ray department, the patient stands behind an X-ray screen and swallows about 300 ml of an emulsion containing barium sulphate. The filling of the stomach is observed, and films are taken at the time and at various intervals during the next 20 minutes. A *follow-through examination* may be requested at the same time (see below). When the examination is completed it is wise for patients suffering from constipation to take a laxative.

Double contrast radiography is a technique for detecting small alterations in the gastric mucosa which may be invisible by ordinary barium meal. It involves the introduction of gas into the stomach (usually from special gas tablets) as well as barium. This provides a double outline which enables small lesions such as early gastric cancer to be seen.

Stomach

If a *gastric ulcer* is present a crater may be seen which will fill with barium, and the small quantity of barium in this crater may be observed some hours after the stomach has emptied of the main mass.

If the ulcer is long-standing, the stomach may be of an 'hourglass' shape, due to scarring and contraction.

If a *growth* is present the stomach outline is often irregular and ill-defined. It may show a filling defect. In early gastric cancer the mucosal folds show an altered pattern.

Pyloric stenosis may be present, leading to dilatation of the stomach, and considerable delay in emptying; this may be due either to an *ulcer* or a *carcinoma*. The normal time of emptying is about 4–5 hours for a barium meal.

If a gastroenterostomy has been performed previously, a barium meal will demonstrate whether it is working satisfactorily.

Duodenum

The first part of the duodenal shadow forms a 'cap' which is often irregular in cases of *duodenal ulcer*. A crater may be seen, or a *duodenal ulcer* may cause *pyloric stenosis*. Adhesions of a *diseased gall bladder* may cause irregularity of the duodenal outline. *Diverticula* of the duodenum may be demonstrated.

'Follow-through' examination

This is a more prolonged method of examination after a barium meal, in which further radiographs are taken during the next 3–6 hours or so, and the course of the barium through the intestinal tract is followed.

Small intestine

In *Crohn's disease* the barium may show a narrowing of the ileum known as the 'string sign'.

Large intestine

The outline of the bowel may show a constant filling defect due to a growth. Diverticula are seen in cases of *diverticulosis*. In *Hirschsprung's disease* the enormously distended colon can be demonstrated. Barium enema, however, provides a much better method of examining the colon (see pp. 155–156).

H. pylori antibodies and peptic ulceration risk

Helicobacter pylori infection of the stomach or duodenum is closely associated with peptic ulceration. The presence of antibodies to *H. pylori* is good evidence of present or past infection by this organism and their absence indicates a very low risk of peptic ulceration. They can be demonstrated using a 5 ml venepuncture sample of blood collected into a plain tube, sent to the laboratory for the Helico G test; or alternatively by means of a near patient test on a finger-prick sample using the Helisal rapid blood test. The latter has 80% of the sensitivity and 75% of the specificity of the former, with a negative predictive value of 58%. It has been used by GPs as a guide to prescribing eradication therapy against *H. pylori* in both investigated and uninvestigated cases of *dyspepsia*.[3]

Gastroscopy

By means of a gastroscope the interior of the stomach may be examined visually, material taken for histological and cytological diagnosis, abnormalities photographed and a sketch made of the findings and of biopsy sites. The fibreoptic endoscope (gastroscope) consists of a firm but flexible plastic tube with a controllable end bearing a light (**Fig. 9.1**). It is passed into the stomach through the mouth and oesophagus (**Fig. 9.2**). A bundle of finely drawn glass fibres (the fibreoptics) passing through the tube connects the eyepiece to the flexible tip, enabling the lining membrane of the stomach to be examined. The tube contains two additional channels: one for introducing air and the other for operative procedures, e.g. biopsy, snaring a polyp or injecting a sclerosing agent. The nature of the examination must be explained to the patient, who will be required to sign a consent form (see p. 2). The examination is often carried out in the morning, with the patient in a fasting condition, nothing having been taken since midnight. He should be told that it usually takes 20–30 minutes and warned that it is slightly uncomfortable. If gastroscopy is to be undertaken in the afternoon, the patient fasts after having a light breakfast of tea and toast at 06.00 hours. One hour before the examination, diazepam (Valium) 10 mg is given; 15 minutes before gastroscopy a tablet of amethocain is given, followed by a second tablet as the patient is taken to the theatre. False teeth, jewellery and glasses should be removed and stored safely.

In skilled hands the passage of the gastroscope into the stomach should cause relatively little discomfort. During the gastroscopy multiple photographs are often taken, e.g. of an ulcer or growth. *Biopsy* material is collected by means of special forceps. Each biopsy specimen should be placed in formol saline in a labelled container with its individual number. A sketch is also made on which the numbered biopsy sites are marked. Material for *cytology* is collected by means of a gastroscopy brush with a protective plastic tube to prevent carryover of cells from one case to the next. Alternatively the whole gastroscope may be withdrawn with the brush still protruding. Material from the brush is immediately smeared evenly on to two to four microscope slides, spray-fixed while still moist and the slides labelled.

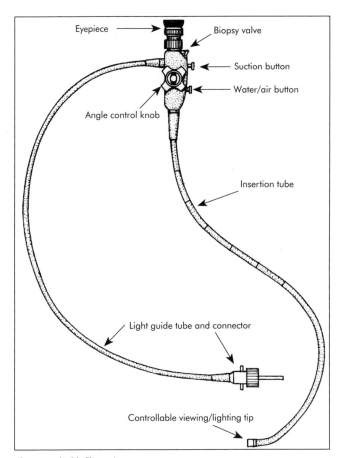

Fig. 9.1   Flexible fibreoptic gastroscope

Following the examination mucus and air may be brought up. Owing to the local anaesthetic, nothing should be allowed by mouth for 1–2 hours, as fluid may be inhaled into the lungs. The patient will require bed rest until fully awake. If the throat is sore following the examination, a simple inhalation may be given.

Gastroscopy is of assistance in the diagnosis of *gastritis, gastric and duodenal ulcers,* and *carcinoma of the stomach.* Atrophy of the mucosa is seen in cases of pernicious *anaemia* and with other *gastric lesions.* Gastroscopy should not be undertaken if there are *oesophageal diverticula,* if perforation is suspected or if the patient is uncooperative.

The gastroscope is also used for obtaining *duodenal biopsies* in suspected coeliac disease (intestinal malabsorption). This is now considered a more reliable technique than the Crosby capsule (see ileal biopsy p. 149).

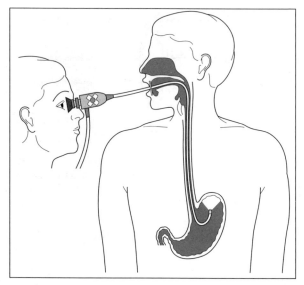

Fig. 9.2 Gastroscope introduced into the stomach with tip flexed to examine the fundus.

Gastrocamera examination

The gastrocamera is introduced into the stomach in the same way as a gastroscope, which it resembles, but it has a tiny camera at its tip, enabling high quality pictures of the gastric mucosa to be taken directly instead of through the fibreoptics of a gastroscope, giving better definition.

Gastric secretion tests

These tests are now seldom used. They should not be undertaken prior to endoscopy, if this is contemplated, because the appearance of the mucosa is affected.

Pentagastrin 'test meal'

Pentagastrin is chemically similar to the normal gastric stimulant hormone gastrin, and has now virtually replaced alcohol, histamine and the gruel test meals. The patient is allowed no food or drink after midnight. At 06.00 hours a Ryle's tube is passed pernasally into the stomach; a mark on the tube shows when it has passed far enough. Resting juice is collected at 15-minute intervals for a period of 1 hour to determine the basal acid output (BAO). Pentagastrin (Peptavlon) is then injected subcutaneously in a dose of 6 μg/kg body weight using a tuberculin syringe. Specimens are collected at 15-minute intervals, usually for a further period of 1 hour. The volume of each sample is measured and it is then filtered through gauze into a bottle. The acidity is estimated in the laboratory. The peak acid output/h (PAO) is 2 (the sum of the two consecutive 15-minute acid outputs giving the largest total). A normal example is shown in **Fig 9.3** and the findings in various conditions in **Table 9.1**. See also gastrin, p. 136.

The success of the test depends on good collections of gastric juice. If these are incomplete, the test is valueless. The absence of acid (achlorhydria) in *pernicious anaemia* may be confirmed by pH measurement which remains at about pH 7 (see p. 73).

Fig. 9.3 Pentagastrin 'test meal'. BAO-basal acid output; PAO-peak acid output

Insulin 'test meal' (Hollander test)

The fasting patient is intubated as for the pentagastrin 'test meal'. The fasting juice is aspirated and discarded. The basal secretion is collected over the next two 30-minute periods. Soluble insulin 15–20 units is then given intravenously. Gastric juice is collected for a further four 30-minute periods. Blood is taken at 30 and 45 minutes after the insulin injection into fluoride tubes for glucose estimation. All the specimens are sent to the laboratory for analysis of volume, and free and total acid secretion.

Insulin stimulation tests the integrity of the vagus nerve and is usually carried out about 1 week after the operation of 'highly selective vagotomy'. The insulin produces a low blood sugar (hypoglycaemia), which causes the vagus nerve to promote the secretion of acid and gastrin. This response is abolished if the operation has been successful.

Alcohol and histamine 'test meals'

The patient is prepared as for the pentagastrin 'test meal' (p. 134), and the resting juice similarly collected. The patient then drinks 50–100 ml of 7% ethyl alcohol.

Table 9.1 Pentagastrin 'test meal' findings in various conditions		
Condition	BAO (mmol/h)	PAO (mmol/h)
Normal subjects	1–8	1–50
Gastric cancer	0–8	0–30
Gastric ulcer	0–8	1–50
Duodenal ulcer	0–25	15–100
Pernicious anaemia	0	0
Zollinger–Ellison syndrome	over 15	15–100

Specimens of gastric juice are collected quarter-hourly. At the end of 1 hour the patient may be given an injection of histamine hydrochloride 0.25–0.5 mg subcutaneously. This is a powerful stimulant of gastric secretion. Further specimens of gastric juice are collected 30 minutes and 1 hour after the histamine injection. If no free acid is detected in the latter specimens, the patient has histamine-fast *achlorhydria*, a typical finding in *pernicious anaemia*. Alternatively, the alcohol may be omitted, the patient being given histamine only, i.e. the histamine 'test meal'. The 'augmented histamine test meal' in which the patient was protected from side-effects of the extra large dose of histamine by an antihistamine drug, is no longer used. Most hospitals now use the pentagastrin 'test meal' instead of any of the above.

Gastrin

This hormone, produced by G cells of the gastric antrum and the duodenum, stimulates gastric secretion. Its normal range in the plasma is 5–50 pmol/litre. Patients with a *gastrin-producing tumour* (Zollinger–Ellison or ZE syndrome) usually have over 100 pmol/litre. However, patients with *hypochlorhydria* may have over 1000 pmol/litre. So a high plasma gastrin only indicates ZE syndrome if there is also a high gastric acid. Collect 8 ml blood into heparin tubes and transport immediately to the laboratory.

Tests for malabsorption of vitamin B$_{12}$

Normal gastric juice contains intrinsic factor which is essential for the absorption of vitamin B$_{12}$. In *pernicious anaemia* intrinsic factor is absent, so that vitamin B$_{12}$ cannot be absorbed. Its absorption may also be impaired by defective intestinal mucosa as in intestinal malabsorption.

Schilling test

A small dose of radioactive B$_{12}$ is given by mouth to the fasting patient, followed by a large dose (e.g. 1000 µg) of non-radioactive B$_{12}$ intramuscularly. All urine for the next 24 hours is collected and sent to the laboratory. (**NB**: complete urine collection is vital.) Normally more than 7% of the radioactive dose is excreted in the urine in 24 hours. In *pernicious anaemia* less than 3% is excreted.

If less than 7% of the dose is excreted in the urine the patient is given a capsule containing 60 µg of intrinsic factor and the test repeated as before. If the amount of radioactive B$_{12}$ excreted now reaches normal levels the diagnosis of *pernicious anaemia* is confirmed. Failure to reach normal levels after the intrinsic factor has been given indicates intestinal malabsorption.

Dicopac test

The pack for this test is produced by Amersham International (Cardiff, Wales). It involves one administration by capsules, one injection and one urine collection. In principle it is similar to the Schilling test but in practice it is more convenient.

Both the above tests have the great advantage that they can be used for treated cases without suspension of treatment.

Liver

Imaging techniques for liver examination: radiology, ultrasound and MRI
The liver may be examined by:

- Straight radiography of the abdomen (see below)
- Ultrasound (see below)
- Radioisotope (p. 22) imaging of liver ('liver scan')
  - (a) Space-occupying lesions can be demonstrated by colloid particles labelled with technetium^{99m} (Tc^{99m}). These particles are taken up by the reticuloendothelial system (Kupffer cells). Alternatively Tc^{99m} labelled millispheres (<10 μm) of albumin may be used.
  - (b) Lesions obstructing the biliary tree can be demonstrated by TC^{99m} labelled HIDA (hydroxy iminodiacetic acid). This is concentrated in the liver cells and is then excreted like bile into the biliary tree, common bile duct, gall bladder and bowel.
- Computerized tomography (CT) scan (see p. 151)
- ERCP (endoscopic retrograde cholangiopancreatography). This enables the biliary tract to be visualized (see p. 144)
- Angiography (see p. 83)
- MRI (magnetic resonance imaging, see p. 21)

NB: For gall bladder see pp. 141-142.

Radiograph of abdomen
A plain X-ray of the abdomen can be most informative, particularly in the investigation of the 'acute abdomen'. The soft tissue shadows of liver, spleen and kidneys can often be identified and their size assessed. Pathological calcifications due to *gallstones* (but see pp. 141, 142), *glandular calcification* or *vascular calcification* are shown. Distension of gut shadows with fluid levels will indicate *intestinal obstruction* and establish whether it involves small or large gut. Air below the diaphragm signifies a *perforation of the gut*.

Ultrasound
See p. 20. Ultrasound examination can decide whether an abdominal mass is solid or fluid-containing, and is of value in demonstrating *aneurysms, gallstones* and *tumours* involving the liver.

Routine liver function tests

The liver carries out many different chemical processes. In any particular liver condition only some of these may be affected. A number of different tests for liver function are therefore necessary. The routine tests on urine and blood will first be described.

Routine urine tests for liver function (ward or clinic tests)
Bile pigments (bilirubin)
Yellow froth on the urine when it is shaken suggests bilirubin. Its presence may be demonstrated by either stick tests or the Ictotest:

Stick tests

Bilirubin is detected by Bililabstix and Multistix (Ames, see p. 163) and also by Bilur-Test (Boehringer–Mannheim, see p. 163).

Ictotest

Five drops of urine are placed on one square of the test mat provided. An Ictotest tablet (Ames) is put in the centre of the moist area. Two drops of water are allowed to flow on to the tablet. The mat turns bluish-purple within 30 seconds if bilirubin is present. The speed and intensity of the colour is proportional to the amount of bilirubin. If no bilirubin is present the mat may turn pink, red or remain unchanged.

Urobilinogen and urobilin

Urobilinogen

This is most readily demonstrated by the stick test Multistix or by the Ugen-Test (see p. 163).

Urobilin

To 10 ml of urine 1 ml of Ehrlich's aldehyde reagent is added. After 3–5 minutes normal urine shows a faint reddish tinge, intensified by heating. If urobilin is increased a red colour is given by the urine, even diluted with about five times its own volume of water.

Routine blood tests for liver function

About 10 ml of blood in a plain sterile container is normally sufficient for all the following tests to be performed by the biochemistry department of most laboratories:

Serum bilirubin
Serum alkaline phosphatase
Serum aminotransferases (transaminases)
Serum gammaglutamyl transferase (γGT)
Proteins and electrophoresis.

Serum bilirubin

Test strip

A quick estimation of bilirubin in a sample of serum can be made by using Bilur-Test (Boehringer–Mannheim). The colour scale for serum provided with this single-test strip permits differentiation between normal and raised values.

Laboratory test

Bilirubin is estimated by the Van den Bergh test. Normally it is less than 17 µmol/litre (1.0 mg/100 ml). When bilirubin has passed through the liver cells it is altered (conjugated) and gives a direct Van den Bergh reaction. In *obstructive jaundice* it regurgitates back into the blood, producing an increase in the conjugated (direct) serum bilirubin. In *haemolytic jaundice* excessive breakdown of red cells causes increased production of the bilirubin which has not passed through the liver cells and so is unconjugated, giving an indirect Van den Bergh reaction.

Serum alkaline phosphatase

See p. 111. The normal values depend on the method used in the laboratory. It should be noted that the serum level is normally raised in infancy, childhood, adolescence (up to 21 years) and also in pregnancy.

Serum aminotransferases (transaminases)
See p. 116.

Serum gammaglutamyl transferase (transpeptidase), gGT
See p. 117.

Serum proteins
See p. 118. Normally about 70 g/litre (7 g/100 ml) of protein is present in the serum, of which 45 g/litre (4.5 g/100 ml) are albumin and 25 g/litre (2.5 g/100 ml) globulin. A reduction in the level of albumin may be due to liver damage.

Interpretation of routine liver function tests
When liver function is sufficiently impaired to interfere with the excretion of bile pigments, jaundice results. It is due to the retention of the bile pigment bilirubin in the blood. (Bilirubin is formed from the breakdown of haemoglobin from destroyed red blood cells.)

Jaundice may be of three types:

- *Obstructive*, due to blockage of the bile ducts, e.g. by gallstones
- *Haemolytic*, due to excessive destruction of the red blood cells (see p. 98), e.g. acholuric jaundice
- *Toxic or infective*, due to chemical or inflammatory damage to the liver cells, e.g. infective hepatitis.

Typical results in the different types of jaundice are presented in Table 9.2.

Additional liver function tests
Plasma ammonia
Ammonia, a toxic breakdown product of proteins and amino acids, is normally converted into urea by the liver. In severe liver failure this fails to happen and the raised ammonia level damages the brain, causing hepatic encephalopathy.[4] The normal plasma ammonia is 12–55 μmol/L. About 5 ml of blood is required, collected into a container with anticoagulant.

Hippuric acid test (oral method)
The patient is given a light breakfast 2–3 hours before the test, then 6 g of sodium benzoate in 30 ml of water, followed by half a tumbler of water. The bladder is immediately emptied completely and the urine thrown away.

Hourly specimens of urine are collected for the next 4 hours and all the urine sent to the laboratory. Normally at least 3.5 g of hippuric acid (expressed as sodium benzoate) is excreted in the 4 hours. This is reduced in liver damage.

The test is not reliable if kidney disease is present or if absorption is impaired. An intravenous method can be used to overcome poor absorption, but the hippuric acid test is now seldom used.

Serum iron
See p. 91. Normal serum iron is 1–3 mmol/litre (60–180 μg/ml). This is increased in toxic and infective liver disease, with values over 3.5 mmol/litre (210 μg/ml). It may help to distinguish these conditions from jaundice due to mechanical obstruction where values below 3.5 mmol/litre are obtained.

Table 9.2 Liver conditions: comparison of laboratory results			
Tests		**Obstructive jaundice**	**Haemolytic jaundice (acholuric jaundice)**	**Toxic and infective hepatitis**
Urine	Bile salts and pigments	Present	Absent	Present
	Urobilin	Absent	Increased, often greatly	Variable
Blood	Bilirubin	Increased direct (conjugated)	Increased indirect (unconjugated)	Increased, mainly direct (conjugated)
	Alkaline phosphatase	Much increased	Little affected	Increased
	Aminotransferases	Often normal May be increased	Increased in 50%,	Greatly increased, (see p.116)
	Gammaglutamyl transferase	Normal or slightly increased	Normal	Greatly increased
	Proteins	Normal	Normal	Low albumin
Liver biopsy		May show changes of large duct obstruction	Normal	Changes of hepatitis or drug damage often present

Serum cholesterol
See p. 111.

Investigation of duodenal contents for bile secretion
See duodenal aspiration tests, pp. 143–144.

ERCP (endoscopic retrograde cholangiopancreatography)
See p. 144.

Liver puncture biopsy
Large bore needle biopsy
This test enables liver tissue to be obtained for histological examination without the dangers of a laparotomy and anaesthesia. *Written informed consent is required* (see p. 2). Before the test is performed, bleeding, clotting, prothrombin times and platelet count must be determined, in order to exclude any bleeding tendency. Vitamin K (phytomenadione, e.g. Konakion) may be given if the prothrombin time is prolonged.

The patient's blood must be grouped and suitable blood may be available for cross-match. Liver function tests should also be carried out. Half an hour before the puncture a mild sedative may be given if required, e.g diazepam (Valium) 5–10 mg. Stronger narcosis prevents the patient from cooperating. The biopsy is usually undertaken in the ward.

A sterile trolley is prepared containing towels, swabs, skin cleaning materials, 2% lignocaine hydrochloride solution with syringe and needles, tenotomy knife, and special liver puncture biopsy set, including 20 ml syringe to fit where required. Collodion dressing should be on the trolley, also specimen containers; one containing formol saline, and a dry sterile container, useful for cryostat work or for culture.

The patient lies on his back on the bed, his right hand under his head and his right side parallel with the edge of the bed. He is told that he must follow the doctor's instructions regarding breathing while the puncture is being performed. By means of the special puncture needle (Trucut or Bard Biopty gun, see p. 4) a small cylinder of liver tissue is removed. This is either placed immediately in fixative or else taken unfixed direct to the laboratory for frozen section. Following the puncture, careful watch must be kept on the pulse rate and blood pressure for any sign of internal haemorrhage. They must be recorded every 15 minutes for the first 2 hours and then hourly for the next 22 hours, any rise in the pulse rate or fall in blood pressure being notified to the physician at once. The liver puncture site should also be checked. The patient may eat and drink as soon as he wishes.

By this procedure many conditions can be diagnosed, including *cirrhosis of the liver*, *neoplasms, amyloidosis, sarcoidosis* and *miliary tuberculosis*.

Fine needle aspiration (FNA)

Using a fine needle, material may be collected from the liver for cytological examination. This may be sufficient for the diagnosis of some *tumours* but, unlike large bore needle biopsy, it provides little information about liver structure which is essential for the diagnosis of *cirrhosis* or assessing the severity of *fatty degeneration*. *Written informed consent is required* (see p. 2). The technique is similar to that for FNA of the breast (see p. 195). It is simpler and safer than a Trucut needle biopsy. It is used for the demonstration of neoplasms and hydatid cysts but does not provide the structural information necessary for the differential diagnosis of *cirrhosis*.

Gall bladder and bile ducts

A straight radiograph of the gall bladder may demonstrate the presence of stones, but only 10% of gallstones are opaque to X-rays. All the following tests require written informed consent (see p. 2).

Cholecystography

This is a much more satisfactory method of examination. It consists of giving the patient an opaque medium which is excreted by the liver and concentrated in the normal gall bladder. If the gall bladder fills with the medium, it is rendered opaque to X-rays. The procedure, which should only be undertaken on patients who are not jaundiced, is as follows.

A light meal free from fat – e.g dry toast and tea – is given at 17.00 hours, and at 18.00 hours the patient is given the medium in the form of tablets, followed by a drink of water to remove the taste. The patient then goes to bed, and no food or drink except water (at least three glasses) are allowed. At 09.00 hours the following morning, a radiograph of the gall bladder region is taken. A meal containing fat is then given, and a further radiograph taken half an hour later.

If the gall bladder is normal, it is shown filled with medium, and empties after the fat meal. If the gall bladder is diseased, it is unable to concentrate the medium, and will not show. This is a rough guide, but many different conditions may exist. Sometimes the medium will outline the gall bladder, and demonstrate stones which were not visible on a straight X-ray. The fact that the medium has not concentrated in the gall bladder may rarely be due to other factors besides the gall bladder itself.

Intravenous cholangiogram

Another opaque medium, e.g. Biligrafin, can be injected intravenously, or infused over 1 hour to outline the bile ducts, the patient having been checked for sensitivity to iodine. Films are taken at 30, 60 and 90 minutes after injection. This may demonstrate bile duct obstruction, e.g. from a growth or stone. It is of no value in jaundiced patients. No breakfast should be taken on the morning of the examination but tea or coffee *without milk* is allowed. The test is usually done in the morning at about 09.00 hours. The patient should be told that it involves having a small drip in the arm and takes about 2 hours.

Percutaneous (transhepatic) cholangiogram

This involves direct injection of contrast medium into the biliary tree for the investigation of obstructive jaundice. Bleeding, clotting, prothrombin times and platelet count are first determined in order to exclude any bleeding tendency. Antibiotic cover is given for 24 hours before the test. The patient is sedated, e.g. by diazepam (Valium) 10 mg, 1 hour before the examination. Metal markers are attached to the skin of the epigastrium and right side. A plain X-ray is taken to check the liver size, position and relationship to the metal markers. Then with full aseptic precautions a long thin needle is introduced between the lower right ribs in the lateral line. The progress of the needle is watched under fluoroscopy. As soon as the lumen of the bile duct is reached, contrast medium enters it, outlining the biliary tree. It enables obstruction from *stone, stenosis* or *carcinoma* to be demonstrated. After the investigation the patient is kept in bed for 12–18 hours and the pulse rate recorded.

T-tube cholangiogram

This is performed 7–10 days after operative removal of gallstones to check whether there are any residual stones. No sedation is necessary. Contrast medium is injected into the T- tube which has been left in the common bile duct to provide drainage, and an X-ray is taken.

Gall bladder scan

The patient should fast for 2 hours before this test, which is performed in the nuclear medicine section of the radiology department (see radioisotopes, p 22). The radiologist injects radionuclide dye and within 60 minutes the gall bladder, common bile duct and duodenum should be visualized. Failure to visualize the gall bladder within 60–120 minutes is virtually diagnostic of cystic duct obstruction which occurs with acute cholecystitis: it is the method of choice for demonstrating this condition in patients with pain in the right hypochondrium.[5]

Pancreas

Tests for pancreatitis

Serum amylase (diastase)

About 5 ml of fresh clotted blood should be sent to the laboratory. In *acute pancreatitis* the serum amylase rises greatly soon after the onset, a figure of 5–10 times the normal value, of 25–180 somogyi units/dL, being considered diagnostic. But it may return to normal limits in a few days even though the disease is not subsiding. A slight rise may occur in *chronic pancreatitis*.

Urine amylase (diastase)

If urgent a single urine specimen will suffice. Otherwise a 24-hour specimen should be collected, and preserved with a little toluene. Normally urine amylase is 130–1300 IU/litre (5–50 Wohlgemuth units). Levels of 25 000 IU/litre (1000 Wohlgemuth units) or more may be reached in acute pancreatitis, falling to normal slightly later than the serum amylase.

Sweat test for fibrocystic disease (mucoviscidosis)

In children with fibrocystic disease of the pancreas (mucoviscidosis) the sodium chloride content of sweat is increased. This may be detected by the following test, which should only be undertaken by an experienced operator, after having obtained *written informed consent* (see p. 2). Sweating is stimulated usually on the forearm, or in babies on the thigh, by means of two pads placed one on each side of the limb, one pad being moistened with 0.2% pilocarpine nitrate solution and the other with N/10 magnesium sulphate. A mild electric current is passed between the two pads for 5 minutes, using an iontophoresis apparatus. The stimulated area is washed with distilled water and dried before the test. An accurately weighed filter paper is placed on the prepared area and covered by a slightly larger polythene sheet which is strapped into position for half an hour. The filter paper is returned to its original container and sent without delay to the laboratory, where the sweat is analysed. In fibrocystic disease the sodium level is increased, usually above 60 mmol/litre (60 mEq/litre).

CT (computerized tomography) scan for cysts and tumours

See p. 151.

Pancreatic function tests

The pancreas has two separate functions:

- The secretion of pancreatic juice into the small intestine
- The secretion of insulin into the bloodstream.

Tests relating to the secretion of pancreatic juice
Examination of stools

Trypsin test

This is suitable only for children. A sample of fresh faeces is sent to the laboratory where the presence and concentration of trypsin is detected by its ability to digest protein (e.g. gelatine or an exposed X-ray film).

Fat in stools

See Faecal Fat p. 150. This is estimated in the laboratory. Increased unsplit fat in the stools suggests pancreatic disease, but is not a constant finding.

Muscle fibres in stools

A marked increase in the number of undigested muscle fibres in the stools may occur in pancreatic disease but is not constant.

Duodenal aspiration tests

These necessitate the passage of a special tube into the duodenum. Written informed consent is required (see p. 2). The tube has a double lumen, one opening into the duodenum and the other into the stomach. Preparation of the patient is similar to that for the pentagastrin 'test meal' (p. 134). The tests are most conveniently performed under fluoroscopic control. The patient then sits with the tube in position while continuous suction at a controlled pressure (25–40 mmHg) is applied to the duodenum for 80 minutes. Suction is also applied to the mouth and stomach to remove saliva and gastric juice.

Pancreatic secretion

- *Secretin test*. Pancreatic secretion is stimulated by secretin. (An injection of 1 clinical unit per kilogram body weight of secretin from the GIH Research Unit of the Karolinska Institute gives maximal stimulation.) Pancreozymin injection is sometimes given as a more specific stimulus of enzyme secretion. The aspirated fluid from the duodenum is collected into ice-cooled flasks containing an equal quantity of glycerol. In pancreatic disease, the enzymes are reduced, particularly amylase. In more severe conditions bicarbonate estimation is the best guide to pancreatic exocrine function.

- *Lundh test*. Instead of using secretin, a special test meal is given to stimulate pancreatic secretion. It consists of milk powder, vegetable oil and dextrose. Fluid from the proximal jejunum is aspirated over the next 2 hours and the mean trypsin level estimated. This test is simpler to perform than the secretin test, but less accurate.

Secretion of bile

Absence of bile from all specimens indicates bile duct obstruction. Stimulation of bile secretion by 25% magnesium sulphate at 37°C injected through the duodenal tube is occasionally used. Pus cells are found in *cholecystitis*. The causative organism may be obtained on culture. Typhoid bacilli have occasionally been isolated from 'carriers' (see also Vi test, p. 16).

ERCP (endoscopic retrograde cholangiopancreatography)

Using a duodenoscope (a larger version of the gastroscope) it is possible to introduce a tube into the ampulla of Vater, under fluoroscopy. This enables the contents and the anatomy of the bile and pancreatic ducts to be investigated. *Written informed consent is required* (see p. 2). For a morning ERCP, no breakfast is allowed. For an afternoon ERCP, a light breakfast may be given. No fluids should be taken for 6 hours prior to the test. Atropine 0.6 mg is injected half an hour before the test and the patient is given an amethocaine lozenge to suck, followed by a second lozenge just before leaving the ward for the X-ray department. Specimens may be collected from the ampulla for chemistry and cytology (for the diagnosis of *pancreatic cancer*). A radioopaque medium is then injected to outline the pancreatic duct and the biliary tract, e.g. to demonstrate the site of a tumour. After the test nothing must be taken by mouth for 3 hours; then a cup of tea may be given.

Tests related to insulin secretion

In diabetes mellitus, glucose and ketones appear in the urine.

Sugar in urine

Stick or strip tests

Quick tests are in routine use for the simultaneous detection and monitoring of urine for glucose and ketones. Specifically designed for these two substances are Diabur-Test 5000 (Boehringer–Mannheim) and Ketodiastix (Ames). These substances may be detected by multiple test strips, e.g. BM-Test-5L (Boehringer–Mannheim), Multistix, Labstix and Bili-Labstix (Ames). Diastix is for glucose only. The method of testing for all stick tests is as described for Labstix on p. 162. Laboratory confirmation is essential. Patients receiving large doses of vitamin C may be given false-negative results.

Clinitest (Ames)
Five drops of urine are placed in a test tube. The dropper is rinsed and ten drops of water added. One Clinitest tablet is dropped in and spontaneous boiling occurs; 15 seconds after the boiling stops the tube is shaken gently and compared with the Clinitest colour scale to estimate the amount of sugar or other reducing substance present.

Benedict's test
Eight drops of urine are added to 5 ml of Benedict's solution in a test tube and boiled for 5 minutes. If sugar or other reducing substance is present the colour changes and is estimated by the degree of change: green = a trace; yellow = +; orange = ++; brick red = +++.

Ketones in urine
Stick or strip tests
Simultaneous testing for ketones and glucose is described under Labstix (p. 162) and BM multitest (p. 163). Ketostix (Ames) and Ketur-Test (Boehringer–Mannheim) test for ketones only (p. 162).

Acetest (Ames)
An Acetest tablet is placed on a clean white surface. One drop of urine is put on the tablet. After 30 seconds the colour is compared with the Acetest colour scale. The test detects acetone and acetoacetic acid. A moderate or strongly positive result indicates a severe ketosis. **NB**: Salicylates and other drugs can give a false-positive test for ketones.

Rothera's test
To 10 ml of urine in a test tube add sufficient ammonium sulphate crystals to make a saturated solution, add three drops of freshly prepared sodium nitroprusside solution and 2 ml of strong ammonia. A purple colour forms at the junction of the two liquids if ketone bodies are present. This is a very sensitive test.

Gerhardt's test
About 5 ml of urine are put in a test tube, and 10% ferric chloride solution added drop by drop. At first a white precipitate forms, which disappears on adding more ferric chloride. A port-wine colour develops if acetoacetic acid is present. A false-positive result may be given if the patient has been taking certain drugs, e.g. aspirin. If Rothera's and Gerhardt's tests are positive in the absence of drugs, the patient has severe ketosis, as in *diabetes* and *severe starvation*.

Blood sugar (glucose)
Blood sugar estimation 2 hours or more after a meal is a simple screening test for *diabetes mellitus*. A glucose tolerance test (pp. 147–148) is a more sensitive form of the test, used for detecting mild diabetes. The normal fasting glucose for *whole blood* is 3.6–5.6 mmol/litre (65–100 mg/100 ml) for adults and 2.2–5.6 mmol/litre (40–100 mg/100 ml) for children. For this estimation 2 ml of blood is taken into a fluoride tube. The fasting glucose for plasma is slightly higher, being 4.2–6.0 mmol/litre (75–107 mg/100 ml). For this estimation 2 ml of blood is also taken into a fluoride tube. Usually estimation is undertaken in the hospital laboratory. There is also a desktop analyser,

Reflotron® (Boehringer–Mannheim), which enables a direct reading of the blood sugar to be made on a small drop of blood serum or plasma. The instrument requires periodic cleaning and checking with a Reflotron® check colour standard.

In *diabetes mellitus* the blood sugar as a whole is higher than normal (*hyperglycaemia*) and may rise to over 28 mmol/litre (500 mg/100 ml). A fasting blood glucose of 12 mmol/litre (214 mg/100 ml) or more is diagnostic of *diabetes mellitus*. So a glucose tolerance test is not indicated. Estimation of the blood sugar is of the greatest importance in *diabetes*; it is a guide to the diet to be given and the amount of insulin required. It is an essential part of the satisfactory treatment of *diabetic coma*.

The blood sugar is also of considerable importance in the diagnosis of '*spontaneous hypoglycaemia*' when the blood sugar falls below normal limits due to the action of insulin. The estimation also enables other conditions (*renal glycosuria, lactational lactosuria*, etc.) which give rise to reducing substances in the urine to be distinguished from *diabetes*.

Approximate blood sugar estimation may be obtained in the ward, casualty department or at home by means of BM-Test-Glycemie 1-44 or Glucostix (Ames):

BM-Test-Glycemie 1-44 (Boehringer–Mannheim)

A large drop of blood is obtained from the finger. This may be done conveniently using the BM Autoclix gadget. This large drop (dabbling with small drops gives erroneous results) is placed over both test zones on the test strip, taking care not to allow the finger to touch the strip, and timing is started. The strip is placed on a flat surface. After exactly 1 minute the blood is wiped off with clean cotton wool. This is repeated twice, using clean areas of cotton wool. After a further minute the colour of the test zones is compared with the colour blocks on the label of the vial. If the reading at 2 minutes is above 17 mmol/litre the reaction is not complete. Leave for a further minute and read again. More accurate readings may be taken by using the Refloflux S, a pocket-sized meter. It is important to store the test strips in a cool place but not in a refrigerator, and not to use strips after the expiry date has passed.

Glucostix (Ames)

Prick finger and apply a drop of blood large enough to cover both reagent pads. Leave blood on pads for exactly 30 seconds. Remove the blood by blotting between folds of absorbent tissue for 1–2 seconds. If blood is not completely removed, repeat using a clean area of tissue. Wait an additional 90 seconds (2 minutes from applying blood) before comparing the pads with colour charts. If there is a matching green, this provides the blood glucose level. If the green pad is darker than the 6 mmol/litre colour block, compare the other pad to the nearest orange colour block and record results.

A more accurate estimation is obtained by measuring the colour with a reflectance meter such as the Ames Glucometer II. Dextro-chek (Ames) control solutions provide a quality control for the reagents and the user's technique.

Self-monitoring of blood sugar

This is now an established part of the management of insulin-dependent diabetes mellitus. Methods used include the BM-Test 1-44 and Glucostix described above. Additional meters are available: Glucometer GX and Hypocount GA, with which the patient starts a timer when blood is applied to the strip and wipes the blood off after a set interval; Accutrend, Hypocount Supreme and One Touch II, where timing is automatic and no wiping is required; ExacTech Companion or Supreme, where the drop of blood applied to the strip produces an electric current proportional to the glucose concentration. Meters need recalibration, e.g. with each new batch of test strips, and each patient's technique needs to be reviewed regularly.

Glycosylated haemoglobin (GHb)

Glucose in the blood combines with some of the haemoglobin in circulating red cells to form glycohaemoglobin. This is an irreversible change and the amount of glyco-haemoglobin formed accurately reflects the blood level of glucose.[6] Since the red blood cells have a life of 120 days, estimation of GHb provides an accurate guide to the blood glucose level in the preceding 2–3 months. Normally the proportion of haemo-globin which is glycosylated is 2.2% in adults and 1.8–4.0% in children. In diabetes mellitus which is under good control the level is 2.5–6.0%, with moderate control it is 6.1–8.0%, but if poorly controlled it is over 8%. This test is of great value in assessing the effectiveness of diabetic treatment and in determining the duration and severity of a newly-diagnosed case of diabetes. The specimen required is 5 ml of fluoridized or sequestrenated venous blood.

Glucose tolerance tests

Glucose tolerance test (oral)

This is a sensitive test for detecting mild diabetes mellitus. It measures the patient's ability to stabilize his blood sugar level after taking a quantity of glucose. The absorption of glucose raises the blood sugar level and the action of insulin lowers it.

Preparation: first explain to the patient the purpose and nature of the test. Tell him that after 3 days on a high carbohydrate diet he will have to fast from 22.00 hours on the eve of the test. He may continue to drink water, but no alcohol, coffee, tea, smoking or strenuous exercise is allowed until after the test. The test is done in the morning, the patient having fasted for about 10 hours. A 2 ml sample of blood is taken into a fluoride container for the fasting sugar estimation, and the bladder emptied. The patient is given 75 g of glucose dissolved in about 300 ml of water to drink, flavoured with diabetic squash. For children, a smaller quantity of glucose is given (2.5 g/kg body weight) with a minimum dose of 15 g. A second 2 ml sample of fluoridized blood for sugar estimation is taken 2 hours later and a specimen of urine collected.

During the test, be alert for signs of *hypoglycaemia*: sweating, weakness, restlessness and excessive hunger. Notify the doctor immediately if they occur. Encourage the patient to drink plenty of water. In normal persons the blood sugar resumes its normal level of about 5.6 mmol/litre (100 mg/100 ml) within 2 hours. Diagnostic values for *diabetes* are a fasting whole blood level of at least 7.0 mmol/litre (125 mg/100 ml) and/or a level of at least 10.0 mmol/litre (180 mg/100 ml) at 2 hours after the glucose. Corresponding plasma levels are 8.0 mmol/litre and 11.0 mmol/litre. In the malabsorption syndrome the glucose is only absorbed slowly, so that a flat curve is produced (see intravenous glucose tolerance test, below).

Extended glucose tolerance test

If *hypoglycaemia* is suspected, e.g. in a child having fits, it is usually necessary to extend the test to 5 hours. For convenience, blood sugar estimations up to 4 hours may be omitted. In *spontaneous hypoglycaemia* the blood sugar may fall to a very low level towards the end of the test, e.g. below 3.6 mmol/litre (65 mg/100 ml).

Intravenous glucose tolerance test

This is only used when the oral glucose tolerance test (p. 147) is unsuitable, e.g. if there is intestinal malabsorption. Patient preparation is as for the oral GTT and the test procedure is similar except that the glucose is given as a 50% glucose infusion over 3–4 minutes. Blood samples are taken pre-infusion and at 2 hours after the infusion. The blood sugar reaches its peak immediately, and normally returns to a fasting level in about 1 1/4 hours. Failure to return within 2 hours generally indicates *diabetes mellitus*. Delayed return also occurs in *starvation, carcinomatosis, cirrhosis of the liver* and *old age*.

Serum (plasma) insulin

Insulin lowers the blood sugar. Its measurement is indicated when there is a low blood sugar with a blood glucose of less than 5 mmol/L. In normal people, as the blood sugar level falls, the insulin level also diminishes. Thus, after fasting overnight the normal insulin level is <186 pmol/L. Following a hypoglycaemic episode with a blood sugar of <2.2 mmol/L the insulin level is <21 pmol/L. In cases of *insulinoma*, however, the insulin level remains high in spite of a low blood sugar. The following assists in the diagnosis of *insulinoma* (islet cell tumour of the pancreas). On each of three successive mornings after a 15-hour fast (18.00 hours to 09.00 hours) two samples of blood are collected: 2 ml into a fluoride tube for glucose and 5 ml clotted blood for insulin. These are sent at once to the laboratory. During the fast the patient may drink tap water. If symptoms of *hypoglycaemia* occur, blood samples must be collected before giving food.

When the results are equivocal the diagnosis of *insulinoma* is supported if the serum insulin remains above 30 mmol/litre when the blood glucose is reduced below 3 mmol/litre (54 mg/100 ml) by the injection of fish insulin. The laboratory will give details of an alternative (porcine insulin) test.

This test has alerted doctors to insulin overdose, which may be accidental or due to criminal intent.

Fructosamine

In uncontrolled diabetes mellitus, the high blood sugar affects the tissues and produces changes in certain proteins. Fructosamine is a product of such changes, and the blood level rises. The normal blood fructosamine level is <285 mmol/L. This assay provides a guide to the blood sugar level over the previous 10–15 days.[7]

Pancreatic and related tumours
Biopsy and aspiration cytology

These tests are used in the diagnosis of pancreatic tumours and other lesions. The advantage of fine needle aspiration cytology (FNA, see p. 5) over tissue biopsy (see p. 3) is that there is less danger of releasing pancreatic enzymes and causing pancreatitis. Since the pancreas is situated deeply on the posterior abdominal wall, biopsy and, usually, FNA are undertaken during laparotomy, for which written informed consent will have been obtained.

Plasma glucagon

Glucagon raises the blood sugar (glucose). Its estimation is only of value in the glucagon test (p. 58) and in the preoperative diagnosis of a *glucagon-producing tumour* of the pancreas, characterized by *wasting diabetes, anaemia* and *skin rash* (*necrolytic migratory erythema*). Normally, fasting levels are always below 100 ng/litre. *Glucagonomas* produce levels of up to 1000 ng/litre or more. Details of this specialized investigation can be obtained from the laboratory.

Plasma vasoactive polypeptide (VIP)

A patient with a *vipoma*, i.e. a tumour secreting VIP, develops a watery diarrhoea with *hypokalaemia* (p. 115) and *achlorhydria*[8] (p. 134). Normally the plasma level of VIP is <30 pmol/L. This is raised in vipoma. For its estimation the laboratory should be consulted.

Plasma pancreatic polypeptide (PP)

A significant proportion of patients with *multiple endocrine tumours* develop *Ppomas*,[8] i.e. tumours which secrete PP. They are clinically silent and can only be detected by the raised plasma PP. The normal plasma PP level is <300 pmol/L. The laboratory should be consulted if its estimation is required.

Small intestine

Tests for intestinal absorption

The commonest condition requiring investigation for intestinal malabsorption is *coeliac disease* (*gluten enteropathy, idiopathic steatorrhoea*).

Biopsy of the small intestine

1. Duodenal biopsy. This procedure is carried out under visual control using a gastroscope. Preparation is as for gastroscopy (p. 132). A sample of duodenal mucosa is obtained using special forceps. It is placed in formol saline and sent for histological examination. In *coeliac disease* there is a flattening of the mucosa. This test has replaced ileal biopsy (Crosby capsule) in many centres.

2. Ileal biopsy. By means of an instrument such as the Crosby capsule it is possible to obtain a specimen of tissue from the ileum for examination. The capsule contains a guarded cutting mechanism actuated via a long, thin, flexible tube. *The nature of the procedure must be explained to the patient, who will be required to sign a consent form* (see p. 2). The instrument is usually swallowed in the morning, the patient having fasted since midnight. From the stomach it gradually progresses through the duodenum to the jejunum, which it reaches in about 1 or 2 hours , the patient lying on his right side. The position of the capsule is checked by X-ray and the biopsy taken from the appropriate site by applying suction to the tube. The ileal mucosal changes in coeliac disease are similar to those in the duodenum. In many centres ileal biopsy has been replaced by duodenal biopsy.

D-xylose excretion test

This is a convenient test for the malabsorption syndromes, e.g. *coeliac disease*. The fasting patient is given 5 g of D-xylose sugar by mouth, dissolved in about 600 ml water. All urine is collected for the next 5 hours and sent to the laboratory. Normally this contains more than 1 g of xylose. If there is malabsorption it is diminished. With children the test is carried out using only 0.33 g/kg body weight; of this one fifth of the dose should be found in the 5 hour urine specimen.

Glucose tolerance test

See pp. 147–148. Typically a 'flat curve' is obtained in intestinal malabsorption, due to slow absorption of the glucose.

Faecal fat

For fat balance the patient is put on the normal ward diet, which should contain 70 g fat per day. After a few days to allow stabilization, all the faeces are collected for an exact period of time, e.g. 3 or 5 days. To make the test more accurate a 'marker' dye may be given by mouth at the beginning and end of the 3-day or 5-day period. With the appearance of the first 'marker' the faeces collection is started, and with the appearance of the second it is stopped. Normally the fat excreted does not exceed 5 g/24 hours and at least 90% of the fat taken is absorbed. Less than 90% suggests malabsorption.

Tests for malabsorption of vitamin B$_{12}$

See p. 136. Defective vitamin B$_{12}$ absorption, indicated by the low urine excretion values, is not rectified by giving intrinsic factor.

Peritoneum

Other abdominal tests (requiring written informed consent)
Ascitic fluid

Ascites is the accumulation of fluid (ascitic fluid) in the peritoneal cavity. It occurs in *failure of the liver, heart and kidneys* and in *abdominal tumours* and *inflammations*. Ascitic fluid is obtained by paracentesis, i.e. the aseptic introduction into the peritoneal cavity of a sterile aspiration needle or a trocar and cannula. Often sterile plastic tubing is introduced through the cannula to facilitate subsequent drainage, the rate of drainage being controlled by a clip. One sample of fluid should be sent to the cytology laboratory for the detection of malignant cells and chylomicrons, which are minute fat droplets seen in thoracic duct lesions. Another sample should be sent to the microbiology laboratory for culture (see p. 11).

Laparoscopy

This is the examination of the peritoneal cavity with a laparoscope (a sort of telescope) through a small abdominal incision under local anaesthesia. Written informed consent must be obtained (see p. 2). It is used occasionally for examination of the liver but more often in the investigation of lower abdominal pain which cannot be diagnosed by other methods. It is also used for examining the peritoneal surface of the female genitalia (p. 196), for sterilization and for ovarian biopsy (see p. 186).

Laparotomy

This is a full surgical operation for examination of the peritoneal cavity, requiring all the usual preoperative preparation. It provides similar but much more extensive information than laparoscopy, under direct vision, and enables appropriate intervention to be undertaken at the same time, if required. As for any surgical operation, written informed consent must be obtained (see p. 2).

Radiograph of abdomen

See p. 137.

Computerized tomography (CT) scan

If facilities are available a CT scan (p. 21) provides an accurate image of the site and extent of lesions such as tumours or cysts of the pancreas, liver or posterior abdominal wall. Patients should fast for 12 hours before the scan. They are also required to drink a watery solution of contrast medium at both 12 and 3 hours before the test.

Gastrointestinal bleeding scan

Finding the exact site of bleeding into the alimentary tract can be very difficult, particularly if it is in the small intestine beyond the reach of gastroscopy (p. 132). The test involves an intravenous injection of labelled sulphur colloid or red cells. They are usually labelled with radioactive technetium. This enables the site of bleeding to be detected by the pooling of radioactive material (see radioisotopes, p. 122). With the patient lying on a couch under a scintillation camera, images of the abdomen are taken, usually every 15 minutes for 1 hour and then hourly for 24 hours. The bleeding site shows up as a focus of radioactivity. This enables the surgeon to operate at the right site to determine and treat the source of the bleeding.[9] The nature of the test must be explained to the patient and *written consent obtained* (see p. 2).

References

1. Zilva, J F and Pannell, P R. *Clinical chemistry in diagnosis and treatment.* London. Lloyd-Luke; 1978: 420–421.

2. Pagana, K D and Pagana, T J. Sialography. In: Pagana, K D and Pagana, T J, (eds). *Mosby's Diagnostic and Laboratory Test Reference.* St. Louis. Mosby Year Book; 1992: 661–662.

3. Delaney, B C, Kenkre, J E and Hobbs, F D R. A whole blood near patient test for antibodies to *Helicobacter pylori*; effect on the management of dyspepsia in primary care. *Family Practice* 1995; 12: 263–264.

4. Johnson, P J. The assessment of hepatic function investigation of jaundice. In: Marshall, W J and Bangert, S K, (eds). *Clinical Biochemistry: Metabolic and Clinical Aspects.* New York. Churchill Livingstone; 1955: 217–236.

5. Pagana, K D and Pagana, T J. Gall bladder scanning. In: Pagana, K D and Pagana, T J, (eds). *Mosby's Diagnostic and Laboratory Test Reference.* St. Louis. Mosby Year Book; 1992: 358–359.

6. Pagana, K D and Pagana, T J. Glycosylated haemoglobin. In: Pagana, K D and Pagana, T J, (eds). *Mosby's Diagnostic and Laboratory Test Reference.* St Louis. Mosby Year Book. 1992: 391–392.

7. Coppack, S. Diabetes mellitus. In: Marshall, W J and Bangert, S K, (eds). *Clinical Biochemistry: Metabolic and Clinical Aspects.* New York. Churchill Livingstone; 1995: 257–280.

8. Hillhouse, E W and Loughlin, T. Metabolic effects of tumours. In: Marshall, W J and Bangert, S K, (eds). *Clinical Biochemistry: Metabolic and Clinical Aspects.* New York. Churchill Livingstone. 1995: 679–703.

9. Pagana, K D and Pagana, T J. Gastrointestinal bleeding scan. In: Pagana, K D and Pagana, T J, (eds). *Mosby's Diagnostic and Laboratory Test Reference.* St. Louis. Mosby Year Book; 1992: 376–378.

CHAPTER TEN

Tests related to eliminating (1)

Lower alimentary tract (the defecatory system)

Index of tests	Page		
Amoebic dysentery	154,156	Organisms and parasites in stools	156
Barium enema	155	Paratyphoid	156
Carriers	156	Polyps	154
Crohn's disease	154	Porphyrins in stools	157
Colonoscopy	154	Proctoscopy	153
Diverticular disease	154,156	Pseudomembranous colitis	157
Duodenal ulcer	156	Radiograph of abdomen	155
Dysentery	156	Roundworms	157
Fat, muscle fibres and trypsin in stools	156	Sigmoidoscopy	154
Food poisoning	156	Stricture	156
Gastric ulcer	156	Tapeworms	157
Growths	154	Threadworm	157
Haemorrhoids	154	Tubercle	157
Hirschsprung's disease	156	Typhoid	156
Hookworms	157	Ulcerative colitis	154, 155, 156
Occult blood test	156		

Introduction

Lower alimentary tract

Many patients are reluctant to complain of problems related to the lower alimentary tract. As a result, tests which can reveal the presence of bowel cancer at an early stage, when it is treatable, are often delayed until it is too late. Tact and sensitivity are required when explaining the tests, gaining consent and giving guidance about patient preparation. Visual and radiological examination of the bowel are undertaken by the gastroenterologist and radiologist respectively. Specimens for occult blood are sent to the Department of Chemical Pathology; those for organisms and parasites to microbiology.

Visual examination of rectum and colon

Proctoscopy

This enables the anal canal and lower 8 cm of the rectum to be examined. It is preferable for the bowel to have been emptied prior to the test. The patient is placed in the left lateral, or knee–elbow position, as for a rectal examination. A warmed and lubricated proctoscope is passed. It is of value for the examination of *haemorrhoids* and growths. From the latter a specimen may be taken for biopsy.

Sigmoidoscopy

The sigmoidoscope is a metal or plastic tube with electric illumination which enables the rectum and sigmoid colon to be examined. It is used in the differential diagnosis of *ulcerative colitis, Crohn's disease, diverticular disease, amoebic dysentery, polyps* and *growths*. The examination may be carried out in the ward, outpatient clinic or operating theatre, without anaesthetic. The nature of the test should be explained to the patient to ensure cooperation. He or she should be warned to expect a slight degree of discomfort and that air will be pumped into the bowel during the procedure to provide a clear view of its lining.

The examination is carried out in a similar way to proctoscopy (see above), the greater the length of the instrument allowing the rectum and sigmoid colon to be visualized. A blanket over the patient minimizes exposure and the presence of a nurse provides reassurance. Written informed consent is required (see p. 2).

Colonoscopy

The colonoscope consists of a long, firm, flexible plastic tube, with a controllable end bearing a light, with which it is possible to examine the entire length of the colon (**Fig. 10.1**). Vision is made possible by fibreoptics, as in the flexible gastroscope (p. 132), but the colonoscope is much longer and the glass fibres are more easily damaged by bending. This limits the number of colonoscopies that can be undertaken before the instrument requires costly repair. Preparation of the patient involves a 3-day regime. On day 1, all constipating drugs are stopped, including oral iron, and a clear fluid diet is started. If the patient is constipated, two Senokot tablets are given in the evening. On day 2, fluids only are continued. In the morning, 1 litre of 10% mannitol in tap water is given, to be drunk over a period of 30–60 minutes. On day 3, no

Fig 10.1   Colonoscope introduced into the colon

breakfast is given, fluids are continued and a rectal washout administered 2 hours before colonoscopy. As an alternative fluid-only regime the patient drinks 100 ml sorbitol 70% followed by 500 ml of water on the first morning. This is repeated 4 hours later and again on morning 2 followed by a rectal washout until clear, with a further rectal washout on day 3 prior to endoscopy. For very constipated elderly patients the sorbitol regime may be started 2 days earlier. At 1 hour before the examination diazepam (Valium) 10 mg is usually prescribed.

Colonoscopy is best undertaken in a special room with a table on which the patient lies in the left lateral position. The colonoscope is introduced through the anus and its progress up the colon is monitored by X-ray. It may cause physical and/or psychological discomfort and the nurse can assist greatly by reassuring the patient. Colonoscopy is used mainly for investigating possible *malignant change* in the colon, e.g. in *polyposis* or chronic *ulcerative colitis*, and enables multiple biopsies to be taken for histology. Written informed consent is required (see p. 2).

X-ray examination of gut
Radiograph of abdomen

See p. 137.

Barium enema

This procedure enables the colon to be visualized radiologically. Written informed consent is required (see p. 2). The preparation requires an empty bowel to allow free passage of the enema. The methods vary between hospitals. A satisfactory regimen is the following.

On the day before the test two sachets of Picolax are given: the powder from one sachet is dissolved in a little water (3 or 4 dessertspoonfuls in a glass). After 5 minutes it is diluted with cold water until the glass is half full and then stirred. It is drunk before a light breakfast (not later than 08.00 hours), e.g. an egg, one slice of white bread with honey and one cup of tea or coffee with milk and sugar if required. Within 3 hours frequent bowel movements should occur. Plenty of water should be drunk, at least a glassful every hour. The contents of the second sachet, prepared similarly, are taken not later than 16.00 hours, about 2 hours after a light lunch of grilled or poached (not fried) chicken or fish with a little white rice followed by plain yoghurt, clear jelly or junket, with milkless tea or coffee which may be sweetened. No potatoes, vegetables or fruit are allowed. For supper at 19.00–21.00 hours, clear soup or meat extract drinks may be taken. No further food is allowed until after the examination but plenty of water may be drunk. **NB**: If the patient is a diabetic the X-ray department must be notified so that a modified regime may be arranged.

In the morning the patient is taken to the X-ray department where an enema of 900–1200 ml of an emulsion of barium sulphate is administered.

The filling of the bowel is watched on the screen, and radiographs of the completed results are taken. The double contrast technique, involving the introduction of gas as well as barium, is now being used with increasing frequency. It enables small mucosal lesions to be detected which might otherwise be missed. If no obstruction is present, the enema will pass as far as the caecum.

A barium enema is used to demonstrate obstructions due to *malignant growths*, the presence of *diverticular disease, strictures,* and the great dilation found in *Hirschsprung's disease.* In *chronic ulcerative colitis* the outline of the bowel has fine irregularities.

Patients may eat and drink normally following a barium enema but may well need to lie down and rest. They should be told that their motions will be white for a while. Constipation may be a problem, sometimes requiring an aperient or enema.

Examination of faeces

Occult blood test

Small quantities of blood in the stools can be detected by this test. The patient is given or advised to have a high residue diet without any red meat for 3 days before the test and during the test period, avoiding any high dose vitamin C supplement during this time. The test now often used is FE-CULT (Gamma Biologicals, Inc.).

An outpatient is given three test envelopes with detailed, easily understood directions for their use and applicators for taking samples of stool. On three consecutive days pea-sized samples are taken from two parts of the stool and spread on to the two red-framed openings inside each test envelope. If the patient does not have a bowel movement on one day the samples are taken from the next stool. The envelopes, with identity label completed, are sent to the laboratory at the end of the test.

In the laboratory the analyst opens the back of the envelope, involving no contact with the stool, and applies at least two drops of developer solution to each stool specimen site. A blue colour at 30 seconds is a positive test. One positive test from the six is a 'positive' result.

HEMA-CHEK (Ames) is a similar test for occult blood. The occult blood test is of great value in *gastric and duodenal ulcers*, as an additional factor in diagnosis and also as a guide to whether the ulcer has healed or not. It is positive in an active ulcer and negative in a healed ulcer. It is usually continuously positive in cases of *carcinoma of the stomach* or in *growths in any other part of the alimentary tract.*

Much blood in the stools renders them black, but it should be borne in mind that black stools may be produced by the patient taking iron, bismuth or manganese.

Fat, muscle fibres, trypsin

See pancreatic function tests (p. 143).

Organisms and parasites in stools

The bulk of normal stools is made up of microorganisms. In *typhoid, paratyphoid, dysentery* and *food poisoning* the organisms carrying the disease are present in the stools. 'Carriers' have such organisms in their stools without having the disease, usually having recovered from it in the recent or distant past.

Where infection is suspected, a specimen of faeces is collected into the appropriate container for laboratory examination, with due precautions against spreading infection (e.g. on the hands or the outside of the container). Collection can be undertaken in an ordinary closet if, after micturition and flushing the pan, six pieces of newspaper are placed on the surface of the water before defecation. Faecal material floating on the paper may then be transferred to the container using a wooden spatula. *A negative culture does not exclude infection* and at least three specimens should always be submitted. If *amoebic dysentery* is a possibility and the patient is in an acute phase, a specimen of faeces containing mucus should be sent to the laboratory while still warm. This greatly increases the chances of finding amoebae. In chronic cases and where *intestinal parasites*, e.g. *schistosomes, tapeworms, roundworms* or *hookworms*, are suspected, at least three specimens should be sent to the laboratory. *Tubercle bacilli* occur in the faeces of some cases of tuberculosis. If suspected, this should be stated on the request form. The same applies to *Cryptosporidium*, which requires a special stain (modified Ziehl–Neelsen) for its demonstration. Causes of diarrhoea and dysentery include the following: *Campylobacter, Salmonella* food poisoning strains, *Shigella* (especially Sonne in the UK), *Yersinia enterocolitica* (infection can mimic acute abdomen) and *Rotavirus* which can cause acute diarrhoea in infants up to 4 years old (this and other viruses can be identified by electron microscopy where available, see p. 14). In *pseudomembranous colitis, Clostridium difficile* or its toxin may be demonstrated. The investigations for food-borne infection are described under Food poisoning (p. 128).

Threadworm infestation may be demonstrated by swabbing the anal region with a bacteriological swab and sending it to the laboratory, clearly indicating the investigation required on the request form. An alternative method is to apply the adhesive side of a portion of sellotape to the anus and then stick the sellotape to a microscope slide, which is labelled and sent with the request form.

Porphyrins

Normally the faeces contain only traces of porphyrins. In *erythropoietic porphyria* (*EP*), porphyrins are raised in the urine (see p. 172) but not in the faeces; however in *hepatoerythropoietic porphyria* (*HP*), raised isocoproporphyrin is found in the faeces as well[1]. The increased amounts of porphyrins present in porphyrias may be detected by laboratory screening, usually on urine (see p. 172).

Reference

1. Adriaans, B. Disorders of haem synthesis and the porphyrias. In: Marshall, W J and Bangert, S K, (eds). *Clinical Biochemistry: Metabolic and Clinical Aspects.* New York. Churchill Livingstone. 1995: 467–481.

CHAPTER ELEVEN

Tests related to eliminating (2)

Urinary system

Index of tests	Page		
Acidity or alkalinity of urine	161	Intravenous pyelogram (urogram) (IVP, IVU)	168
Adrenaline and catecholamines in urine	170	Inulin clearance test	167
Amino acids in urine	170	Ketones in urine	162
Amylase in urine	143	Laboratory examination of urine	163
Bacterial counts in urine	164	Labstix	162
Barbiturates in urine	170	Leukocytes in urine	164
Bence–Jones protein in urine	171	Magnesium in urine	171
Bilirubin in urine	163	Microscopical examination of urine	164
Blood in urine	162	Multitest strip	163
Blood urea	165	Parasites in urine	165
Cannabis in urine	208	Phenol red test	167
Calcium in urine	171	Phenylketonuria	163
Casts in urine	165	pH of urine	161
Catecholamines in urine	55	Porphyrins and related substances in urine	172
Chemical analysis of urine	170	Potassium in urine	172
Chloride in urine	171	Protein in urine	162, 173
Collection of urine	160	Protein selectivity	167
Colony counts	164	Pyuria	164
Clinic examination of urine	161	Radiology of the urinary tract	168
Creatine in urine	171	Red cells in urine	165
Creatinine clearance test	167	Reducing substances in urine	173
Creatinine in urine	171	Renal biopsy	167
Crystals in urine	165	Renal function tests	165
Cystine in urine	171	Retrograde pyelogram	168
Cystogram	169	Serotonin in urine	172
Cystoscopy	170	Sodium in urine	172
Cytology of urine	165	Specific gravity of urine	161
Dye excretion test	167	Steroids in urine	52
Electrolytes in urine	171	Sugar chromatography	173
Electrophoresis of urine	172	Sugar in urine	162
Glomerular damage	167	Transport outfits	164
Glomerular filtration rate	167	Tubercle bacilli in urine	164
Glutamine in urine	170	Urea clearance test	166
Glycine in urine	170	Urea in urine	173
Haematuria (blood in urine)	162	Urinalysis	160
5-hydroxyindoleacetic acid in urine	172	Urobilin in urine	173
5-hydroxytryptamine (serotonin) in urine	172	Urobilinogen in urine	163, 173
Indigo carmine test	167		

Index of tests	Page		
Volume of urine	161	Water dilution and concentration test	166
Ward examination of urine	161	White cells in urine	164

Introduction

Apart from the information it provides about other body systems, examination of the urine is a key factor in the investigation of the urinary tract. Screening is generally by means of stick tests, usually undertaken by the nurse. *The tests must be carried out on urine that is fresh, with test sticks that are not time expired.* When an abnormality has been detected or is suspected, it is confirmed by sending a specimen to the laboratory: microbiology for suspected infection; chemical pathology for an abnormal chemical substance. If neoplasia is suspected, a specimen should be sent to the cytology laboratory for the detection of abnormal cells. A useful test for renal function is blood urea estimation, for which a near patient test is available, although the creatinine clearance test is more sensitive. Radiology provides a valuable method for investigating various parts of the urinary tract, and renal biopsy is also usually performed by the radiologist. Cytoscopy enables the bladder to be examined directly and biopsies to be taken by the urogenital surgeon. When 12 or 24 hour specimens are needed, e.g. for electrolyte or porphyrin estimation by chemical pathology, accurate and complete collection over the specified period is critical. A correction can be made for deviation from the correct timing, provided the exact timing is stated on the request form. If a specimen is missed, collection should be restarted.

Urinalysis

The patient may be told that examination of the urine provides information about general body functions as well as that of the kidneys and urinary tract. Apart from checking that no medication is being taken that could affect the results, no preparation is necessary.

Collection of urine

The precautions necessary when collecting a urine specimen depend on the purpose for which it is required. The following types of specimen are collected:

- **(a)** *Urine for ward or clinic testing.* This should be a reasonably fresh specimen collected into a clean container. No special precautions are required unless the patient has a transmissible infection such as *typhoid*, *brucellosis*, etc., or is Australia antigen-positive, when the specimen container should only be handled with protective gloves and tests performed by the laboratory with appropriate precautions (see high-risk specimens, p. 12).

- **(b)** *24-hour urine collection.* The bladder is emptied and the urine discarded immediately before commencing the 24-hour collection. During the 24-hour period all urine must be collected, including any passed at the time of defecation. If a specimen is missing or spilt, the only correct thing to do is to start an entirely new 24-hour collection. At the completion of exactly 24 hours the bladder is emptied, this specimen being included in the 24-hour collection. (Appropriate large containers with the correct preservative for the urine collection are available from the laboratory.)

- (c) *12-hour urine collection*. The technique of collection is the same as for (b) but only for a period of exactly 12 hours.

- (d) Occasionally a *random sample of urine* may be used for quantitative estimation by the laboratory, in which case the report is made with respect to the creatinine concentration in the urine (excretion of creatinine is approximately constant, provided that renal function is normal).

- (e) *Routine laboratory examination of urine*. This is usually a midstream specimen of urine (MSU) collected as described on p. 163. Precautions required if the patient has a transmissible infection are referred to in (a) above. The specimen should be collected shortly before it is sent to the laboratory accompanied by an inoculated Dipspoon (Medical Wire) or Dipslide (Oxoid) if used.

- *Urine for bacterial counts*. The specimen is collected as for (e) but must be sent immediately to the laboratory, accompanied by an inoculated Dipspoon or Dipslide if used.

- *Urine for tubercle bacilli*. At least three complete consecutive early morning specimens of urine (EMU) are required (see p. 164) with the precautions for a transmissible infection, as in (a).

Ward (or clinic) examination of urine
General appearance
Note colour, turbidity and presence of blood. Smell is only rarely of value.

Volume
This may provide vital information concerning fluid balance, e.g. in relation to operations, *shock*, *dehydration*, *oedema*, *renal failure*, *diabetes*, steroid therapy, etc.

Specific gravity
This is measured by floating a urinometer in the urine (the calibrations to be checked periodically). This may give information of the kidneys' ability to concentrate or dilute urine (see also p. 166).

Stick or strip tests
These have become the urine testing methods of choice. It is important to *check that the expiry date has not passed*.

pH (acidity or alkalinity)
1. Universal test papers. These are convenient, merely requiring to be dipped into the urine and the colour compared with the colour scale provided.
2. Stick or strip tests. Protein, pH, glucose, ketone and blood may be tested for simultaneously by BM-Test-5L (Boehringer–Mannheim) or by Labstix, etc. (see pp. 162–163).

Tests for protein

1. Albustix or Uristix (Ames). The end of the test strip is dipped quickly into the urine and the colour compared with the colour scale. It is a quick test but unsuitable for very alkaline urines, for which 2 or 5 should be used.
2. Albym-Test (Boehringer–Mannheim). The strip test is as sensitive as the boiling test and is unaffected by pH in the range pH 5–9. Albumin causes the colour to change from yellow to green.
3. Multitests (see p. 163) or Labstix (see below).
4. Sulphosalicylic acid (25%) for acid urine. Here 5 ml of urine and 0.5 ml of reagent produce a white precipitate if protein is present. If urine is alkaline the boiling test should be used.
5. Boiling. Add a few drops of acetic acid to the urine in a test-tube and boil. Protein gives a white precipitate.

NB: Tolbutamide, cephalosporins and other drugs can give a false-positive test for protein.

Tests for sugar

1. Diastix is a quick preliminary test for glucose only.
2. Multitests (see p. 163) or Labstix (see below).
3. Clinitest is described on p. 145.
4. Benedict's test is described on p. 145.

Tests for ketones

1. Acetest (p. 145) and Ketostix (Ames p. 144). These will detect both acetone and acetoacetic acid in urine.
2. Ketur-Test (Boehringer–Mannheim). This strip test gives a violet colour with acetoacetic acid and acetone (to be distinguished from an orange red colour with phenylketones).
3. BM multitest strip (see p. 163) or Labstix (see below).

NB: *Monitoring the urine for ketones is very important in the management of both juvenile and maturity-onset diabetics,* especially if infection or other illness develops. Salicylates and other drugs can give a false-positive test for ketones.

Tests for blood

1. Haemastix (Ames). The end of the test strip is dipped briefly into the urine and after 30 seconds compared with the colour chart provided.
2. Sangur-Test (Boehringer–Mannheim). This strip test is similar. It is extremely sensitive to blood in urine and is specific for haemoglobin and myoglobin.
3. Multitest (see p. 163) or Labstix (see below).

Labstix (Ames)

This reagent strip tests simultaneously for acidity (pH), protein, glucose, ketones and blood. The test area of the strip is dipped into fresh, clean urine (free from antiseptics, detergents or acid). It is immediately withdrawn and the edge tapped against the side of the container to remove excess urine. The colours of the test areas are then compared with the corresponding colour charts at the times specified: immediately, 10 seconds, 15 seconds and 30 seconds. Any abnormal result should be checked by sending the urine to the laboratory.

NB: *This test does not detect bilirubin* (see tests for bilirubin, below), *nor does it detect galactose or other reducing substances. These must be tested for in young children* (see Clinitest or Benedict's test, p. 145, and sugar chromatography, p. 173).

Tests for bilirubin

1. Bilur-Test (Boehringer–Mannheim). This is a single test strip for bilirubin. Its presence indicates obstructive jaundice (see pp. 139–140).
2. Bililabstix. This test is the same as Labstix (p. 162) but also includes a test area for bilirubin.

Tests for urobilinogen

1. Ugen-Test (Boehringer–Mannheim). This is a single test strip for estimating urobilinogen.
2. Multistix (Ames). This has all the test areas of Bililabstix (see above) and in addition a test for urobilinogen.

BM multitest strip (Boehringer–Mannheim)

In addition to test areas previously mentioned, viz. pH, protein, glucose, ketones, blood, bilirubin and urobilinogen, this also has test areas for leukocytes and nitrites. Leukocytes are an indication of inflammatory change in the urinary tract (see p. 164). Nitrites are an indication that pathogenic bacteria are present in the urine (only significant if the urine is freshly voided).

Test for phenylketonuria

Phenistix will detect the presence and concentration of phenylketone (phenylpyruvic acid) in urine. The test end is dipped into the urine and removed, or moistened against a wet napkin. After half a minute the colour is compared with the chart on the Phenistix bottle. In 2–4-week-old infants the urine phenylketone level should be below 0.5 mmol/litre (8 mg/100 ml). To avoid false-negative results the test paper must not be dropped into the urine and left there, nor pressed too firmly or too long against a wet napkin, nor be placed in the napkin while it is on the baby. This test was previously performed routinely on all babies but has been replaced by the blood phenylalanine test (phenylketonuria, p. 193).

Results should be checked by sending a blood specimen to the laboratory for phenylalanine estimation. Any abnormality should be noted on the request form.

Routine examination of urine in the microbiology laboratory

In addition to the tests described above, the urine is allowed to sediment and the deposit examined microscopically. The deposit is composed of the heavier elements such as cells, casts, bacteria and crystals. The urine may also be cultured to determine the type of bacteria present. Colony counts (see below) are now a routine procedure. If there is evidence of infection (pus cells more than 5/hpf in urine deposit) the bacteria are tested for their sensitivity to the different antibiotics.

For this investigation a midstream sample of urine (MSU), collected into a sterile container after the urethral orifice has been carefully cleansed, is usually found to be satisfactory in both males and females. The first portion of urine passed should be discarded and only the middle portion collected for sending to the laboratory. Catheterization has long been considered the only satisfactory method of obtaining a suitable sample of urine (CSU) from females. Catheterization, however, carries with it the danger of introducing infection. With care it is usually possible to obtain a suitable non-catheter specimen of urine even from females. This should be routine practice whenever feasible. Catheterization should be reserved for selected cases where adequate information cannot otherwise be obtained (see white cells below).

Urine for bacterial counts (colony counts)

To detect cases of *hidden urinary infection, e.g. pyelonephritis*, increasing use is being made of bacterial counts. The urine specimen must be transferred to the laboratory immediately or else placed in the refrigerator prior to transfer on the same day. If immediate refrigeration is impracticable, special containers with collection medium can be used (see transport outfits, below). According to Kass, under 10 000 organisms/ml indicates absence of infection; 10 000–100 000 organisms/ml is doubtful; and over 100 000 organisms/ml in three consecutive urine specimens indicates definite infection.

Transport outfits

In an effort to improve the accuracy and reliability of bacteriological results of urine testing and to eliminate, as far as possible, the problems created by multiplication of contaminating organisms while in transit, many laboratories now offer dip inoculum transport outfits, e.g. Dipspoons or Dipslides. The spoon/slide is dipped into the urine and then returned to its container and transported to the laboratory together with the urine sample. The outfit is incubated overnight and colonies are counted so that an interpretation of any growth can be assessed. Counts of over 105/ml are usually regarded as significant and counts below 104/ml are usually due to contamination.

An alternative transport method is the use of universal containers with boric acid. These are obtainable from the microbiology laboratory.

Urine for tubercle bacilli

When *tuberculous infection* of the urinary tract is suspected, at least three complete consecutive early morning specimens of urine should be sent to the laboratory. The urine should be passed in a normal manner into a clean container. The *tubercle bacilli* are isolated by culture on special media. Normally this takes 4–6 weeks.

Microscopical examination of urine
Interpretation of findings in deposit
White cells (leukocytes)

Occasional white cells are normally of no significance. When present in sufficient numbers to suggest infection (such as five or more per high power field) they are usually reported as 'pus cells'. If in addition to pus cells, a reasonably pure culture of *Escherichia coli* is isolated, the findings indicate an *E. coli* urinary infection. Organisms grown from urine in the absence of pus cells are usually contaminants, except in the very debilitated (when catheterization may be necessary to exclude contamination). A mixed growth of organisms also suggests the possibility of contamination. The finding of pus cells without a causative organism is called 'sterile pyuria'. It occurs for a short time after any urinary infection has been treated. In *nephritis*, too, pus cells are seen, usually in small numbers, but casts are also present. Sterile pyuria occurs in tuberculosis of the urinary tract (see above), but it also occurs in about 50% of healthy young females for various minor causes.

Red cells

The presence of blood in the urine is known as haematuria. It may be due to *injury, stones, infection* or *a growth*, affecting any part of the urinary tract. *Nephritis* is also an important cause of haematuria. A few red cells may be found in normal urine, especially following catheterization. A non-catheter specimen collected during menstruation may contain red cells as contaminants.

Casts

These are microscopic structures with parallel sides somewhat resembling elongated sausages. They result from semisolid material taking on the shape (i.e. forming a cast) of the kidney tubule while passing through. An occasional hyaline (glass-like) cast may be present in urine of normal people. The number of these hyaline casts increases in states of *dehydration*, e.g. *diabetic coma*. In *nephritis* a number of granular, cellular and hyaline casts are seen which incorporate elements of damaged renal tubules, together with a variable number of white cells and often some red cells.

Epithelial cells

These are found in normal urines, usually due to vaginal contamination, and also after catheterization with inadequate lubrication.

Parasites

These may be found in the urine in certain tropical diseases, e.g. *schistosomiasis* (*bilharziasis*).

Crystals

Crystals of various salts, e.g. urates and phosphates, are frequently seen and usually reflect the reaction of the urine and the previous diet, e.g. oxalates following strawberries and rhubarb. Cooling is also a factor. Most crystals are of little significance.

Urine cytology

Freshly voided urine should be sent at once to the cytology laboratory. If this is not possible it should be immediately preserved by the addition of 50% alcohol. It is a sensitive method of detecting cancer cells of the urinary tract. It may also be used to detect the abnormal cells of inclusion body disease.

Renal function tests

Renal function tests only demonstrate gross disease, and more than half of the kidney substance has to be destroyed before inefficiency is evident. The creatinine clearance test is now the generally preferred test.

Blood urea

Urea is the main end product of protein breakdown. If renal function is sufficiently impaired for the blood urea to rise above the normal level of 2.5–7.5 mmol/litre (15–45 mg/100 ml), the condition is called *uraemia*.

1. Laboratory estimation. About 2 ml of clotted blood is sent to chemical pathology (clinical biochemistry) laboratory.
2. Azostix (Ames). A large drop of capillary or venous blood is freely applied over the entire reagent area of the printed side of the strip. After exactly 60 seconds the blood is quickly washed off with a sharp stream of water. Comparison of the colour with the chart provided gives a measure of the blood urea. Any abnormal result is checked by laboratory estimation.

3. Blood urea and BUN (Blood urea nitrogen). This may also be estimated in a clinic or sideroom using an instrument such as Reflotron® (Boehringer–Mannheim).

In *uraemia* the blood urea may be raised considerably, to 33 mmol/litre (200 mg/100 ml), 50 mmol/litre (300 mg/100 ml) or even 100 mmol/litre (600 mg/100 ml). If over 50 mmol/-litre (300 mg/100 ml) the case is often fatal, though not necessarily so. In surgical cases the estimation is of value in considering the question of operation on the genitourinary system, e.g. prostate cases and renal cases. About 8 mmol/litre (48 mg/100 ml) or more in a patient with *hypertrophy of the prostate* may indicate the advisability of the operation being done in two stages. The blood urea also rises considerably in cases of:

- *Gastrointestinal lesions* with obstruction or haemorrhage
- *Severe shock*, especially following crushing injuries, burns and obstetrical conditions, e.g. eclampsia.

Water dilution and concentration test

On the first day, the patient, after passing urine, drinks 1.8 litres of water within half an hour. Urine is passed at half-hourly intervals for the next 4 hours, and the volume and specific gravity of each specimen is measured. Normally the 1.8 litres are excreted within the 4 hours and the specific gravity falls to 1002 or less.

On the second day the fluid intake is limited to 600 ml for the 24 hours. Foodstuffs with a high water content should be avoided, e.g. fruit. Urine may be passed whenever the patient desires, each specimen being collected separately, and the volume and specific gravity measured.

Normally the urine volume does not exceed 900 ml for the second 24 hours and the specific gravity reaches at least 1027.

In *renal insufficiency* the volume on the first day is too little, and on the second day too great, and the specific gravity remains in the region of 1010 for both days.

Urea clearance test

There is a great reserve of kidney tissue. Tests of renal function, such as the urea concentration test, indicate extensive kidney damage. The urea clearance test indicates roughly the amount of healthy functioning tissue remaining in the presence of renal disease. The results are read as the percentage of available functioning renal tissue; 80–100% is a normal reading. Percentages lower than this indicate damage to the functioning kidneys, decreasing to 10% where the tissue remaining is insufficient, and the patient is in a state of *uraemia*.

The test is carried out in the following manner.

The patient has a normal breakfast, but without coffee or tea. Between breakfast and the midday meal:

1. Completely empty the bladder and note the exact time. Discard this specimen.
2. The patient drinks a glass of water.
3. A specimen of blood for urea estimation is taken immediately.
4. One hour after emptying the bladder, empty the bladder again. Label this 'specimen 1' and on it note the exact time interval from 1 above.
5. One hour later, take another specimen of urine, label this 'specimen 2' and on it note the exact time interval from 4 above.

6. Send the two urine specimens and the blood to the laboratory.

It is important that the bladder be completely emptied on each occasion. The time of collection of the specimens must be accurately measured in minutes, and recorded on the label, e.g. 1st, 1 hour and 3 minutes; 2nd, 58 minutes.

Creatinine clearance test

This is a renal efficiency test. It is more sensitive to impairment of renal function than the blood urea, and easier to perform than any of the other renal function tests. All that is required is a 24-hour urine collection (see p. 160) and 10 ml of clotted blood taken at some time during the 24 hours. It is expressed as the volume of blood cleared of creatinine in 1 minute, and is approximately equal to the *glomerular filtration rate* (GFR). Normally this is 70–140 ml/minute. It is related to the body area and so the result has to be multiplied by a correction factor for children and fat people. The normal body area is taken to be 1.73 m^2. The patient's body area (a) can be estimated from height and weight tables. The correction factor is then (a ÷ 1.73). In severe renal failure the creatinine clearance or GFR may fall to 5 ml/minute.

Glomerular filtration rate

A more accurate method of measuring the glomerular filtration rate (see above) is by intravenous injection of radioactive chromium (^{51}Cr). A 10 ml sample of blood is collected 1 hour before the injection, and at 2, 3 and 4 hours after the injection. See 'Radioisotopes' (p. 22) for the usual precautions. The patient should be told to empty the bladder frequently. ^{51}Cr has a biological half life of about 4 hours. The test is comparable with the inulin clearance test; this is seldom used clinically.[1]

Dye excretion test

About 10 ml of 0.4% solution of indigo carmine are injected intravenously, and the time observed before the appearance of the dye in the bladder. Normally it should appear in about 5–10 minutes, and excretion should be complete in about 12 hours. If the dye does not appear within 20 minutes or excretion is prolonged beyond 15 hours, the kidney is inefficient.

The time of appearance may be observed through a cystoscope (see cystoscopy, p. 170). Similar tests may be done with other dyes, e.g. phenol red.

Protein selectivity

This is a test of glomerular damage as in *acute nephritis*. Two proteins of different molecular size, e.g. transferrin (90 000) and IgG (160 000), are estimated in serum and urine. The clearance for the larger molecule should be significantly less than for the smaller molecule. If not, the prognosis for recovery by steroid therapy is poor.

Renal biopsy

Renal biopsy is used to elucidate the nature of kidney disease when the diagnosis cannot be made by the usual methods, provided the patient has two functioning kidneys and there is no bleeding disorder or kidney infection.

Puncture biopsy allows kidney tissue to be obtained for microscopy without open operation. Informed written consent is required (see p. 2). A preliminary pyelogram (see IVU/IVP, below) establishes the position of the kidneys. The patient lies in the prone position with a sandbag under the abdomen. The bony landmarks are marked out, also the measurements obtained from the pyelogram. The sterile trolley includes sterile towels, swabs, skin cleansing lotions, local anaesthetic, syringe and needles, together with the renal puncture needle (e.g. Trucut needle or Bard Biopty gun, see p. 4) and a fine exploratory needle. The biopsy specimen is collected into fixative (e.g. neutral formol saline) and sent for histology. The patient is kept in the prone position for 30 minutes to maintain pressure on the kidney and minimize bleeding, and confined to bed for 24 hours, blood pressure and pulse rate being recorded frequently and all urine examined for blood staining. Any backache, shoulder pain or dysuria should be reported to the doctor.

Radiology of the urinary tract (all the tests require informed written consent, see p. 2)

Radiograph of abdomen

A plain X-ray of abdomen (p. 137) provides soft tissue shadows of the kidneys and renal tract. It reveals calculi and foci of calcification very clearly, but renal cysts and tumours are much more readily demonstrated by kidney ultrasound (p. 169).

Intravenous urography (IVU)

This is also called intravenous pyelography, IVP. When a suitable contrast medium is injected intravenously it is excreted by functioning kidneys, rendering the urinary tract opaque to X- rays. Since the medium contains iodine it is important to exclude iodine sensitivity before arranging the test. If the patient is iodine-sensitive or is pregnant, a kidney sonogram should be used instead (see p. 169).

The night before the examination the patient should be given liquid extract of cascara, and the following morning a high enema about an hour or so before the examination. This procedure eliminates gas in the intestines which interferes with the definition of the radiograph. In addition, fluids are not given for some hours prior to the examination (to render the urine more concentrated). For outpatients it is advisable for laxatives to be taken for 2 days before the examination. On the day of the test, if it is a morning appointment no breakfast should be taken, not even a cup of tea: if it is an afternoon appointment a light breakfast should be taken at 08.00 hours consisting of only one cup of tea or coffee and two pieces of toast (with butter and jam if desired), but no lunch. The bladder is emptied just before the commencement. A contrast medium, e.g. 15–40 ml of sodium diatrizoate (45% w/v) is injected intravenously and films are taken after 5 minutes, 10 minutes, and 20 minutes.

When the urinary tract is obstructed, delayed films may be required, possibly on the following day, as the obstructed kidney only excretes slowly. The test can be used in *acute* or *chronic renal failure* but the patient should not be dehydrated beforehand and high doses of contrast medium may be required.

The IVU is a valuable *test of kidney function*. It also demonstrates *hydronephrosis, hypernephroma, calculi*, etc.

Retrograde pyelogram

The preparation of the patient is similar to that for an intravenous pyelogram but without restriction of fluids.

A cystoscope is passed, and a ureteric catheter inserted into each ureter. A solution of Hypaque is then injected up each ureteric catheter. The quantity that the renal pelvis will hold varies according to the condition present, and the injection is stopped when the patient complains of a pain in the loin. Sodium iodide is opaque to X-rays and when a film is taken the ureter, renal pelvis and calyces will be shown. This procedure is useful for demonstrating *calculi, hydronephrosis, hypernephroma,* etc.

Cystogram

This usually forms part of the IVU/IVP (see p. 168), as the contrast medium is collected in the bladder, providing an outline of the organ on a radiograph. More controlled bladder filling is obtained using a catheter, retrograde cystography. This can be of particular value to see whether there is fluid reflux up the ureters during micturition (micturating cystogram), which may be an important factor in producing recurrent *pyelonephritis.*

An outpatient attending for a micturating cystogram should follow the regime recommended for intravenous urography (p. 168) and, in addition, go to the appropriate ward for insertion of a catheter before the test.

Kidney ultrasound (sonogram)

Ultrasound (see p. 20) provides a much clearer picture of the kidneys than straight X-rays. It also obviates irradiation, which is of importance if the patient is pregnant and, unlike an intravenous pyelogram, it can be used when the patient has *renal failure* or hypersensitivity to iodine (present in the contrast medium used for an IVP). A kidney ultrasound demonstrates *cysts, tumours, hydronephrosis* and *calculi.* It is also of value in guiding a percutaneous needle for the aspiration of cysts or obtaining a biopsy from a *renal tumour.* No fasting or fluid restriction is required, but gas or barium in the alimentary tract impairs the clarity of the ultrasound picture.[2]

Kidney scan

Radioisotopes (see p. 22) may be used to study the structure, blood circulation and excretory function of the kidneys. A scan is of value in demonstrating *infarction, renal arteriosclerosis,* a tumour and evidence of *rejection or trauma.* It should not be arranged within 24 hours of having an IVU. The patient should drink 2–3 glasses of water and empty the bladder before the test. Otherwise no preparation is required, but the patient must give informed consent (see p.2) after being reassured that only tracer doses of radioisotope are used, excreted from the body within 6–24 hours of the test. The radioisotope is given by simple intravenous injection at the beginning of the test. A perfusion study is completed in about 20 minutes and functional scans in less than an hour, but structural scans may take 30 minutes to 4 hours.[3]

Renal angiography

This involves injecting radioopaque material, usually by passing an angiocatheter into the femoral artery and thence up the aorta so that the injected material enters the renal arteries. This is of value in delineating vascular abnormalities, e.g. demonstrating the exact site of arteriosclerotic narrowing of a renal artery prior to surgical intervention. The patient should be tested for iodine sensitivity and the radiologist notified if sensitivity is suspected. A laxative may be required, so that the X-ray picture is not obscured by gut contents. Nothing should be taken by mouth after midnight preceding the test. The patient must be told the nature of the procedure and warned that when the dye is injected a warm flush will be felt and also that bladder distension may cause some discomfort; written consent must be obtained (see p. 2). Prior to the test, the groin is prepared to provide sterility of the arterial puncture site. Following the test, the patient's TPR (temperature, pulse and respiration) should be recorded at regular intervals, the arterial puncture site checked for haemorrhage or inflammation, and the legs checked for evidence of *ischaemia*.[4]

Cystoscopy

By means of a cystoscope it is possible to examine the inside of a patient's bladder, take tissue biopsies to diagnose *tumours* and *schistosomiasis*, and treat such lesions with diathermy. Informed written consent is required (see p. 2).

The cystoscope consists of a hollow tube, like a small telescope with a light attached. Prior to the examination a sedative is given. The procedure is carried out in the theatre but usually without a general anaesthetic. Local anaesthetic is introduced into the urethra prior to the passage of the cystoscope.

In addition to examining the bladder wall for the presence of tumour or inflammation, cystoscopy enables the ureteric orifices to be seen, and if necessary ureteric catheters to be introduced. Careful sterilization of the cystoscope is important.

Excreted substances

Chemical analysis of urine
Adrenaline and like substances
See catecholamines, p. 55.

Alcohol
See p. 208.

Amino acids
Normally relatively small amounts of certain amino acids (e.g. glycine and glutamine) are present in the urine. Abnormal amounts and types of amino acid appear in the urine in *liver failure* and in a number of *congenital metabolic diseases*.

1. Total amino acid nitrogen. Urine normally contains 100–400 mg per 24 hours (as estimated by the formol method). This is greatly increased in the conditions mentioned. For this test an exact 24-hour specimen of urine is required (see p. 160), collected into brown bottles containing preservative.

2. Chromatography. Three separate specimens of midstream urine (MSU, p. 163 (e)) are required, each collected into a universal container. Chromatography identifies the individual amino acids and the approximate amount of each. Usually 6–10 amino acids are present, glycine predominating.

3. Cystine. A screening test will detect *cystinuria*, a congenital disorder with excess cystine in the urine. The normal excretion is 0.1–0.4 mmol/24 hours.

Amylase
See p. 143.

Barbiturates
About 100 ml of urine is usually required. It is a useful screening test for suspected poisoning but blood levels are more satisfactory if available (see p. 206).

Bence–Jones protein

In the diseases of *multiple myeloma* and *secondary carcinoma of bone*, an abnormal protein appears in the urine, where it can be detected 2–3 years before blood or bone changes are found. A 24-hour specimen is required (see p. 160).

Calcium and magnesium

On an average diet 2.5–7.5 mmol (100–300 mg) of calcium are excreted in the urine daily. Nearly three times as much is excreted in the faeces. Excretion is greatly increased on a diet rich in milk and cheese. Diseases causing an increased excretion, e.g. 7.5–15 mmol/24 hours, are *hyperparathyroidism, hyperthyroidism* and *multiple myeloma*. Urine calcium is low in *rickets* and *defective intestinal absorption*. A complete 24-hour specimen of urine is required for the estimation, collected into a container provided by the laboratory (see p. 160). Magnesium, normally 7–11 mmol/24 hours (168–268 mg/24 hours), may be estimated on the same specimen. *Renal calculi* may be associated with raised calcium or magnesium levels.

Cannabis

See p. 208.

Catecholamines

See p. 55.

Creatine

This test is seldom used. Normally there is little, if any, creatine in adult urine.

Creatinine

The normal daily excretion of creatinine is about 10 mmol (1 g) for women and 20 mmol (2 g) for men. Its excretion is very constant from day to day for a given individual. This constancy provides a check that 24-hour urine collection is complete when a series of such samples is required for chemical or microbiological assay. The creatinine clearance test is described on p. 167.

Cystine

The presence of an increased amount of the amino acid cystine in the urine is characteristic of *cystinuria*, one of the congenital metabolic diseases (see amino acids, p. 170).

Electrolytes (chloride, sodium and potassium)

To estimate daily electrolyte excretion a complete 24-hour urine collection is required (see p. 160). Chloride, sodium and potassium may be estimated on the same specimen. The amount of each excreted is normally just sufficient to keep the blood level within normal limits.

Chloride

A normal adult excretes 120–250 mmol (7–15 g) (expressed as sodium chloride, NaCl) daily in the urine. This is reduced or absent in *salt depletion* and also in *salt retention with oedema*. Depletion occurs in excessive *sweating, vomiting* or *diarrhoea*. Retention occurs in *renal or cardiac failure* and in *excessive steroid therapy*. For chloride estimation a specimen of urine should be sent to the laboratory. To estimate daily excretion, a complete 24-hour specimen of urine is required (see p. 160).

An approximate estimate, only to be used when laboratory facilities are not available, is by the method of Fantus: 10 drops of urine are placed in a test tube; 1 drop of 20% potassium dichromate is added; 2.9% silver nitrate is added drop by drop. The number of drops needed to give a brick-red precipitate gives the number of grams of sodium chloride per litre (g/NaCl/l) of urine. The pipette must be washed out with distilled water between each stage. In view of its doubtful reliability, this test is almost obsolete.

Sodium
Normally 130–220 mmol (3–5 g) are excreted daily. This is reduced in sodium retention, which is usually associated with chloride retention (see above). In *Addison's disease* sodium continues to be excreted in spite of a low blood level. This can be controlled by steroid therapy.

Potassium
Excretion varies with diet. Usually it is 25–100 mmol (1–4 g) daily. In *Addison's disease* there is diminished excretion in spite of a high blood level. Steroid therapy increases potassium excretion so that the blood level is lowered.

Electrophoresis
An early morning specimen of urine is usually required. The test is useful for identifying abnormal proteins, e.g. *myeloma* protein.

5-hydroxyindoleacetic acid and 5-hydroxytryptamine (serotonin)
These substances are increased in the urine of many patients with *carcinoid tumours*. Normal urine contains about 100 mg/litre of each (10–47 μmol/24h) and the screening test may detect none or a trace only. Urine is collected as for catecholamine estimation (p. 155).

NB: Any drugs taken must be noted on the request form.

Porphyrins and related substances
Porphyrins are formed during the biosynthesis of haemoglobin; 50–250 mg are excreted in the urine daily. This amount is too small to be detected by the screening test. Increased excretion occurs in *haemolytic anaemias, polycythaemia, liver diseases, fevers* and as a result of some *drugs* and *poisons* (e.g. *lead*). There is also a group of diseases with a hereditary factor known as the *porphyrias* in which there is increased excretion of porphyrins and related substances. Normally a 24-hour urine contains only traces of these: coproporphyrin <240 nmol (<240 mg), uroporphyrin <30 nmol (<30 mg), porphobilinogen (PBG) <45 mmol (<2 mg), g-amino laevulinic acid (ALA) <15 mmol (<7 mg) and delta-aminolevulinate 8–53 μmol/24 hours. In *acute porphyria* the excretion of PBG and ALA is usually increased. A negative urine test for PBG virtually excludes *porphyria*; if the test is positive, *lead poisoning* must be excluded before *porphyria* can be diagnosed.[5] For accurate estimation of porphyrins, etc., a complete 24-hour collection of urine is required (see p. 160), preferably on several successive days. Examination of a single fresh specimen can be of value as a rough guide.

The following points should be noted when investigating suspected *porphyria*:

• Tests are negative before puberty in children who will later develop *porphyria*.

• Screening tests on urine are negative during the latent phases of intermittent *porphyria*.

- Faecal porphyrin estimation should also be done (see p. 157).
- Positive tests must be confirmed by quantitative analysis and typing of the porphyrins.

Proteins

The routine ward tests for protein in urine are given on p. 162. These give a rough guide.

For a more accurate estimation, a complete 24-hour collection of urine should be sent to the laboratory (see p. 160). Normally the total protein excretion is <0.2 g/24 hours, of which albumin is <30 mg/24 hours. Other tests for protein are electrophoresis (see above) and the test for Bence–Jones protein (p. 171).

Reducing substances

Tests for reducing substances are Clinitest, p. 145 and Benedict's, p. 145. The nature of a reducing substance is determined in the laboratory by chromatography (see below) and other methods.

Steroids

See urine tests for steroids, p. 52.

Sugar chromatography

This is a method of separating and identifying sugars present in the urine. Thus it will distinguish between lactose (associated with lactation) and glucose even if both are present. A fresh early morning specimen is required.

Urea

Urine urea estimation is usually part of a renal function test, e.g. urea clearance test (p. 166). Estimations may occasionally be made on single specimens. A high concentration of urea indicates that the kidney has good concentrating power and is evidence that renal failure is not present. The average concentration of urea over the day is about 2%, and the total daily excretion about 30 g. With normal kidney function it is a measure of the breakdown of protein from both food and body.

Urobilin and urobilinogen

The bile pigment bilirubin is altered in the intestine to urobilinogen. Some of this is reabsorbed and then excreted by the kidney, the urobilinogen gradually changing into urobilin. The urobilin and urobilinogen in urine, normally 2–5 mg/24 hours (1.7–5.9 μmol/24 hours), are increased in *haemolytic jaundice*, up to 10 mg daily, and reduced in *simple obstructive jaundice*, usually to less than 0.3 mg daily. A fresh sample of urine in a universal container is sufficient for a rough guide (see also p. 138). For accurate estimation a complete 24-hour specimen of urine (see p. 160) is collected into a brown bottle containing appropriate preservative obtainable from the laboratory.

References

1. Marshall, W J. The kidneys, renal function and renal failure. In: Marshall, W J and Bangert, S K, (eds). *Clinical biochemistry: Metabolic and Clinical Aspects*. New York. Churchill Livingstone. 1995: 117–142.

2. Pagana, K D and Pagana, T J. Kidney sonogram. In: Pagana, K D and Pagana, T J, (eds). *Mosby's Diagnostic and Laboratory Test Reference*. St Louis. Mosby Year Book. 1992: 446–447.

3. Pagana, K D and Pagana, T J. Renal scanning. In: Pagana, K D and Pagana, T J, (eds). *Mosby's Diagnostic and Test Reference*. St Louis. Mosby Year Book. 1992: 634–637.

4. Pagana, K D and Pagana, T J. Renal angiography. In: Pagana, K D and Pagana, T J, (eds). *Mosby's Diagnostic and Test Reference*. St Louis. Mosby Year Book. 1992: 627–630.

5. Adriaans, B. Disorders of haem synthesis and the porphyrias. In: Marshall, W J and Bangert, S K, (eds). *Clinical Biochemistry: Metabolic and Clinical Aspects*. New York. Churchill Livingstone. 1995: 467–481.

CHAPTER TWELVE

Tests related to mobilizing

Index of tests	Page
Angiography	176
Arthritis	176
Arthrogram	176
Arthroscopy	178
Bone biopsy	179
Bone cysts	176
Bone growths	177
Bone scans	176
Cardiothoracic patient tests	179
Cineradiography	176
Computerized tomography (CT) scan	176
Dislocations	177
Fractures	177
Goniometry	178
Intensive care, tests used in	179
Joint fluid examination	178
Lower motor neurone disease, tests used in	180
Musculoskeletal disorders, tests for	179
Nervous system lesions	177
Osteomyelitis	177
Periostitis	177
Physiotherapy assessment	179
Rickets	177
Rheumatoid disease, tests used in	180
Scurvy	177
Skull lesions	177
Subluxations	177
Tenogram	178
Tuberculosis of bones and joints	178

Introduction

The use of radiology or other imaging techniques is an essential part of the investigation of many diseases of bone and joint. Bone biopsy may be required for a diagnosis to be reached, performed by the orthopaedic surgeon and interpreted by the histopathologist. Physiotherapy, for which assessment is essential, provides the road to recovery in many medical and surgical conditions.

Skeletal system

X-ray and MRI examination of bone joints and tendons

The following methods of examination are used:

- Straight radiograph.

- Arthrogram. This is the injection of radioopaque material or air into a joint to outline the joint cavity on the X-ray.

- Bone scans (see radioisotopes, p. 22). These are used mainly for detecting *secondary tumours*, but they are also much more sensitive than X-rays at detecting *small fractures*, especially in ribs, spine, facial bones and the small bones of hands and feet.[1]

- Cineradiography. A cinefilm of the X-ray appearance of the joint in movement provides accurate information concerning its function. Tendon function may similarly be studied (see tenogram, p. 178).

- Computerized tomography (CT) scan. Usually no preparation of the patient is required before a CT scan of bones, joints and soft tissue (see p. 21). It is often of particular value in the total assessment of *spinal lesions*. It can also provide high resolution images of joints and *soft tissues, e.g. cruciate ligaments of knee*. With *complex fractures*, three-dimensional imaging provides an additional method of assessment. Three-dimensional measurements of the *bone density of the lumbar spine* can be made using quantitative CT, but it is less precise, more expensive and involves a higher radiation dose than DXA[2] (below).

- DXA (dual energy X-ray absorptiometry) involves exposure to only low doses of X-rays and permits bone density measurements of sites such as lumbar spine and proximal femur for the diagnosis of *osteoporosis*.[2]

- Single photon absorptiometry has similar advantages to DXA with less expensive equipment, but bone density measurements for detecting *osteoporosis* are limited to sites such as the distal forearm or calcaneum.[2]

- Quantitative ultrasound measurement of bone density for detecting *osteoporosis* is being developed[a].

- Magnetic resonance imaging (MRI). Lesions of soft tissues, including spinal cord and brain, may be more clearly demonstrated by MRI than by X-ray (see pp. 21, 38).

- Angiography is sometimes used to investigate problems of mobility, particularly if there is an abnormality of the blood vessels (see p. 83).

Conditions which may be demonstrated

Bone cysts

Bone cysts are readily visible on X-ray but often require biopsy in order to be distinguished from certain other lesions, e.g. *eosinophilic granuloma* of bone.

Arthritis

This can be both acute and chronic. In *acute arthritis* the bones will be decalcified. In *chronic arthritis* the erosion of bone and new formation of bone is seen. Ankylosis of the joint may be demonstrated.

Dislocations and subluxations
The abnormal position of the bone is seen. After the *dislocation* has been reduced, an X-ray will confirm the fact that the position is now correct.

Fractures
An X-ray will demonstrate a *fracture*, and also its type, e.g. *comminuted, greenstick, impacted, spiral,* etc. Skill is required to place the part in such a position that the *fracture* will be visible, e.g. head of radius, scaphoid, etc. After a *fracture* has been reduced, a further X-ray will show whether or not the position is satisfactory. Subsequently, an X-ray will show whether or not the *fracture* is united.

In a compound *fracture* with delayed healing due to infection, an X-ray may show the presence of a sequestrum. An X-ray can also reveal that a *fracture* has occurred at the site of a secondary growth, the presence of which was not previously recognized. This is known as a *pathological fracture. Complex fractures* may require a CT scan (see p. 21).

NB: It is most important that all cases of injury where there is any possibility of a *fracture* should have an X-ray examination.

Bone growths
Bone growths are visible on X-ray examination. They may be benign or malignant. A *benign growth* may be a *chondroma, osteoma,* etc. *Malignant growths* may be *primary,* e.g. *osteosarcoma,* or *secondary,* e.g. a *secondary growth in the femur from carcinoma of the breast.*

Osteomyelitis
In *acute osteomyelitis* some days must elapse after the onset of the disease before changes are visible on X-ray examination. In *chronic osteomyelitis,* a sequestrum is often visible or a Brodie's abscess may be seen.

Periostitis
Periostitis is visible on X-ray examination after the condition is well established.

Rickets
The changes of rickets are well shown on X-ray examination. Evidence is often obtained from the lower end of the radius.

Scurvy
In this condition haemorrhage occurs under the periosteum of bones in the neighbourhood of joints. This is visible in X-ray examination. The epiphyseal line is irregular.

Skull lesions
Most fractures of the skull are visible on X-ray examination. Bony conditions giving rise to *Jacksonian fits* may be demonstrable. An enlarged pituitary fossa is suggestive of a *pituitary tumour,* or *chronic raised intracranial pressure.*

Lesions of the nervous system
Brain, spinal cord and nerve lesions often cause problems of mobility, e.g. nerve and cord compression, which may be readily identified by CT and MRI and occasionally by angiography.

Tuberculosis of bones and joints

These conditions may be diagnosed by the X-ray picture. The course of the disease is verified by X-ray examinations at various stages of the illness. The formation of *abscesses, necrotic bone,* and the ultimate *bony ankylosis* are all demonstrable.

Osteoporosis

This condition, which particularly affects elderly females and is now treatable, can be diagnosed by DXA (dual energy X-ray absorptiometry), single photon absorptiometry or CT scan (see p. 176).

Other bone diseases

Various bone diseases show diagnostic changes on X-ray examination. Among these may be mentioned *achondroplasia, fibrocystic disease, fragilitas ossium, Paget's disease, Perthe's disease* and *osteomalacia.*

Measurements of female pelvis

See p. 189.

Other tests related to joints and bones

Tenogram

Injections of radioopaque material into a tendon sheath enables the tendon and its sheath to be clearly visualized on X-ray, and its function studied by cineradiography.

Goniometry

The angle of mobility of a joint is measured by means of a goniometer. This enables small changes in the amount of movement in an arthritic joint to be measured.

Joint fluid examination (arthrocentesis)

Fluid from a joint effusion may be aspirated with a needle and syringe after the overlying skin has been cleaned with a skin antiseptic. Part of the aspirated fluid should be placed in a sterile container for bacteriological culture and part sent for cytological examination. Cytoanalysis of the fluid often assists in determining the type of arthritis present, e.g. pus cells in *septic arthritis.* Culture enables the causative organism in *septic arthritis* to be identified.

Arthroscopy

This is an endoscopic examination of the structure of a joint by means of an arthroscope, usually performed under general anaesthesia. It is used in the diagnosis of joint disease, both directly from its endoscopic appearance and indirectly by collecting tissue for histological examination. It is also used in treatment, as in the removal of loose bodies ('joint mice').

The patient is usually admitted to hospital the day before the arthroscopy. Pulse, temperature and respiration are recorded, also weight and urinalysis findings. Preliminary investigations include: medical examination, preinvestigation physiotherapy assessment, X-rays of affected joint (usually knee), and full blood count. Written consent for the test must be obtained (see p. 2) and the affected limb must be marked by a doctor. No food or drink is allowed for 4–6 hours before the test.

Preparation and premedication are as for general anaesthesia. Arthroscopy is performed with full asepsis. A tourniquet is applied to the thigh. The cannula of the arthroscope is introduced through an incision below the patella. Viewing is facilitated by irrigating the joint with physiological saline. Biopsy forceps may be introduced through a second trocar and cannula. Any tissue removed is normally placed in formol saline in a labelled container and sent to the histopathology laboratory. After the examination the wound is sutured, the tourniquet removed and the circulation to the toes checked. Postoperative care is as usual for minor surgery, including physiotherapy, the patient usually leaving hospital 1 or 2 days after the test. Sometimes arthroscopy is performed as an outpatient procedure under local anaesthetic but with full aseptic precautions.

Conditions that can be diagnosed by this technique include *rheumatoid arthritis, osteoarthritis, tuberculosis, villonodular synovitis* and *malignant synovioma*.

Bone biopsy
This is used in the diagnosis of bone tumours and other bone diseases, e.g. *cysts, Paget's disease* and *osteomalacia*. The bone specimen is usually obtained by open operation and collected into formol saline. Sometimes a small cylinder can be obtained using a trephine through an aspiration biopsy needle (as for bone marrow puncture, p. 93). Where osteomalacia is suspected the specimen should be collected into neutral formol saline (ordinary formalin, if acid, tends to remove calcium from the bone and prevents an accurate measurement of bone calcification). To obtain material for bone cytology a special drill can be used.

Physiotherapy assessment

General
The assessment of a patient's condition is based on the doctor's notes, including operation records, site of incision, any peri-operative problems and X-ray findings. Additional assessment is required for the patients as listed below.

Tests for cardiothoracic (including intensive care) patients
1. Lung function tests (see p. 67)
2. Exercise tolerance test (see p. 79)
3. ECG findings (see pp. 79–81)
4. Blood gases and pH (see p. 73).

Tests for patients with musculoskeletal disorders
Particular consideration should be given to the following:
1. Static and dynamic posture; movement patterns, gait, etc.
2. Orthopaedic appliances
3. Structural deformities
4. Skin colour, condition, sensation (see p. 36) and temperature (local and general)
5. Blood changes.

Creatine phosphokinase (see p. 117) is raised in most diseases of muscle. Muscle antibodies are raised in autoimmune conditions such as dermatomyositis (5 ml of clotted blood are required) (see fluorescent antibody technique, p. 103).

Movement is assessed as follows:

1. Active and passive range of affected and unaffected joints
2. Reasons for limitation of active and passive movements
3. Accessory and trick movements
4. Muscle power (see p. 40), tone, wasting and, if relevant, electrical responses (see p. 40)
5. Assessment of demands of lifestyle and aids needed, short term and long term.

Tests for patients with lower motor neurone disease
These are as for musculosketal disorders (p. 179) and also:

1. Soft tissue mobility and extensibility
2. Sweat test (p. 143)
3. Strength duration curve (muscular electrical reactions similar to those on p. 40).

Tests for patients with rheumatoid and other rheumatic diseases
These are as for musculoskeletal disorders and also:

1. Gold tolerance assessment (based on history)
2. Blood changes in rheumatoid disease. These are tested by the following: differential agglutination test (see p. 101) and Hyland RA test (see p. 101); haemoglobin (see p. 88) – anaemia is common in rheumatoid disease; ESR (see p. 89) – the degree to which the ESR is raised is a guide to the activity of the disease
3. Other rheumatic diseases (see autoantibody tests, p. 102).

Reference

1. Pagana, K D and Pagana, T J. Bone scan. In: Pagana, K D and Pagana, T J, (eds). *Mosby's Diagnostic and Laboratory Test Reference*. St. Louis. Mosby Year Book. 1992:120–122.

2. Eastell, R and Peel, N. Osteoporosis. *Journal of the Royal College of Physicians*. London. 1998: 32 (1): 14–18.

CHAPTER THIRTEEN

Tests related to sexuality

Reproductive systems

Index of tests	Page		
Acid phosphatase	185	Genetic 'fingerprinting'	184
AIDS (acquired immune deficiency syndrome)	201	Gonadal biopsy	188
Alpha-fetoprotein (AFP) in amniotic fluid	192	Gonadal endocrine function	187
Amniocentesis	191	Gynaecological cytology	197
Assessment of fetal lung maturity	192	Hepatitis B	16
Beta subunit human chorionic		Heredity	183
gonadotrophin (b-HCG)	189	Human chorionic gonadotrophin (hCG)	189
Bilirubin in amniotic fluid	191	Human placental lactogen (HPL) assay	190
Blood groups	184	Hydatidiform mole	189
Breast biopsy	195	Infertility	185
Breast, excision biopsy of	195	Laparoscopy	196
Breast, fine needle aspiration (FNA) of	195	Lecithin in amniotic fluid	192
Breast, frozen section biopsy of	195	Malignant gonadal teratoma therapy	
Breast, mammography of	194	monitoring	189
Breast, self-examination of	194	Mammography	194
Breast, thermography of	194	Neural tube defect detection	192
Breast, xeroradiography of	194	Oestradiol-17b	187
Breast, Trucut needle biopsy of	195	Oestrogen (oestriol) excretion	190
Cervical cytology	197	Oestrogens, total non-pregnancy	187
Cervical scrape	197	Ovarian biopsy	186
Chancre	200	Paternity	184
Choriocarcinoma	189	Placental monitoring	189
Chorionic villous sampling (CVS)	192	Post-coital test	186
Chromosome study	183	Pregnancy tests	188
Colposcopy	197	Pregnancy, ultrasound in	189
Ectopic pregnancy	189	Pregnancy X-rays	189
Encephalocoele detection	192	Pre-implantation genetic diagnosis	184
Endocervical scrape	198	Premature rupture of membranes, test for	193
Fetal blood sample examination	192	Progesterone	187
Fetal cell chromosome studies	190	Prostate, fine needle aspiration (FNA) of	185
Fetal cell sexing	190	Prostatic biopsy	185
Fetal distress assessment	192	Prostatic specific antigen (PSA)	185
Fetal heart monitoring	192	Radiography of uterus, tubes and ovaries	196
Fetal monitoring	189	Salpingogram	196
Frei test for lymphogranuloma venereum	201	Sex chromatin	183

Index of tests	Page		
Sexually transmitted disease	199	Ultrasound of uterus	196
Spina bifida detection	192	Urethral discharges	199
Syphilis, blood tests for	200	Uterine curettings	196
Testicular biopsy	186	Uterine swab	193
Testosterone and other androgens	188	Vaginal aspirate	198
Tissue enzyme study	183	Vaginal discharges	198
Toxaemias of pregnancy	192	Vaginal wall scrape	198
Threatened abortion	189	Vaginal vault smear	198

Introduction

Sexuality is primarily related to reproduction but has many ramifications, with a correspondingly wide range of tests related to the reproductive systems. Testing for fetal genetic disorders by chromosome and tissue enzyme studies is of growing importance. Where in-vitro fertilization is being used, pre-implantation genetic diagnosis (PGD) has been developed to ensure that the implanted ovum is free from an inherited disorder. In cases of disputed paternity, 'genetic fingerprinting' gives many more conclusive results than blood groups, although only a limited number of haematologists or serologists are prepared to participate in this medicolegal procedure. Fine needle aspiration of the prostate enables prostatic cancer to be detected by the cytologist in material aspirated by the urogenital surgeon. Infertility studies are mainly undertaken by the gynaecologist, who is also usually responsible for organizing gonadal hormone estimations and pregnancy (placental and fetal) monitoring to be done by chemical pathology, for pregnancy tests to be done in the relevant department of pathology (which, like fertility tests, varies in different hospitals), and for radioimmune assays to be done by the Supraregional Assay Service (SAS) via chemical pathology. Tests for, and monitoring of, toxaemia of pregnancy are usually done by the nurse.

Breast screening for cancer, using mammography, has now become a specialized service with a designated director, radiologist, surgeon, histopathologist and cytologist. Imaging of the uterus, tubes and ovaries is done by the radiologist; curettage of the uterus and colposcopy by the gynaecologist; and cervical (and vaginal) cytology by the gynaecologist or by the nurse, for example in a well woman clinic, the slides being examined in the department of cytology. Collection of vaginal and urethral discharges is done by the gynaecologist, the venereologist or the nurse, the specimen then being examined in the microbiology department. With regard to cervical neoplasia and sexually transmitted diseases, the need for tact and confidentiality cannot be overemphasized, particularly with HIV testing and AIDS, where patient counselling is mandatory.

Heredity

Sex chromatin examination

This is a structure present in the nuclei of normal female cells. It is related to the presence of two X chromosomes and enables the nuclear sex to be determined by microscopic examination of cells from hermaphrodites and other intersex conditions, using one or more of the following: buccal squames, blood films, and tissue sections.

Buccal squames

The inside of the cheek is scraped with a wooden spatula and smeared across a prepared albuminized glass slide. This is placed in alcohol fixative and sent to the cytological department.

Blood films

In females more than 1% of the polymorphs contain 'drumstick' structures. The required blood smears are collected and examined by the haematology department. Occasionally the results of this method do not agree with the others.

Tissue sections

This test is carried out in the histology department on biopsy material. Good histological sections of almost any tissue may be used, e.g. skin biopsy (p. 8).

Chromosome study

This gives much more detailed information of the chromosome structure than sex chromatin examination, but can only be done in special centres. A tissue culture from blood or bone marrow is often used. Cells from the unborn fetus, obtained by amniocentesis, chorionic villous sampling or cordocentesis are also being used with increasing frequency to detect congenital abnormalities such as Down's syndrome (see pp. 190–192).

Tissue enzyme study

The SAS (Supraregional Assay Service) tissue enzyme service has three main aims:

- Diagnosis of *inherited metabolic diseases* by assay of relevant enzymes in the appropriate cells, tissue or fluid.

- Identification of *carriers of the disease*s by demonstration of partial enzyme deficiencies.

- *Prenatal diagnosis* in high-risk pregnancies for those diseases where adequate techniques are available.

Appropriate specimens include amniotic fluid (ideally from 15 weeks' gestation), blood, skin and other tissues (obtained as above under 'Tissue sections' and 'Chromosome study'), depending on the enzymes to be studied. The SAS centre should be contacted and the case discussed before any tissues are collected.

Pre-implantation genetic diagnosis (PGD)
Inherited disorders are the cause of much distress to their sufferers and to their families. With the development of in-vitro fertilization (IVF) and more refined DNA examination, it is possible to check that an embryo does not carry the gene for an inherited disorder before implantation into the uterus. For example, there is an abnormal gene which promotes the development of *Alzheimer's disease in the third decade of life*: by using PGD it has been possible to ensure that the daughter of a mother carrying this gene will not suffer from the same disability.[1] PGD has progressed from a research technique into the clinical field and is due to become more widely available to prevent the perpetuation of a familial genetic disorder.

Paternity

There are two main methods of paternity testing in current use: blood groups and genetic fingerprinting. For both methods it is necessary to have signed and witnessed documentary evidence of the parties concerned (including photographs) and of the blood samples obtained from them. Preliminary arrangements are usually undertaken by solicitors. All the relevant samples should be collected on the same day and tested with the same reagents. For example, it is convenient for the blood sample from the putative father to be collected at 09.30 hours and those from the mother and child to be collected at 10.00 hours, the tests being undertaken as soon as practicable thereafter.

Blood groups
Clotted blood is required: 5–10 ml from the putative father and the mother and a 1–2 ml finger prick sample from the child are sufficient. An outline of blood groups is given on pp. 103–104. Many additional blood group types are tested for paternity investigations. If the baby's blood contains a blood group which is absent from the mother's blood and this group is also absent from that of the putative father, he cannot be the father of the child. Using blood groups it is possible to prove that a man is not the father of a child but it is never possible to prove that he is. In some instances it is possible to say that there is a strong probability that he is the father, but this is only when one or more of the rarer blood groups are present in both baby and father but absent from the mother.

Genetic 'fingerprinting'
Anticoagulated blood is required. Special tubes containing EDTA (sequestrene), together with protective containers, labels and documents, are supplied by Cellmark Diagnostics, who undertake the testing of the samples. Two 2.5 ml venepuncture samples are required from the child and two 5 ml samples from each of the adults. The blood is very gently mixed with the sequestrene, without shaking. The labelled samples from each individual with the relevant photographs and completed documents are placed in the separate bags supplied and together sent to Cellmark Diagnostics without delay. There the DNA is extracted and analysed. The results enable a positive recognition or exclusion of the child's paternity to be made. Immigration authorities already accept this technique as proof of familial relationships. Its acceptance in paternity disputes requires ratification but time will establish its reliability.

Prostate

Prostatic tumours: cytology and biopsy
Prostatic specific antigen (PSA)

PSA is a glycoprotein produced by the prostate gland cells. It is detectable in the serum of most men,[2] the normal level being <4 µg/L. A raised level is far more specific for *prostatic carcinoma* than acid phosphatase, but there is some overlap with the raised level which occurs in *benign prostatic hypertrophy*. Because of this overlap it was originally not considered suitable for population screening. It is now however being used for screening men of 65 and over and for patients with prostatism (particularly those on a long waiting list). A 5 ml sample of clotted blood is required, sent to chemical pathology early in the day.

Acid phosphatase

About 5 ml of blood are sent to the laboratory in a dry tube. The normal figure depends on the method used in the laboratory. In *carcinoma of the prostate* it rises, especially when *secondary growths* are present, but prostate specific antigen is more reliable and has become the routine test for this condition.

Fine needle aspiration (FNA) cytology

Prostatic carcinoma often arises in the posterior lobes of the gland. Material may be aspirated from this site by using a special long needle (e.g. Franzen needle). No anaesthetic is required. The patient is placed in a suitable position for a rectal examination. The gloved index finger, with the special needle attached, is well lubricated and introduced into the rectum. When suspect nodules are felt the needle is advanced into the prostate and cells aspirated, using a syringe. Apart from the special needle, the materials required and the preparation of the smears are similar to those for FNA of the breast (see p. 195). Informed written consent must be obtained (see p. 2).

Prostatic biopsy

Prostatic biopsy is taken through a cystoscope (see p. 170) with the patient under a general anaesthetic (requiring informed written consent, as on p. 2). It is usually undertaken primarily to relieve urinary obstruction resulting from prostatic enlargement. The fragments of tissue are collected into formol saline in a labelled container and sent with a completed request form to the histopathology department. The commonest finding is benign *prostatic hyperplasia* but in a significant minority of cases *prostatic carcinoma* is found.

Infertility

A general medical examination may reveal a cause for infertility in either sex, e.g. endocrine disturbance or debilitating infection. Special investigations are set out below.

Tests in females

1. *Pelvic examination* to confirm that the reproductive organs are anatomically normal. Abnormalities may be an indication for nuclear sexing (sex chromatin, p. 183) or occasionally chromosome study (p. 183).

2. *Tests for ovulation.* (a) Temperature. Take the temperature on each day of the cycle. A rise in temperature in mid-cycle strongly suggests ovulation. (b) Blood progesterone (p. 187). If ovulation has taken place the blood level rises during the luteal phase (20–25th day of cycle).

3. *Tests for patency of fallopian tubes* (see salpingogram, p. 196).

4. *Uterine curettings* (see p. 196). This may reveal *tuberculosis* or functional disturbance of the endometrium.

5. *Blood progesterone estimation* (see p. 187).

6. *Test for antispermatozoal antibodies in serum.* A 7–10 ml sample of blood is collected into a plain tube and sent to the department of the laboratory dealing with fertility tests (which varies in different hospitals). Their presence is an occasional factor in infertility.[3]

7. *Ovarian biopsy.* A small portion of ovarian tissue is removed either during laparoscopy (p. 196) or laparotomy (open abdominal operation), placed in formalin fixative and sent for histology. It often provides diagnostic information (as in *Klinefelter's syndrome*) in the investigation of infertility and gonadal endocrine dysfunction. Informed written consent is required (see p. 2).

Tests in males

1. *Examination of the genitalia* to confirm that they are anatomically normal.

2. *Examination of seminal fluid.* Fresh seminal ejaculate collected directly into a clean glass container (never into a condom) is examined in the laboratory for the number of spermatozoa, and also their motility and microscopic structure. Seminal culture, including investigation for tubercle, may be required as part of the infertility investigation or in suspected epididymo–orchitis.

3. *Testicular biopsy.* A small portion of testis is removed under local anaesthetic, collected into formalin fixative and sent for histology. This reveals whether *spermatogenesis* is normal and can detect testicular damage or disease, including *tumours*. Informed written consent is required (see p. 2).

4. *Test for antispermatozoal antibodies in serum.* A 7–10 ml sample of blood is collected into a plain tube (as in test 6 in females). Such antibodies can occur as a result of reabsorption of sperm from a blocked duct or following a vasectomy.[3]

Post-coital test

The female partner attends for examination optimally 6–10 hours (maximum 18–24 hours) after coitus. She is examined in the left lateral position with the aid of a speculum and an Anglepoise lamp.

1. With a Pasteur pipette a few drops of fluid are taken from the vagina, put on a slide, covered by a coverslip and examined microscopically for spermatozoa.

2. With a sterile platinum loop a drop of mucus is collected from the cervical canal and similarly prepared for microscopy. If fertility is normal the mucus is penetrated by actively motile spermatozoa. In cervicitis, pus cells are seen.

3. A swab for bacteriological culture should also be taken from the cervical canal.

Gonads

Gonadal endocrine function investigations – urine
Total non-pregnancy oestrogens
Complete 24-hour urine specimens are required (see p. 160). The normal ranges are as set out in Table 13.1.
Multiple assays are needed to detect ovulation. Excretion is increased in *precocious puberty* and *gynaecomastia*. It is reduced in *amenorrhoea* due to *hypogonadism*. In *primary hypogonadism* serum FSH (p. 57) values are high but in the *secondary form* they are low. Cyclical FSH and LH (pp. 56–57) changes may be seen in precocious puberty. For oestrogen excretion in pregnancy (see p. 190).

Oestradiol-17b
This provides an assessment of ovarian function similar to the total non-pregnancy oestrogens. It can be estimated from a 24-hour urine and from a 5 ml heparinized sample of blood. Several samples at weekly intervals are recommended for assessment of ovarian activity, e.g. in dysfunctional uterine haemorrhage. High levels occur with *oestrogen-secreting tumours* which can arise in ovary, testis and adrenal glands.

Gonadal endocrine function investigations – blood
Progesterone
Progesterone, produced by the corpus luteum in the ovary, prepares the endometrium for pregnancy during the second half of the menstrual cycle and, if fertilization of the ovum occurs, maintains this change as the decidua of pregnancy. The reduction in blood progesterone at the end of the cycle provokes menstruation. Plasma progesterone assay provides evidence of luteal function. Levels of 0.3–2 nmol/L are normally present during the proliferative phase, rising to >30 nmol/L during the luteal phase, reaching a peak value of up to 60 nmol/L by about the 24th day of the cycle. If infertility is due to failure of ovulation the normal rise does not occur. After consultation with the laboratory, one sample is taken on the 8–10th day and a second sample on the 20–23rd day of the menstrual cycle: 5 ml blood is collected into a lithium heparin tube and placed in the refrigerator until it can be taken to the laboratory.

Oestradiol
Oestradiol is the main circulating oestrogen. Oestrogens cause the endometrium to thicken during the follicular phase of the menstrual cycle, promote cervical mucus

Table 13.1 Non-pregnancy oestrogens: normal ranges	
	nmol/24 hours
Children under 10 years	0–80
Women:	
Follicular phase	20–150
Mid-cycle peak	60–300
Luteal phase	45–290
Post-menopausal	10–55
Men	5–40

secretion at ovulation and cause mammary duct growth and enlargement of the breasts at puberty.[4] The normal adult serum (or plasma) level in males is <180 pmol/L; in females it is 200–400 pmol/L in the follicular phase, 400–1200 pmol/L at mid-cycle, 400–1000 pmol/L in the luteal phase and <100 pmol/L after the menopause. Its measurement is of value in *monitoring superovulatory treatment of infertility*. The blood oestrogen level is raised in *oestrogen-secreting tumours* which can arise in the *ovary, testis or adrenal gland.*

Testosterone and other androgens

The main circulating androgen is testosterone.[4] The normal adult serum (or plasma) level is 10–20 nmol/litre (280–600 mg/100 ml) in males and 1–2.5 nmol/litre (27–70 mg/100 ml) in females. It is increased in *women with virilizing tumours*, in *XYY males* and in *boys with precocious puberty*. Male testosterone levels in a patient with a female appearance characterizes the *testicular feminization syndrome*. Decreased levels occur in *hypogonadism* (including *Klinefelter's syndrome*), *hypopituitarism, undescended testes* and *post-traumatic impotence*. About 5 ml of blood is required in either a plain or a heparin tube, best collected at about 09.00 hours in view of circadian variation. This applies to all the androgens.[4]

Dihydrotestosterone is at least twice as active in its biological effects as testosterone but there is ten times as much of the latter in the circulating blood.[4] An increase in this ratio to 30:1 is diagnostic of a syndrome, called *5α-reductase deficiency*, in which affected males have undescended testes, hypospadias and a micropenis so that they are usually brought up as females until puberty when virilization occurs.[4] The normal adult serum levels of dihydrotestosterone are 9–35 nmol/L in males and 0.3–9.3 nmol/L in females.

Other androgens are androstenedione and dehydroepiandrosterone (and its sulphate), whose androgenic effect is probably due to their peripheral conversion to testosterone. They are secreted by the adrenal glands and an increase in this secretion starts at about 7 years of age in both sexes and continues for the next 7 years (the 'adrenarche').[5]

Androstenedione levels in the blood are usually raised in *idiopathic hirsutism*.[4] The normal adult serum levels are 1.6–8.4 nmol/L in males, 0.6–8.8 nmol/L in females and 0.9–6.8 nmol/L in post-menopausal females. The normal dehydroepiandrosterone serum levels are 7–31 nmol/L and dehydroepiandrosterone sulphate 2–10 μmol/L in males and 3–12 μmol/L in females.

Gonadal biopsy

Testicular or ovarian biopsy may assist in the investigation of gonadal endocrine dysfunction and infertility (see pp. 185–186).

Pregnancy

Pregnancy tests

During pregnancy there is a hormone in the blood called *human chorionic gonadotrophin* (hCG). This passes into the urine and can be detected by the following tests, which become positive earlier in pregnancy than the older biological tests using mice, rabbits or toads. They can also be used in the detection of *hydatidiform mole* and *chorion epithelioma.* Early morning specimens of urine are more concentrated and therefore contain more HCG, but any reasonably fresh specimen of urine is suitable.

Haemagglutination inhibition tests

These include Prepuerin and Pregnosticon. The tests take about 2 hours to perform. Sheep red cells coated with hCG are used, and when exposed to rabbit anti-hCG serum are agglutinated. Pregnancy urine prevents this agglutination, its hCG blocking the anti-hCG serum. The tests detect pregnancy about 8 days after the first missed period would have occurred (about 36 days after the last monthly period).

Slide tests

These include Gravindex and Prepurex. The tests take about 3 minutes to perform. A drop of the urine is added to a drop of anti-hCG serum. Pregnant urine contains hCG and neutralizes the antibody, preventing it from agglutinating latex particles coated with the hCG. The tests detect pregnancy about 37–40 days after the last normal monthly period (LMP).

These tests are very sensitive and become positive early in pregnancy.

Radioimmunoassays

The following sensitive tests are undertaken by the SAS following discussion and arrangement with the department of medical biochemistry.

Human chorionic gonadotrophin (hCG)

An ordinary urine sample is required. It is of value for the following:

1. *Missed abortion, threatened abortion, ectopic pregnancy and early pregnancy*: hCG values are lower than usual during pregnancy but above the normal range.

2. *Hydatidiform mole.* Assays (including βhCG, see below) should be done 3 weeks after evacuation of the uterus, then every 2 weeks, until values are in the normal range, then monthly for 1 year and 3 monthly for the next year.

3. *Choriocarcinoma, other trophoblastic tumours and gonadal teratomas*, but see βHCG (below).

Beta subunit human chorionic gonadotrophin (βhCG)

Serum assays for βhCG are more sensitive than urine hCG. About 5 ml clotted blood suffices for this and AFP. It is of value for:

1. Detection and monitoring therapy of *hydatidiform mole, choriocarcinoma*.

2. Monitoring malignant *gonadal teratomas*.

Placental and fetal monitoring

Ultrasound and X-rays

The use of X-rays during pregnancy has been greatly reduced as a result of the recognition that irradiation may be harmful to the growing fetus, occasionally promoting leukaemia. They are no longer used to demonstrate fetal bones in doubtful cases of pregnancy. Measurement of the diameters of the pelvis (pelvimetry) by means of X-rays has been reduced to the minimum (although it may be conveniently undertaken between pregnancies using a CT scan, see p. 21) in favour of ultrasound (p. 190).

However, in carefully selected cases X-rays are still occasionally of value. They can be used to clarify severe abnormalities of the fetus such as *anencephaly*, and fetal death by the overlapping of the cranial bones.

Obstetric ultrasound (p. 20) is now being used to replace X-rays in estimating *fetal maturity*, measuring the *biparietal diameter* and for detecting *multiple births*, *fetal abnormalities* and the *placental site*. Pelvic organs can be seen better when the bladder is full. So the patient is given three glasses of water to drink 1 hour before the examination. She should be asked not to empty her bladder.

Oestrogen (oestriol) excretion

Estimation of the oestrogen excretion in a 24-hour urine provides an assessment of both *placental and fetal function*. Oestrogen excretion gradually increases during pregnancy, but before the 28th week the level is so low that its estimation is a lengthy process. After the 28th week more rapid methods of estimation are practicable.

The normal range is very wide, e.g. 35–115 mmol/24 hours (10–33 mg/24 hours) at 36 weeks. A sudden drop in a series of readings provides a clearer guide than a single low reading in reaching a decision to terminate pregnancy.

Exactly timed 24-hour urine (see p. 160) is collected into dark Winchester bottles without acid or preservative, initially on two consecutive days and then, if indicated, twice weekly. For non-pregnancy oestrogen excretion, see Table 13.1.

Human placental lactogen (HPL) assay

This has been used to monitor the *health of the placenta and fetus* (and occasionally the *growth of certain tumours*, e.g. *teratomas*; see tumour markers, p. 119). About 10 ml of clotted blood are required. Request forms should include the diagnosis and must state the stage of a pregnancy.

HPL is a peptide normally produced by the placenta (abnormally, by tumours). Its blood level increases most during the first 3 months of pregnancy when placental growth is greatest, and then rises gradually until the 38th week. During the first 6 months, levels lower than normal for the stage of gestation are associated with an increased risk of abortion. Levels less than 4 mg/litre after the 34th week indicate serious fetal risk, especially if the level is falling. In *diabetes* the HPL level is raised and so less than 5 mg/litre indicates fetal risk. In cases of *rhesus immunization* levels above the normal range at the 26th week suggests a severely affected fetus.

Serial estimations are of much more value than a single sample. More commonly used tests for monitoring *fetal health* are ultrasound and urinary oestrogen excretion (see above).

Sampling of fetal material

Methods of obtaining samples of fetal material, using ultrasound visualization, include amniocentesis, chorionic villous sampling (CVS) and cordocentesis (see **Fig. 13.1**). All require informed written consent (see p. 2). During delivery, direct visualization is used to obtain fetal scalp blood samples (see assessment of fetal distress, p. 192). Examination of fetal cells is required for:

- Chromosome studies (karyotyping) and DNA analysis, for detecting *Down's syndrome* (mongolism) and *other congenital abnormalities*. The list of inherited disorders which may be diagnosed by DNA studies is growing rapidly.[5] Before the material is obtained, practical arrangements must be made with the tissue culture laboratory for its collection.

- Sexing (tissue culture is not required; see p. 183). This is of value for example if *Duchenne's muscular dystrophy* (affecting males) is suspected.

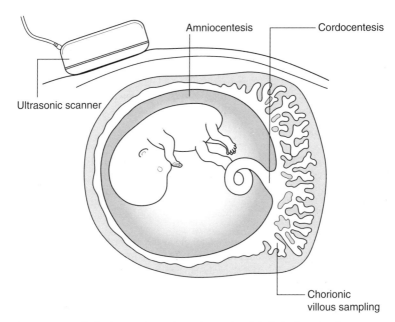

Fig. 13.1 Sites of collection: amniocentesis, cordocentesis and chorionic villous sampling

If fetal abnormality is suspected, sampling should be performed as early as possible; cell culture for chromosome studies usually takes from 72 hours to approximately 2 weeks,[5] but may take longer. Abortion after 24 weeks is undesirable and is preferably done before 18–20 weeks (quickening).

Amniocentesis

Amniocentesis may be undertaken from the 14th week of pregnancy until term. It is used for determining the *severity of haemolytic disease in the fetus*, estimating *fetal lung maturity*, *sexing* and for detecting whether certain *fetal defects* may be present. The technique involves the introduction of a lumbar puncture needle through the abdominal wall into the uterine cavity for the removal of liquor amnii.

 Before the operation the patient must empty her bladder. Full aseptic precautions are required as to gowns, masks, etc. The position of the back of the fetus is determined by palpation. The use of ultrasound minimizes the risk of puncturing the placenta. The skin is cleansed with weak iodine solution BP and anaesthetized with 0.5% procaine hydrochloride. The needle is then introduced below the umbilicus of the mother, behind the fetal back **(Fig. 13.1)**. A 20 ml syringe is used for extracting the liquor and the fluid placed in a dark brown bottle. It is immediately sent to the laboratory where, if it is bloodstained, it requires to be centrifuged and decanted into another dark bottle.

Bilirubin

A spectrophotometer is used to study the optical density deviation produced by the liquor amnii on light (wavelength 450 nm). This gives a guide to the amount of bilirubin-like substances present. For example, at the 34th week a deviation of 0.03–1.8 from linearity indicates moderate to severe *haemolytic disease*.

Assessment of fetal lung maturity

This is done by estimating the total lecithin level and the ratio of lecithin to sphingomyelin. Lecithin enables respiratory epithelium to function normally. It acts like a detergent.

Alpha-fetoprotein estimation

This is for detecting *open neural tube defects*, e.g. *spina bifida, anencephaly* or *encephalocele* (see also AFP in blood, pp. 119–120).

Chorionic villous sampling (CVS)

The genetic make-up of fetus and placenta is identical in the vast majority of cases, and so chromosome and DNA analysis of chorionic villi (**Fig. 13.1**) can be used to provide information about the fetus. CVS can be undertaken after the 10th week. It requires surgical anaesthesia and there is a risk of precipitating miscarriage in about 2.5% of cases.[5]

Cordocentesis

From the nineteenth week of gestation, fetal blood can be obtained from the umbilical cord (**Fig. 13.1**) as an outpatient procedure. Using real time ultrasound the site of the umbilical cord insertion into the placenta can be visualized.[5] After cleansing the skin surface with a spirit swab, followed by local anaesthetic, a lumbar puncture needle is introduced into the umbilical cord and the fetal blood sample aspirated. The risk of miscarriage from this procedure is about 1%.

Toxaemias of pregnancy

In cases of toxaemia of pregnancy the urine is tested for protein as described on p. 162, and specimens are sent to the laboratory for confirmation and routine examination. In addition, frequent estimation of the blood pressure is carried out, and fetal heart rate checked.

Assessment of fetal distress

An abnormal fetal heart rate and meconium staining of the liquor amnii indicate fetal distress. More accurate assessment of the fetal state is provided by:

1. *Fetal heart monitoring*, using electronic equipment This records the fetal heart beat in relation to uterine contractions by means of two transducers which are attached to the patient's abdomen.

2. *Fetal scalp blood sample examination* collected through an amnioscope. This is a slightly conical hollow tube with a light, the narrow end being introduced with aseptic precautions through the vagina and cervix after the membranes have ruptured, with the patient in the lithotomy position. The fetal scalp is cleansed with antiseptic, dried with sterile cotton wool and a small amount of petroleum jelly applied to the fetal scalp to cause the droplets of fetal blood to bead.[6] Blood is collected from the fetal scalp using a special instrument with a small blade, into heparinized capillary tubing (5 cm without bubbles), mixed by drawing a small needle through the tube by a magnet, sealed with gum or wax, placed on ice and sent immediately to the laboratory for estimation of blood gases, pH (see p. 73) and lactate. Of these, the most useful is the pH. Normally the pH is 7.25–7.35 during labour. If the fetus is suffering from a lack of oxygen more lactic acid is produced, causing acidosis with an abnormally low pH.[6]

Test for premature rupture of membranes

Sometimes the membranes surrounding the fetus rupture before term. If this is suspected a sample of vaginal fluid should be sent to the laboratory in a plain universal container. Microscopic examination will detect the presence of lanugo hairs or vernix caseosa cells (staining red or orange with 0.05% aqueous Nile blue sulphate). If these are found, a diagnosis of *ruptured membranes* can be made.

Uterine swabs

To take a uterine swab, the patient should be prepared as for a cervical swab (see vaginal discharges, p. 198), but in addition the cervical canal is swabbed clean, and a throat swab passed into the uterine cavity.

Uterine swabs may be taken in cases of *puerperal infection* and *septic abortion*. Swabs from the throat of the patient should also be taken to see if she is a carrier of *haemolytic streptococci* (see pp. 62–63).

Neonatal screening for inborn errors of metabolism

Screening criteria

Screening of newborn babies for inborn errors of metabolism enables treatment to be instituted before irrevocable damage is caused by the condition. In 1969, mass screening for *phenylketonuria (PKU)* was introduced in the UK and the criteria for such mass screening were defined:[7]

- The disorder has serious consequences, preventable by early treatment
- Screening allows diagnosis to be made before symptoms develop
- Screening is feasible to organize
- The methods are simple, quick, inexpensive and reliable
- The programme is justified on economic grounds.

Phenylketonuria (PKU)

By estimating the blood level of phenylalanine on all babies at the age of 1 week it is possible to detect *phenylketonuria (PKU)* before the brain is damaged. The phenylalanine used to be estimated by Guthrie's test (by the amount of bacterial growth (*B. subtilis*) that it promotes), but a chemical method is now more frequently used. For either method, a few drops of blood are collected on to thick filter paper from a heel-prick, the collection usually being done by the district nurse (see also p. 163). Normal blood contains less than 0.25 mmol/litre (4 mg/100 ml). A greater level than this requires further investigation. Phenylalanine is present in all food protein. In *phenylketonuria* the liver lacks an enzyme needed to control the blood level of phenylalanine and it rises, e.g. to 1 mmol/litre (16 mg/100 ml) and above. This leads to mental deficiency unless treatment is started very early in life. Uncontrolled phenylalanine levels in phenylketonuric mothers can damage infants *in utero*.

Congenital hypothyroidism (CH)

Screening for CH has now been accepted in most developed countries. In the UK, the Guthrie card blood spots collected for the detection of PKU (see above) are also used to screen for CH, using the plasma TSH (thyroid stimulating hormone) concentration.[7] Normally after birth the TSH rises rapidly, reaching a plateau of about 100 mU/L in 3–4 hours and then falling gradually over the next 48 hours. The test should be performed during the next few weeks when the level in babies with CH fails to fall below the accepted cut-off figure. The cut-off for babies requiring full thyroid profile (p. 45) depends on the method used, but is usually about 15 mU/L. All infants found to have CH need to be re-evaluated after 1 year. This is done by replacing the L-thyroxine (T$_4$) used in their treatment by liothyronine (T3) for about 4 weeks and then stopping all treatment for 10 days before repeating the full thyroid profile.

In America most babies are screened within 48 hours of birth, when the TSH levels are still high, even in babies with CH. Instead total plasma T$_4$ (thyroxine, p. 45) levels are used as a screening test. This also detects cases of CH which are not due to intrinsic thyroid disease and so it is recommended that when the T$_4$ is low, TSH analysis is also performed (in the early postnatal period a higher cut-off level is appropriate).

Galactosaemia

The aim of screening is to detect the most severe form of *galactosaemia*. This may be done using a dried blood spot (as for PKU and CH), using either a fluorescent spot test or a semiquantitative test. In its acute form *galactosaemia* presents with *vomiting, diarrhoea* and *hepatic dysfunction*, often with an *E. coli septicaemia*. Dietary galactose restriction can reverse these acute symptoms but may not prevent long-term failure to thrive,[7] probably due to galactose being produced in the body.

Breast examination

Self examination

Finding a lump in the breast is often the first indication that a tumour is present; so regular and careful breast palpation is now a recognized screening procedure. The Women's National Cancer Control Campaign have produced booklets which explain clearly and simply how to undertake self-examination. A tumour has to reach a certain size before it becomes palpable. This technique cannot detect the very earliest lesions demonstrable by mammography. However, it is of undoubted value and if the finding of a lump is followed up with mammography and fine needle aspiration (see breast biopsy, p. 195) it is often possible to distinguish between benign and malignant lumps before admission to hospital. The majority of lumps found by palpation prove to be benign.

Mammography

Soft tissue X-rays are passed through the breast only, with the patient in the erect and supine positions. By using low kilovoltage X-rays a clearer picture of soft tissue changes is obtained. Microcalcification can be detected in a *small cancer* before it can be detected clinically by palpation.

Xeroradiography (xerography)

This is a medical application of the photocopying process. It enables the clarity of soft tissue X-rays to be enhanced, with the production of a blue photocopy.

Thermography

Heat given out from the body in the form of infrared emission can be recorded to detect 'hot spots'. These indicate possible sites of cancer. Thermography is not sufficiently specific to be a diagnostic technique, but may be used for screening, prior to mammography.

Breast biopsy
Fine needle aspiration (FNA)

The use of a fine needle to obtain cells from a breast lump is almost painless. It is of great diagnostic value and is simple, quick and cost-effective. It may eliminate the need for hospital admission or provide a clear indication that admission is urgent, if *malignant cells* are found. The nature of the test must be explained to the patient and her written consent must be obtained by the clinician undertaking the fine needle aspiration (see p. 2).

The materials required are:

- Swabs with spirit or skin sterilizing solution.

- Disposable syringe (10 or 20 ml) with fine needle (swg 21–23 or 0.8 mm diameter) as used for venepuncture. A pistol-grip syringe holder provides greater control but is not essential.

- Microscope slides, preferably with frosted ends for ease of labelling with a pencil (not pen or ball point).

- Fixative. Carnoy's fixative or 70–90% alcohol in Coplin jars is preferable to spray fixative. Formol saline should also be available in case any tissue fragments are obtained (glutaraldehyde if electron microscopy is contemplated).

- Small transport box such as that provided for cervical smears.

- Completed laboratory request form with full details.

Even with a good collection technique only a small amount of material is obtained. It should be sufficient to spread evenly on two slides. While still wet, one slide is immersed in fixative for at least 30 minutes. The other is waved in the air to air-dry. The slide labels should indicate which is air-dried and which is fixed. Completed request forms must accompany the slides to the cytology laboratory.

Triple diagnosis is the combination of clinical examination, mammography and fine needle aspiration. If all three are in agreement that a lesion is benign or malignant, the diagnostic accuracy is over 99%.

Trucut needle biopsy

By using a large bore needle a small cylinder of tissue can be obtained from a breast lump. It differs from FNA (above) in that it preserves the tissue structure in the specimen and so provides more diagnostic information. Because of its large bore it causes more pain and so the skin must be anaesthetized by local anaesthetic before introducing the Trucut needle. The nature of the test must be explained to the patient and her written consent must be obtained by the clinician undertaking the biopsy (see p. 2). One or more tissue portions are obtained which are collected into formol saline and sent to the histopathology department. A *positive diagnosis of breast cancer* may be made by this technique, but a *negative result does not exclude cancer*.

Frozen section biopsy

If there is a suspicion that breast cancer may be present but a definitive diagnosis has not been made before the patient reaches the operating table, frozen section biopsy is frequently undertaken. It is important to arrange the time so that the histopathologist can deal with the specimen without delay. After the patient has been anaesthetized the surgeon makes an incision over the suspect lesion. Unfixed tissue from the lesion is sent to the laboratory where a small portion is selected by the pathologist. The tissue is frozen, sectioned, processed, examined microscopically and the *report telephoned to the waiting surgeon*. He will then decide what additional tissue, if any, needs to be excised. As for any surgical operation, written informed consent must be obtained (see p. 2).

Excision biopsy

In cases where there is a high probability that a breast lump is benign or, if malignant, small enough to be excised completely without mastectomy, it is common for 'lumpectomy' (excision of the lump) to be performed. This is placed in formol saline and sent routinely to the laboratory where the histopathologist selects as many portions of tissue as may be necessary for a diagnosis. *Fibroadenoma* and *fibroadenosis* are lesions which are frequently managed in this way. Occasionally an *unexpected cancer* may be found which may or may not require further treatment. As for any surgical operation, written informed consent must be obtained (see p. 2).

Female genital tract

Laparoscopy

By means of a laparoscope (p. 150) the peritoneal surface of the ovaries, tubes, uterus and vagina may be examined. This assists in the diagnosis of *ovarian cysts and tumours*, *endometriosis* and *adhesions*. It is used in the investigation of infertility (p. 186) and for female sterilization. The procedure must be explained to the patient and written consent obtained (see p. 2). Similar but more extensive information may be obtained by the operative procedure of *laparotomy* (p. 151).

Radiography and ultrasound of uterus, tubes and ovaries

Because of the possible damaging effects of radiation to the developing fetus, abdominal radiography on female patients of child-bearing age is now avoided except in the first 10 days of the menstrual cycle (the 'ten-day rule'). A straight X-ray may show a *dermoid cyst*, containing teeth or bony structures. A *calcified fibroid tumour* may also be seen.

Ultrasound and pregnancy
See p. 190.

Salpingogram
In the female, sterility may be due to the fact that the fallopian tubes are blocked. To test the patency of the tubes, a special syringe is inserted into the cervical os, and contrast medium injected. An X-ray photograph is then taken from which it can be seen whether the passage of the medium is obstructed in the tube or is dripping through the fimbriated end into the abdominal cavity.

Uterine curettings

All curettings from the uterus should be examined microscopically. Conditions which may be so diagnosed include residual *products of conception*, *hydatidiform mole*, *chorion epithelioma*, *anovulatory cycles*, *cystic hyperplasia*, *atypical hyperplasia* and *carcinoma*. The material removed from the uterus should be placed immediately in a small jar or tube containing fixative, preferably Masson's, Bouin's or Susa's fluid, and correctly labelled. This is sent to the laboratory, where it is mounted in wax and sections cut for microscopical examination.

Gynaecological cytology
Cervical cytology

The examination of material collected from the cervix is invaluable in the *early diagnosis of cancer*, and is useful for detecting *trichomonas* and *human papillomavirus* (*HPV*, not infrequently a precursor of cancer) infections and other conditions. Its main advantage is that it can detect *changes which are likely to progress to cancer* long before any symptoms are produced. By screening well women regularly, most cancers of the cervix can be prevented. Cells with significantly abnormal nuclei are reported as *dyskaryotic*. Women with severe or moderate *dyskaryosis* should be referred to a gynaecologist, preferably for colposcopy (see p. 198). Women with mild *dyskaryosis* and even borderline changes should also be referred if the changes persist for more than 6 months.

Cervical scrape

The collection technique for cervical cytology is undergoing radical change. The traditional technique is used in many centres, but increasingly it is being superseded by LBC (liquid based cytology):

1. *Traditional technique.* The cervical scrape is obtained under direct vision provided by a good light, with a vaginal speculum in position. With the point inserted into the external os, an Ayre's spatula (or one of its modifications, e.g. the Aylesbury spatula) is gently but firmly rotated through 360°, particular attention being paid to obtaining material from the squamocolumnar junction. The material obtained is spread on a glass slide, the frosted end of which has previously been labelled *in pencil* with the patient's name and number. Care should be taken to spread the smear evenly but not too thickly, and to fix while still wet. Fixatives are of several kinds. Some are sprayed on, some are poured on, and some the slides are immersed in, e.g. alcohol fixative. With the latter there must be at least sufficient fixative to cover all the smear, and the lid must be replaced on the container to prevent evaporation. At least 30 minutes must be allowed for the slides to fix before removal from the fixative.

2. *Liquid based cytology* (LBC). Several different systems are currently on trial. Details of the system in use in a particular area can be obtained from the local cytology laboratory. Currently in Cardiff, material is obtained from the cervix using a plastic broom instead of a spatula. The central bristles of the broom are inserted into the endocervical canal deep enough to allow the shorter bristles to gently push against the ectocervix. Since the broom has soft fronds it must be rotated 5 times (as opposed to 1 or 2 with Ayre's spatula) and is immediately rinsed vigorously in the special phial provided, so that no material remains on the broom, which is discarded. The cap on the phial is then tightened fully.

Whichever technique is used, a completed cervical cytology request form must be sent, together with the fully labelled material from each patient, to the cytology laboratory.

Endocervical scrape

In older women an Ayre's spatula may fail to reach the squamocolumnar junction because it has receded up the endocervical canal; so neoplastic change may be missed. To prevent this a special spatula with a longer point (e.g. the Aylesbury spatula) should be used. Alternatively a nylon brush (Medscand) or an endocervical swab may be used. A smear is made as for a cervical scrape.

Upper third vaginal wall scrape

A scrape from the upper third of the vaginal wall with the rounded end of an Ayre's spatula provides the most suitable material for evaluating hormonal response cytologically.

Vaginal aspirate

Specimens obtained by vaginal aspirate are usually of much less diagnostic value than those from a cervical scrape, and are only indicated on rare occasions when the cervix cannot be visualized.

Vaginal vault smear

A vault smear is indicated at appropriate intervals (e.g. annually) following hysterectomy for cervical neoplasia. The rounded end of an Ayre's spatula is used to collect the material, which is then spread and fixed as for a cervical scrape.

Colposcopy

Colposcopy is the examination of the cervix, vagina and occasionally vulva by means of a colposcope. This is a binocular microscope with a central illuminating device. The main indication for colposcopy is the finding of dyskaryotic cells in the cervical smear, with an apparently normal cervix. Usually no anaesthetic is required but the patient should be warned to expect some discomfort when a biopsy is taken. Informed written consent must be obtained (see p. 2) A special colposcopy couch enables the patient to take up a lithotomy position with her feet resting comfortably on the supports provided. Hibitane in watery solution (not spirit!) is used to lubricate the speculum before its insertion. The colposcope enables the cervix to be examined at various magnifications (4–40 times). Biopsy is taken from the site of greatest colposcopic abnormality and the tissue sent, in formol saline, for histological examination. Before she leaves, the patient should be given reassurance and clear guidance concerning the anticipated management. If the degree of abnormality revealed histologically is appropriate, the lesion may be treated on an outpatient basis, using laser, cautery or cryosurgery under colposcopic control. This reduces the number of patients requiring admission to hospital for cone biopsy.

Discharges
Vaginal discharge

In cases of vaginal discharge, it is important to discover the organisms present, and for this purpose several different types of specimen may be collected.

In children vulvovaginitis may be present, and in this case a vaginal swab is taken.

In adults a vaginal discharge is often associated with *Trichomonas vaginalis*. This is a protozoon a little larger than a leukocyte. In order to recognize its presence, a drop of discharge is examined on a glass slide, in a fresh, warm condition under the microscope. Alternatively it may be preserved temporarily by using a vaginal swab put in a transport medium which is then transmitted to the laboratory without delay (see pp. 11–12).

A specimen taken with a dry swab should be collected at the same time. *T. vaginalis* can also be detected by cervical cytology (p. 197).

In pregnancy, a vaginal discharge is often due to the presence of thrush caused by a yeast, *Monilia albicans*, and this can be recognized by examination of a vaginal swab or by cervical cytology.

Provided the patient is not pregnant a *cervical swab* should be taken for microbiological examination. The vaginal fornices are swabbed dry and a throat swab passed into the cervical canal. If urethral discharge is present a urethral smear and culture should also be collected (see below).

Sexually transmitted diseases

Urethral discharge and sexually transmitted disease
Urethral discharge
In the female the patient should be placed in the lithotomy position, the vulva separated and swabbed down. A finger is then inserted into the vagina, and the urethra 'milked' from behind forward by pressure on the anterior vaginal wall. A sterile mounted loop of platinum wire (sterilized by heating in a flame and then allowed to cool) is then passed into the urethra, and the material obtained spread thinly on a sterile glass slide, dried without heat, and fixed by adding a few drops of alcohol. Sometimes the material obtained may be transferred to a culture tube.

In the male the urethral orifice is cleaned, and a platinum wire loop inserted as described. If the discharge is scanty it may be necessary to massage the prostate by a gloved finger in the rectum prior to taking the swab.

Gonococci are frequently found in urethral discharges. Repeated examinations may be necessary to prove or disprove their presence. The organisms may be cultured by collecting the discharge on a swab. When delay is anticipated a special swab is used and placed in Stuart's transport medium for dispatch to the laboratory (see pp. 11–12).

Chlamydia trachomatis is a common cause of non-gonococcal urethritis; it has been isolated from the cervices of nearly 50% of consorts of males with non-gonococcal urethritis and from one-third of all women attending VD clinics. It is a cause of infertility and ectopic pregnancy. Diagnosis can be made on cervical smears, using monoclonal antibodies to reveal the organisms as extracellular elementary bodies.[8]

Herpes genitalis
This is caused by the *herpes simplex virus type 2* (HSV2), to be distinguished from HSV1 which causes herpetic sores affecting the mouth. *Herpes genitalis* is characterized by vesicular lesions on the penis, scrotum, vulva, vagina, cervix, perineum or perianal region. A lesion in the birth canal at the time of delivery is likely to infect the baby, with serious, and sometimes fatal, consequences. In the male, material is collected from the urethra as described under urethral discharge (above). In the female, the patient is placed in the lithotomy position, a vaginal speculum is inserted and cervical mucus is removed with cotton wool. A sterile swab is then introduced into the endocervical canal and gently agitated to provide material for culture. In pregnant women with *herpes genitalis* this should be done with extreme care and should be undertaken weekly, starting 4–6 weeks before delivery. Vaginal delivery should only

be considered if the two most recent cultures are negative, if the woman is symptom-free with no visible herpetic lesions in the birth canal and she has not had more than one positive culture throughout the pregnancy during which she was symptom-free.[9]

Chancre

At the site of primary syphilitic infection, a hard nodule forms. This breaks down to form a shallow ulcer, from the surface of which serous fluid is exuded. This is highly infectious, therefore rubber gloves should be worn when collecting a specimen.

The surface of the sore should be cleaned with a swab soaked in spirit. The sore should be squeezed until serum exudes. A drop is taken with a platinum loop or capillary tube, and diluted with a drop of saline on a slide.

The specimen is sealed with a cover slip, and examined immediately under a microscope, using dark ground illumination to detect the spirochetes of *syphilis* (*Treponema pallidum*).

Blood tests for syphilis

The blood tests most commonly used for screening for syphilitic infection are the VDRL (venereal disease reference laboratory) slide test and the TPHA (*Treponema pallidum* haemagglutination) test. The Wassermann reaction (WR) and the Reiter protein complement fixation test (RPCFT) are now usually replaced by the above tests. For the tests, 5 ml of clotted blood is sufficient. If an equivocal or unexpected result is obtained the tests are repeated on a later sample. If necessary, blood may be referred to the VD reference laboratory, in order to demonstrate the syphilitic reagin.

VDRL (venereal disease reference laboratory) slide test

This test usually becomes positive 7–10 days after the appearance of the chancre. It is a satisfactory and rapid screening test. It has taken the place of the Wassermann reaction for monitoring treatment, and like the WR, it can give a false biological positive reaction, e.g. in pregnancy and certain infections.

TPHA (*Treponema pallidum* haemagglutination) test

This is a sensitive test for antibody in all stages of syphilis. It cannot be used for monitoring treatment because it remains positive for a very long time, even after cure. In this respect it resembles the *Treponema immobilization test* (TIT or TPI) and the *fluorescent treponemal antibody test* (FTAT).

The TPHA test rarely gives rise to a false biological positive reaction. The FTAT only very rarely gives such a reaction.

Wassermann reaction (WR)

This usually becomes positive 6–8 weeks after infection. Successful treatment early in the disease usually causes it to become negative fairly quickly. Long-standing cases however may never become negative. The test may also be done on cerebrospinal fluid but has been virtually replaced by the VDRL and TPHA tests (above).

The result may be classified as positive (+), doubtful (±) or negative (-). Sometimes the result may be given according to the titre, i.e. dilution of serum at which antibody can just be detected. With much antibody the titre is high, e.g. 1 in 40. With less antibody the titre is lower, e.g. 1 in 5.

The test may give a false-positive reaction temporarily during pregnancy or in the course of various diseases in persons who have not had syphilis.

Reiter protein complement fixation test (Reiter protein CFT or RPCFT)

This test is being replaced by the VDRL and TPHA tests (p. 200) as screening tests. The antigen used is Reiter treponema group antigen from the organism which causes syphilis, and so in theory this is a more specific test than the others. In practice the use of the above two screening tests is found to detect more cases of syphilis than any one test alone.

Confirmatory tests for syphilis

The most important are the treponema immobilization test and the fluorescent treponemal antibody test (see p. 200).

Other blood tests used in infections

AIDS (acquired immune deficiency syndrome)

It is generally accepted that AIDS is caused by a virus called the human immunodeficiency virus, of which there are at least two types (HIV 1 and HIV 2). Infection may occur during sexual intercourse or as a result of accidental inoculation of infected blood and other body fluids. Inoculation may be due to a stick wound from needle or scalpel or from a blood transfusion. Usually from 3 weeks to 3 months after a person has been infected, antibodies to the virus appear in the blood, but antibody response may be delayed by several months in some cases. A positive blood test implies that the person has developed antibodies to the virus. The infected person becomes a carrier weeks before becoming antibody-positive, and is capable of infecting other people through blood, semen, vaginal fluid and possibly other body fluids. The acquired immune deficiency syndrome (AIDS) does not usually develop for several years after infection, and a negative test does not exclude infection if undertaken within 3 months, in some cases up to 1 year, of possible infection.

The patient must give his/her written consent before the test is undertaken (see p. 2), and at the same time be given counselling (by a recognized counsellor). The 5 ml of clotted blood required must be collected with great care, preferably into a vacuum container, and the needle discarded safely (see p. 12). The microbiologist should be consulted on how to preserve confidentiality when labelling the HIGH RISK specimen and completing the request form. If the result is positive, the patient must receive further counselling when he/she is informed.

Frei test for lymphogranuloma venereum

Lymphogranuloma venereum is a venereal disease occurring in tropical climates which may also be found in those returning from such areas. An antigen prepared from the causal organism is generally available from the local public health authority. Some of this antigen is injected into the patient intradermally. In a positive case a papule with a necrotic centre appears in about 48 hours.

References

1. Hawkes, N. Woman has baby designed free of Alzheimer's gene. *The Times* No. 67385 (Feb. 27). London. 2002: 1.

2. Beastall, G. H. and McAllister, E. Jean. Tumour markers. In: Marshall, W J and Bangert, S K, (eds). *Clinical Biochemistry; Metabolic and Clinical Aspects*. New York. Churchill Livingstone. 1995: 705–716.

3. Pagana, K D and Pagana, T J. Antispermatozoal antibody. In: Pagana, K D and Pagana, T J, (eds). *Mosby's Diagnostic and Laboratory Test Reference*. St. Louis. Mosby Year Book. 1992: 58–59.

4. Hughes, I A. Abnormal sexual development. In: Marshall, W J and Bangert, S K, (eds). *Clinical Biochemistry: Metabolic and Clinical Aspects*. New York. Churchill Livingstone. 1995: 375–391.

5. Bradley, R and Crook, D. Pregnancy, oral contraception and hormone replacement therapy. In: Marshall, W J and Bangert, S K, (eds). *Clinical Biochemistry: Metabolic and Clinical Aspects*. New York. Churchill Livingstone. 1995: 413–422.

6. Pagana, K D and Pagana, T J. Fetal scalp pH. In: Pagana, K D and Pagana, T J, (eds). *Mosby's Diagnostic and Laboratory Test Reference*. St. Louis. Mosby Year Book. 1992: 345–346.

7. Mayne, P and Hancock, M. Paediatric clinical biochemistry. In: Marshall, W J and Bangert, S K, (eds). *Clinical Biochemistry: Metabolic and Clinical Aspects*. New York. Churchill Livingstone. 1995: 423–451.

8. Colemann, D V and Evans, D M D. *Chlamydia trachomatis*. In: Colemann, D V and Evans, D M D, (eds). *Biopsy Pathology and Cytology of the Cervix*, 2nd edn. London. Arnold. 1999: 139–148.

9. Pagana, K D and Pagana, T J. *Herpes genitalis*. In: Pagana, K D and Pagana, T J, (eds). *Mosby's Diagnostic and Laboratory Test Reference*. St. Louis. Mosby Year Book. 1992: 410–411.

CHAPTER FOURTEEN

Tests related to drug taking

Toxicology

Index of tests	Page
Alcohol	208
Asthma	204
Aminophylline	204
Barbiturates	206
Benzodiazepines	206
Cannabis	208
Carbamazepine	205
Carbon monoxide	207
Cardiac drugs	204
Cocaine	207
Cytotoxic drugs	204
Depression	205
Digoxin	204
Drug addiction	207
Drug overdose	206
Drunkenness	208
Epilepsy	204
Gammaglutamyl transferase (gGT)	208
Heroin	207
Lead	207
Lithium	205
LSD	207
Methadone	207
Malignancy	204
Morphine	207
Paracetamol	205
Phenytoin	204
Poisoning	206
Substances of abuse	208
Tricyclic antidepressants	206

Introduction

Toxicology is the study of drugs and poisons; their identification and measurement is the main function of a hospital toxicology laboratory, which is usually part of the department of chemical pathology. Measurement of drugs and poisons falls into three groups:

1. Therapeutic drug monitoring
2. Overdose and poisoning
3. Drug addiction and substances of abuse.

Therapeutic drug monitoring

The estimation of drug levels for monitoring therapy is a rapidly growing field. The indications include:

- Drugs with a narrow 'therapeutic window' whose serum levels need very careful control
- Difficult cases, for example, with poor intestinal absorption of a drug
- Altered drug distribution, for example, following leg amputation
- Subclinical toxicity, for example, in lithium or digoxin treatment
- A check on patient compliance
- Suspected drug interaction.

For several groups of drugs monitoring is particularly important. They include: cardiac drugs used in the control of *heart failure* (e.g. digoxin, digitoxin, quinidine), *asthma* (e.g. theophylline, aminophylline), *epilepsy* (anticonvulsant drugs, e.g. phenytoin, carbamazepine, ethosuximide), *depression* (e.g. lithium), *schizophrenia* (e.g. respiridone), *immunosuppression* (e.g. cyclosporin), *infection* (e.g. gentamycin) and *malignancy* (cytotoxic drugs).

The effect of drugs can also be studied by PET (see p.23).

Heart failure
Digoxin

Digoxin estimation is performed in cases of suspected digoxin intoxication. About 10 ml of clotted (or heparinized) blood is required, collected at least 6 hours after the last dose. A concentration of 1–2.5 nmol/litre is within the accepted therapeutic range. If therapy is prolonged the patient may develop tolerance, requiring an increased blood level. Over 3.0 nmol/litre is associated with digoxin toxicity.[1]

Asthma
Theophylline and aminophylline

Theophylline is a bronchodilator which requires careful monitoring because the toxic blood level is not very much greater than the therapeutic level,[1] which in adults is 55–100 µmol/L (10–18 mg/L). In the newborn it is 25–80 µmol/L (5–15 mg/L). For intravenous therapy, which must be given very slowly, *aminophylline* is used, the therapeutic range being 10–20 µg/ml, which must not be exceeded. About 5 ml of heparinized blood is required.

Epilepsy
Phenytoin

The accepted therapeutic range for serum phenytoin is 40–80 µmol/L, but should be modified according to the severity of the *epilepsy*. Levels of 20 µmol/L may control a 'mild' epileptic. Levels as high as 90 µmol/L may be appropriate in other patients. Any level above this can cause acute depression of the CNS, e.g. *drowsiness* and *nystagmus*.[1] Monitoring blood levels enables the appropriate dosage to be determined.

The effects of chronic toxicity, e.g. *gum hyperplasia*, are not directly related to serum drug levels. A 5 ml sample of clotted blood is required.

Carbamazepine

This is used for temporal lobe epilepsy and also for cases of grand mal and petit mal where phenytoin proves unsatisfactory.[1] It is effective at plasma levels of 20–40 μmol/L (5–10 mg/L). At levels over 45 μmol/L, *nystagmus, ataxia* and *drowsiness* occur, with more severe toxic effects as the level increases. About 5 ml of heparinized blood is required.

Ethosuximide

Ethosuximide is used in the control of petit mal. The accepted therapeutic range for the plasma level is 280–710 μmol/L. Toxicity is readily detected clinically, by *anorexia, nausea, vomiting* and *dizziness*. It is therefore only necessary to monitor the plasma levels if the patient is receiving multiple drug therapy, or to check compliance.[1] A 5 ml sample of heparinized blood is required.

Depression
Lithium

The use of lithium carbonate in the treatment of depression is controlled by the estimation of serum lithium, the accepted therapeutic range being 0.6–1.2 mmol/litre. It is important that the level should be checked on a regular basis, e.g. every three months. About 10 ml of clotted blood is required, collected at least 3 hours after the last dose.

Schizophrenia
Respiridone

One effect of respiridone is to raise the blood level of prolactin. This provides a useful method of checking compliance, since the degree of elevation of prolactin is related to the amount of respiridone taken. Ideally the prolactin level should be assayed (see p. 57) before starting treatment in order to establish a baseline. Estimating the blood level of respiridone is less helpful, since this will only confirm that a recent dose of respiridone has been taken, but does not confirm that the drug has been taken regularly to control the *schizophrenia*.

Immunosuppression
Cyclosporin

Cyclosporin is widely used in transplant surgery for immunosuppression. If the blood level is too high, the kidneys will be damaged; if too low, the transplant will be rejected.[1] Close cooperation between clinician and laboratory is essential. Although a blood level of 100–150 μmol/L is generally accepted, there are significant local variations, depending on reagents used. The laboratory should be consulted if assay is required.

Infection
Gentamycin

Gentamycin is frequently effective against anaerobic organisms which are resistant to other antibiotics. It is, however, essential that the blood concentration is sufficient, with a peak level of 5–7 μg/ml, but avoiding any rise above this level. Toxic levels cause damage to the kidneys, which is reversible, and to the ears, which is irreversible.[1] The laboratory should be consulted if assays are required.

Overdose and poisoning

Drug overdose

Estimation of the serum drug level is of great importance in a suspected overdose. Suspected salicylate or paracetamol overdose in particular must be investigated as an emergency. Both conditions are due to easily available drugs and are potentially lethal, but are readily treatable in their early stages.

The laboratory should be given detailed information about the patient, the circumstances of the suspected poisoning and any drugs likely to be available. Barbiturates, benzodiazepines and tricyclic antidepressants may be demonstrated by a quick screen. Other drugs take longer. About 10 ml clotted blood should be sent to the laboratory (heparinized blood in paracetamol poisoning, see below). In cases of suspected overdose, urine (at least 50 ml), stomach contents, vomit and/or gastric washings (see next section) should also be sent where relevant, but should not delay submission of the blood sample.

NB: Many apparent overdose cases are simply drunk. This is shown by blood alcohol estimation (see p. 208). On the other hand, *apparent drunkenness may be due to drugs or to illness such as cerebral haemorrhage or diabetic ketosis.*

Poisoning

In a case of suspected poisoning it is first necessary to exclude corrosive poisoning. The lips, upper surface of tongue and pharynx are examined for the marks of strong corrosives. If there is no evidence of corrosive poisoning a stomach tube should be passed and the stomach emptied (normally only up to 4 hours after taking the drug unless it is slowly absorbed). The stomach is then washed out with successive small quantities of water (about 250–300 ml). It should be repeated at least six times or until the washings are clear. Charcoal may be left in the stomach to prevent further absorption of some drugs. The stomach contents and first washings are kept for subsequent examination. Any vomit, urine or faeces should be kept in case required. It is also important to find, if possible, the glass or bottle from which the poison has been taken.

Antifreeze and herbicidal toxins such as Paraquat and Diquat require urgent attention and specialist clinical treatment. The assays needed for monitoring are only available in specialized toxicology laboratories but qualitative tests can be undertaken in most hospitals.

Investigation for bacterial food poisoning is described on p. 128. In suspected poisoning and drug overdose a 10 ml sample of clotted (heparinized for paracetamol) blood should be sent to the laboratory.

Paracetamol

In cases of paracetamol overdose the blood level of the drug determines whether treatment with an antidote is necessary. Some 4 hours after the overdose or as soon as possible thereafter, 10 ml of blood is taken into a heparin container and sent to the chemical pathology (clinical biochemistry) department for urgent estimation of the blood paracetamol level. The result is plotted on a graph (**Fig 14.1**), and the area in which it falls determines the treatment.

NB: Figure 14.1 outlines a recommended procedure, but there are regional variations.

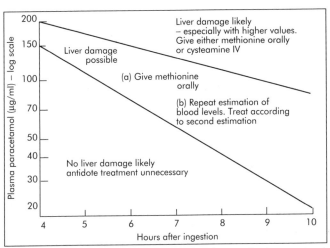

Fig. 14.1 Management of paracetamol overdose; liver damage related to paracetamol concentration and number of hours

Carbon monoxide

This is found in poisoning from a car exhaust, coal gas or products of incomplete combustion from oil heaters, fires and smouldering material. In fatal poisoning 30–95% of the haemoglobin is in the form of carboxyhaemoglobin. In non-smokers the figure is <2%, but in smokers it is 3–15%. See also last paragraph of 'abnormal haemoglobins', p. 100.

Lead

Minute quantities of lead are excreted by normal individuals. In cases of suspected lead poisoning the following examinations may be carried out:

1. *Haemoglobin and blood film.* Lead poisoning produces *anaemia* and *stippling of the red cells.*

2. *Urine for lead and coproporphyrin.* A complete 24-hour urine is collected. Lead excretion of over 1 mg per day suggests lead poisoning. There is also increased coproporphyrin excretion. (see p. 112).

3. *Blood lead level.* This should be less than 2 mmol/litre (40 mg/100 ml). Blood lead assay detects subclinical poisoning. Clinical effects only become evident with levels of 3–4 mmol/litre (60–80 mg/100 ml). Levels of 5–8 mmol/litre (100–160 mg/100 ml) are seen in lead encephalopathy and can be fatal.

Drug addiction and substances of drug abuse

'Hard drugs' include morphine, methadone (morphine substitute), heroin, cocaine and LSD. 'Soft drugs' include cannabis, barbiturates, benzodiazepines and tricyclic antidepressants. The last three mentioned and alcohol, with which many drugs are taken, can be measured accurately. Most of the other tests used are qualitative only and are carried out on urine. At certain centres, such as Tricho-Tec, Cardiff, hair may be used to detect whether certain drugs, e.g. heroin and methadone, have been taken within the previous few months. International bodies set limits for performance-enhancing drugs, e.g. anabolic steroids.

Substances of abuse

These include glue, felt pens and dry cleaning solvents. In cases of suspected abuse both urine and blood should be sent to the laboratory.

Alcohol (ethanol)

Blood alcohol estimation, as undertaken for legal reasons, is usually carried out by forensic laboratories, but when there is a clinical reason, e.g. *coma*, it can be undertaken by clinical laboratories.

About 5 ml of blood are sent to the laboratory in a fluoride oxalate (blood glucose) tube with a minimum of air space. Alcohol (ethanol) is usually measured enzymatically. Gas chromatography can also detect other alcohols such as methanol. The figures for urine alcohol are usually higher than those given by blood and are less reliable.

Blood levels in alcoholic intoxication:

slight	0.8–1.0 g/litre (80–100 mg/100 ml)
obvious	1.5 g/litre (150 mg/100 ml)
stupor	3.0 g/litre (300 mg/100 ml)

(*Urine levels are usually slightly higher.*)

In alcoholics the blood level of gammaglutamyl transferase (γGT, p. 117) is increased when there is no other evidence of liver damage, and the MCV (mean cell volume, p. 90) is raised, both changes persisting after the blood and urine alcohol have returned to normal.

Drunkenness

Evidence may be gained from the patient's appearance and behaviour. There may be abnormalities in the clothing, speech and gait. Injection of the conjunctiva and tremors may be present. Questions may be asked as to date, place and time, and an account of various happenings. Tests may be given in respect of coordination and writing. The smell of alcohol in the breath is not very reliable in itself. Conditions somewhat resembling drunkenness may be produced by illness, e g *diabetic precoma*, and by some drugs and therapeutic agents such as insulin. With the patient's permission, blood and urine may be collected and sent to the laboratory for alcohol estimation. Using a breathalyser the subject's breath can be analysed for its alcohol content.

Cannabis

In cannabis intoxication urine levels of cannabis derivatives usually exceed 100 mg/litre. About 5 ml of freshly collected urine is sent to the laboratory for urgent transmission to the Supraregional Assay Service (SAS) centre for radioimmunoassay. Samples more than 24 hours old are not acceptable.

Reference

1. Stewart, M J. Therapeutic drug monitoring. In: Marshall, W J and Bangert, S K, (eds). *Clinical Biochemistry: Metabolic and Clinical Aspects*. New York. Churchill Livingstone. 1955: 641–658.

CHAPTER FIFTEEN

Tests related to dying

Brain death | **autopsy**

Index of tests	Page
Autopsy	212
Body temperature and brain death	211
Diagnostic tests for brain death	210
Electroencephalography (EEG) and brain death	211
Informing the coroner	211
Obtaining relatives' permission	212
Organ donation and brain death	211
Post-mortem examination (autopsy)	212
Preconditions for brain death testing	209
Spinal reflexes in brain death	211

Introduction

Departments of intensive care are now so effective that they can keep a patient's body alive long after the brain is dead. Hence the need to test for brain death. This has medicolegal implications, both in relation to organ donation and in determining when it is appropriate to switch off life-sustaining equipment. Also included in this chapter is the autopsy examination, whose value should not be underestimated: for investigating the cause of death, the exact nature of a disease process, the effectiveness of certain forms of treatment and also in providing nurses with a realistic understanding of human anatomy.

Tests for brain death

Preconditions

Tests for brain death are only undertaken after all the following preconditions are met:

1. The patient is deeply comatose
   (a) There should be no suspicion that this state is a reversible depression of the nervous system due to *drugs* such as alcohol, narcotics, hypnotics or tranquillizers. The drug history should be reviewed and time allowed for the persistence of drug effects to be excluded.
   (b) *Primary hypothermia* as a cause of coma must be excluded.
   (c) *Metabolic and endocrine disturbances* which can cause or contribute to coma must be excluded. There should be no significant abnormality of blood electrolytes, acid–base balance or blood sugar.
2. The patient is being maintained on a ventilator because of apnoea (absent breathing)

The possibility that failure to breathe may have been caused by neuromuscular blocking drugs such as curare must be excluded. This may be done on the basis of the history and by the elicitation of spinal (deep) reflexes (p. 35) or the use of a nerve stimulator to check whether there is a neuromuscular block. Persistence of hypnotics and narcotics should also be excluded as a cause of *respiratory depression*.

3. There should be no doubt that the patient has suffered irreversible brain damage. The diagnosis of the cause should be firmly **established**.

It may become obvious within hours of a primary intracranial event such as *severe head injury, cerebral haemorrhage* or following neurosurgery that the condition is irreversible. However, after a *cardiac arrest, cerebral anoxia* of uncertain duration, *air or fat embolism* it may take much longer to determine the diagnosis and be certain of the prognosis.

Diagnostic tests for the confirmation of brain death

Five brainstem reflexes are tested and only if there is no response is the ultimate test undertaken, which is for the respiratory centre, also situated in the brainstem.

1. The pupils are fixed in diameter and do not respond to a bright light.

2. There is no corneal reflex (see p. 34).

3. The vestibulo-ocular reflexes are absent. Both ears should be examined to ensure that the external auditory canals are patent. About 20 ml of ice-cold water is then syringed into each ear in turn. There is no deviation of the eyes. This test may be contraindicated on one or other side by local injury.

4. No motor response within the cranial nerve distribution can be elicited by adequate stimulation of any somatic area, e.g. firm supraorbital pressure or a pencil pressed down firmly with the thumb against the patient's fingernail. There is no grimacing or screwing up of the eyes in response to such stimuli.

5. There is no gag reflex or response of any kind to stimulation of the air passages by a suction catheter passed through the larynx and trachea as far as the main bronchi.

6. The ultimate test. No respiratory movements occur when the patient is disconnected from the mechanical ventilator for long enough to raise the arterial carbon dioxide tension ($paCO_2$) above the threshold for stimulating respiration. To prevent *hypoxia* the patient breathes 100% oxygen for 10 minutes before testing and diffusion oxygen is maintained by continuing to deliver endotracheal oxygen at 6 litres/minute while the ventilator is disconnected. To ensure an adequate $paCO_2$ level the rate of the ventilator may be slowed or, preferably, the patient breathes 5% CO_2 in 95% oxygen for a further 5 minutes. The patient is then disconnected from the ventilator for 10 minutes. A $paCO_2$ of more than 6.65 kPa (50 mmHg) should by then have been reached, which is above the threshold for stimulating the respiratory centre. The final $paCO_2$ should be checked whenever possible (see pp. 73–74).

NB: Patients with *chronic respiratory deficiency*, who may be unresponsive to a raised $paCO_2$ and depend on *hypoxia* to stimulate the respiratory centre, are special cases requiring expert investigation and blood gas monitoring. Unless the evidence of irreversible brain damage is very obvious (see precondition 3) it is customary always to repeat the tests to ensure that there has been no observer error. The time interval between testing depends on medical judgement and may be as long as 24 hours. The diagnosis of brain death should be made by two doctors who have expertise in this field; one should be a consultant and the other either a consultant or senior registrar, not on the same firm. Neither should be a member of a transplant team.

Other considerations
Spinal reflexes
Spinal reflexes may persist, or disappear and then return after brain death has occurred.

Electroencephalography (EEG)
This may well be of value in assisting in the diagnosis of the underlying brain condition. However, it is now widely accepted that it is not necessary for the diagnosis of brain death.

Body temperature
Body temperature may be lowered either by drugs or by brainstem damage. It is recommended that it should not fall below 35°C. A low-reading thermometer should be used.

Organ donation
After the tests for brain death have been repeated the patient would usually not be reconnected to the ventilator unless organ donation is contemplated. In this case it is advisable for a death certificate to be issued at the time of reconnection, making it clear, particularly to relatives, that further ventilation is no longer treatment for the patient but is being done to ensure that organs are in the best possible condition for a recipient.

Investigating the cause of death

Informing the coroner
Her Majesty's coroner should be informed whenever the cause of death is unknown or when the cause of death may be due or partly due to other than natural causes. Conditions which could be due to occupational or accidental exposure to dust or chemicals, however long previously, should be reported. *Mesothelioma of the pleura*, for example, could be the result of exposure to asbestos 40 years previously and the occupation in which exposure was sustained may not be mentioned in the case notes. A chance word from a relative may be the only clue to occupational exposure initially, and should not be dismissed without enquiry. Although the responsibility for informing the coroner normally lies with the doctor looking after the patient, it may well be a nurse who gleans the relevant information.

Unnatural causes of death such as *drug overdose* should not be overlooked even though the terminal event may be a 'natural' condition such as *bronchopneumonia*. Similarly, death following any operative interference should be reported, even if the patient is dying from a 'natural' condition such as pulmonary embolism. Referral of the death certificate by the registrar of births and deaths, with the resultant delay in funeral arrangements, may cause much more distress to the relatives than referring the matter to the coroner in the first instance. Once a death has been reported to the coroner he or she may or may not order that an autopsy shall be undertaken, depending on the circumstances.

Obtaining relatives' permission

The relatives should only be requested to give permission for an autopsy (post-mortem examination) in cases where the death is not being reported to the coroner (or where the coroner has decided that he does not need to order an autopsy to establish the cause of death). It follows that such a request should only be made when death is due to natural causes and when the cause of death is already sufficiently well understood for the doctor (or the coroner) to complete the death certificate in the event of a refusal. The coroner should not be put in the position of having to order a post-mortem after the relatives have refused to grant permission.

Legislation concerning autopsies and retention of organs is being reviewed in the UK. When it is likely that there will be a need to retain any tissues, body fluids or organs, for all autopsies (including those ordered by the coroner) it is essential that relatives are involved in the decision:[1]

- Where a child has died, written parental consent to the removal, storage and use of such material for research must be obtained.

- Where an adult has died, reasonable efforts should be made to ascertain what the person would have wanted, for example by discussing the issues with their relatives or representatives, and reading any 'living will' or other statements made by that person, and then obtaining written permission.

- Clear information must be given to the family or representatives concerning the amount of material involved and, as far as possible, the nature of the research for which it will be used. Honesty and due consideration for the relatives' feelings are essential.

The decision to request permission for an autopsy is normally made by the doctor in charge of the case, usually the consultant or his deputy. The autopsy findings provide definitive 'quality control' on the diagnosis made and the treatment given during life. They may also extend scientific knowledge about disease processes and the effects of a particular form of therapy

Scope and types of autopsy

A full autopsy includes an external examination, and internal examination of the thoracic and abdominal viscera, the brain and, if indicated, the spinal cord and musculoskeletal system. Small portions of tissue may be collected into fixative (usually 10% formol saline) for histological examination, e.g. to determine the exact nature of a *tumour*. Blood, urine, CSF, stomach contents and tissues may be collected for chemical analyses, e.g. for drugs.

Relatives may request that only a limited post-mortem be undertaken, e.g. examination of the thoracic viscera only. In certain instances this may be adequate to provide the required information but insufficient to provide a complete picture of the disease processes.

For a coroner's post-mortem a full autopsy is almost invariably undertaken. Depending on the circumstances it may be necessary to make a detailed examination of any wounds or marks present or undertake special forensic tests on samples of semen, blood or hair which may have come from another person. It may be necessary to visit the site where the body was found so that the circumstances of the death may be more fully understood. All the relevant information is reported to the coroner, who will then decide whether an inquest needs to be held. In certain cases there will also be a police inquiry and perhaps further legal proceedings. However, the great majority of sudden deaths are the result of natural causes, such as *coronary atheroma*, with no necessity for an inquest.

Reference

1. General Medical Council. Research: the role and responsibility of doctors. London. General Medical Council. 2002: 13–14.

INDEX

Page numbers in bold indicate figures and tables.

Abdomen, X-ray examination, 137, 168
Abdominal reflex, 35
ABO blood groups, 103–104
Abortus fever, 16
Abscesses
  infection, tests for, 11
  lung, 64
Absolute values, blood investigations, 90
Accommodation, pupil reflexes, 33
Acetest, 145, 162
Acholuric jaundice, 99
Acid phosphatase, prostatic tumours, 185
Acidosis, 73
Acquired haemolytic anaemias, 99
Acquired immune deficiency syndrome (AIDS), 201
Acromegaly, 46, 56, 57, 58
Actinomycotic sinuses, 11
Activated partial thromboplastin time (APTT), 96
Activities of living, 1
Acute nephritis
  complement components C_3 and C_4, 112
  glomerular damage, 167
Acute pancreatitis, 142, 143
Addison's disease, 51, 53, 172
Adrenal gland, 50–53
  adenoma and carcinoma, 57
  cortex, 50–51
  hyperplasia, 57
  medulla, 55
Adrenal hyperplasia, congenital, 52, 53
Adrenocortical insufficiency, 52
Adrenocorticotrophic hormone (ACTH)
  assay, anterior pituitary assessment, 57
  stimulation test, 53–53
Adult mental function, 41
Adult-onset congenital adrenal hyperplasia, 52
Agglutination tests, 16
Agranulocytosis, 93
Air contamination, 10
Air encephalography, 39, 40
Airway resistance and conductance, 73
Alanine aminotransferase (ALT), 116
Albumin, 118, 162
Albustix, 162
Albym Test, 162
Alcohol, blood level estimation, 208
  see also Drunkenness
Alcohol test meal, 135, 136
Alcoholics, gammaglutamyl transferase and mean cell volume, 208
Aldolase, 116
Aldosterone assay, 51–52
Aldosteronism, 52
Alimentary tract investigations
  foreign body localization, 22

lower, 153–155
  oesophagus, 129–130
  stomach and intestines, 130–136, 149–150
  upper, 128–129
Alkaline phosphatase, 111, 138
Alkalosis, 73
Allergies, 8, 9–10
  white blood count, 92
Alpha, antitrypsin, 110
Alpha hydroxybutyrate dehydrogenase (aHBD), 117
Alpha-fetoprotein, 119–120
  amniocentesis, 192
Alzheimer's disease in third decade of life, 184
Ambulatory monitoring, cardiac, 80, 81
Amino acids
  blood analysis, 110
  urine, 170
Aminophylline, 204
Aminotransferases, 116
Ammonia, plasma, 130
Amniocentesis, 190, 191, 192
Amniotic fluid embolism, DIC, 97
Amoebic dysentery, 156–157
Amylase, 142–143
Anaemias, 88, 89
  absolute values, interpretation, 90
  anaplastic, 92, 93
  haematocrit, 90
  haemolytic, 98–101, 172
    see also Haemolytic disease of the newborn
  reticulocytosis, successful treatment response, 91
Anaesthetic areas, malingering, 36
Anaplastic anaemia, 92, 93
Androstenedione, 188
Anencephaly, 189
Aneurysms, 83
Angina, 81
Angiography, 83
  angiocardiography, 83–84
  brain studies, 39
  coronary, 84
  mobility, problems of, 176
  pulmonary, 64
  renal, 169–170
Anion gap, 115
Ankylosing spondylitis, 102
Antenatal blood tests, 104–105
Anterior pituitary function, 56–59
Antibacterial drugs, assay, 12
Antibodies, tests for, 17–19
  acquired haemolytic anaemias, 99
  antiglobulin (Coombs' test), 107
  antispermatozoal, 186
  autoantibodies, rheumatic disease, 102
  fluorescent antibody technique, 103
  haemolytic disease of the newborn, 105
  thyroid, tests for, 48
  viral or rickettsial infections, 13
Anticoagulation, prothrombin ratio, 95, 128

Antidiuretic hormone see Vasopressin (antidiuretic hormone)
Antifreeze ingestion, 206
Antigen tests, 14, 17
Antiglobulin (Coombs') test, 107
Antinuclear factor (ANF), 103
Antispermatozoal antibodies in serum, 186
Aphasia, 26
Apical heart rate, 79
Arterial disease, 85
Arthritis, 176
Arthrocentesis, 178
Arthrography, 176
Arthroscopy, 178–179
Articulation disturbance, tests for, 26
Ascitic fluid, 150
Ascorbic acid saturation test, 127
Ashby's method, red cell survival, 101
Aspartate transferase (AST), 116
Aspergillosis, antibody test, 17
Asthma
  drug monitoring, 204
  exercise-induced, 72
  skin tests, 9
  sputum, examination of, 65
  white blood count, 92
Atrial fibrillation, 79, **80**
Atrial septal defect, cardiac catheterization, 84
Audiometry, 29–30
Auditory nerve, examination, 34
Aural thermometers, 19
Autoantibody tests for rheumatic diseases, 102
Autoclaves, check on functioning, 10
Autohaemolysis, 99–100
Autoimmune disease, 94
  fluorescent antibody technique, 103
  see also Rheumatoid arthritis
Autopsy, 212–213
Aylesbury and Ayre's spatulae, 197, 198
Azostix, 165

Babinski's sign, 35
Bacteraemia, 16
  DIC, bacterial septicaemia, 97
Bacteria
  CSF, 32
  infections, 11
  sputum, 65
  urine, bacterial counts, 161, 164
Bactericidal activity, 103
Barbiturates, urine, 170
Barium studies
  enema, 155–156
  follow-through, 131–132
  meal, 131
  swallow, 130
BCG (bacille Calmette-Guérin), 15
Bell's palsy, 33
Bence-Jones protein, 171
Benedict's test, 145, 173
Benign prostatic hyperplasia, 185
Bernstein, Baker and Earlam test, 129

Beta subunit human chorionic
  gonadotrophin, 189
Bicarbonate(CO₂), 73, 113
Bile
  duodenal aspiration test, 144
  urine tests for pigments, 137–138
Bilharziasis, antibody test, 18
Biliary obstruction, cholesterol levels,
  112
Bililabstix, 163
Bilirubin
  amniocentesis, 191
  serum, 99, 138
  urine, 137–138, 163
Bilur Test, 138, 163
Biopsy, 3–4
  bone, 179
  breast, 195–196
  bronchoscopy, 74
  colposcopy, 198
  duodenal, 133
  frozen section, 4
  gastroscopy, 132
  gonadal, 188
  laryngeal, 27
  liver puncture, 140–141
  lymph node, 93
  needle, 4–5
  ovarian, 186
  parathyroid, 50
  pleural needle biopsy, 75
  prostate, 182, 185
  renal, 167–168
  salivary gland, 129
  skin, 8–9
  small intestine, 149
  thyroid, 49
  see also Fine needle aspiration
    (FNA) cytology
Biopty gun, 4
Bladder, cystoscopy, 170
Blanket contamination, testing for,
  10–11
Bleeding time, 94
Blood chemistry, 109
Blood counts, 88
  and related investigations, 88–93
Blood cultures, 16
Blood films
  haemolytic anaemias, 98
  sex chromatin, 183
Blood gases, 73–74
  fetal scalp blood, 192
Blood groups, 103–104
  blood group labels, **106**
  haemolytic anaemia of the
    newborn see Haemolytic
    disease of the newborn
  paternity, tests related to, 184
Blood pressure, 77–78
Blood samples
  collection, 5
  renin-angiotensin system, 78
Blood sugar, 145–147
Blood tests
  alcohol, 208
  allergies, 9–10
  anterior pituitary function
    assessment, 56, 57
  antibody and antigen tests, 16–19

ascorbic acid, 127
blood grouping, 103–108, 184
calcium, 49, 50, 110–111
chemical analysis, 109–121
copper and caeruloplasmin, 112
drug overdose, 206, 206–207
glucose and insulin levels,
  145–147, 148
gonadal endocrine function,
  187–188
haemolytic anaemias, 98–101
haemorrhagic disorders, 93–98
infections, 16–19
lead, 207
liver function, 138–139
microbiology, 16
neonatal screening, 193–194
pancreatic and related tumours,
  149
parasites, 92
paternity, 184
phenylalanine, 193
placental and fetal function, 190
serum amylase, 142
sexually transmitted diseases,
  200–201
steroids, 51–52
theraputic drug monitoring,
  204–205
urea, 165–166
see also Haematology
Blood transfusion, 103–108
  essentials of, 105–108
  grouping, crossmatching and
    storage, 105–106
  multiple, 91
Blood in urine see Haematuria
BM Autoclix, 146
BM Reflotest-Glycemie, 146
BM Test Glycemie 1–44, 146
BM multitest strip, 163
Body plethysmography, 71
Body temperature
  artificial, malingering, 37
  and brain death tests, 211
  infection, 19
Boiling, urine, 162
Bone biopsy, 179
Bone cysts, 176
Bone density measurements, 176,
  178
Bone disease, radiological
  demonstration of, 177–178,
  179
Bone marrow puncture, 4, 93
Bone scans, 176
Bones and joints
  other tests related, 178–179
  skeletal system imaging, 176–177
Bowie-Dick test, 10
Brain biopsy and smear, 40
Brain damage, irreversible, 210
Brain death tests, 209–213
  blood gas estimates, 73–74
  confirmation of brain death,
    210–211
  preconditions, 209–210
Brain scans, radioisotope, 38
Brain and spinal cord, detailed
  studies, 38–40
Brain tumour, visual field, 28

Brainstem reflexes, brain death tests,
  210
Brainstem response audiometry,
  30
Breast examination, 194–196
  biopsy, 195–196
  screening, 182
British ratio (BR) (prothrombin
  ratio), 95
Bronchial brushings, 74
Bronchiectasis, 64
Bronchography, 63
Bronchoscopy, 74
Browne's tube, 10
Brucellosis, 16
Buccal squames, 183
BUN (blood urea nitrogen), 166

C-reactive protein, 112–113
Ca 19–9, 120
Ca-125, 120–121
Caeroplasmin, 112
Calcitonin, 111
Calcium
  blood analysis, 110–111
    hypoparathyroidism, 50
    parathyroid investigation, 49,
      50
  urine, 171
Caloric test, 34
Candidiasis, antibody test, 17
Cannabis, 208
Capillary microscopy, 94
Capillary resistance test, 94
Carbamazepine, 204, 205
Carbon monoxide poisoning, 207
Carboxyhaemoglobin, 207
Carcinoembryonic antigen (CEA),
  119
Cardiac catheterization, 83–84
Cardiac function, tests of, 79–83
Cardiac infarction, enzymes:CPK,
  γGT, LDH, γHBD, 117
Cardiac monitoring, 80, 81, **82**
  fetal, 192
Cardiothoracic patient, physiotherapy
  assessment, 179
Cardiovascular system imaging,
  83–86
Carotid angiography, 39
Carriers
  diphtheria, 62–63
  organisms and parasites in stools,
    156
  streptococci, 63
  typhoid, 16
Casoni test, 14
Casts, urine, 165
Cat-scratch fever
  antigen test, 14
  lymph node biopsy, 93
Catecholamines, 55
Catheterization, obtaining urine
  sample, 163–164
Central venous pressure, 85–86
Cerebral tumour, perimeter and field
  analyser tests, 28
Cerebrospinal fluid (CSF)
  examination of, 30–32
  findings, **32**

pressure, 31
routine investigation, 31
Cerebrospinal meningitis, 32
Cervical cytology, 197
Chancre, 200
Chemical markers
myocardial ischaemia, 81–83
tumour markers, 119–121
Chemistry (chemical pathology), 109-122
Chest X-rays, 63–65
Chest pain, oesophagitis, distinguishing from other causes, 129
Children
AFP, raised, 120
calcium, blood levels, 110
consent forms, 2
cortisol levels, 51
glucagon test, 58
mental development tests, 41
peak flow rate (PFR), **69**
vulvovaginitis, 198
Chinitest, 145
Chlamydia trachomatis, 199
Chloride, 113
CSF examination, meningitis, 32
urine, 171–172
Cholangiography, 142
Cholecystography, 141
Cholesterol, 111–112
Cholinesterase levels, 116
Choriocarcinoma, 189
Chorion epithelioma, 189
Chorionic villous sampling, 190, 192
Christmas disease, 94, 96
Chromatography, urine, 170
Chromosome studies, 182, 183
fetal material, 191
Chronic myeloid leukaemia, 92
Chronic nephritis, 111, 112, 113
Chronic pancreatitis, serum amylase, 142
Chronic respiratory deficiency and brain death tests, 210–211
Chvostek's sign, 50
Cineradiography, musculoskeletal system, 176
Circulation, tests related to, 77–86
Cisternal puncture, CSF examination, 31
Clinitest, 173
Clomiphene test, 58
Clonus response, 35
Closed circuit helium rebreathing method, 71
Clostridium botulinum, 128
Clostridium perfringens, 128
Clot retraction, 94
Clotting factors, 88
Clotting time, 94
Coagulation factor assays, 96–97
Coccidioimycosis
antibody test, 17
coccidioidin test, 14
Coeliac disease, 150
blood calcium levels, 111
small intestine biopsy, 149
Colonoscopy, 154–155

Colour tests, 27
Colposcopy, 197, 198
Complement C_1 esterase inhibitor, 112
Complement components C_3 and C_4, 112
Complete spinal block, cysternal puncture, 31
Computerized tomography (CT), 21
abdomen, 151
brain and spinal cord, 38
foreign body localization, 22
musculoskeletal system, 176
oesophageal tumour, 130
pituitary gland, 56
thoracic, 84
thyroid, 48
Congenital abnormalities
alpha antitrypsin deficiency, 110
chromosome studies, 183
congenital adrenal hyperplasia, 52, 53
hypothyroidism, 193–194
inborn errors of metabolism, 193–194
urine, amino acids, 170
Conn's syndrome, 52
Consent, 2–3
skin biopsy, 8
Coombs' test, 107
Coordination, 35–36
Copper
blood levels, 112
excessive zinc intake, 121
Cordocentesis, 190, 192
Corneal reflex, 34
Coronary angiography, 84
Coroner, informing the, 211–212
Coroner's post-mortem, 213
Cortical evoked response audiometry, 30
Cortisol
combined anterior pituitary function tests, 59
plasma levels, 51
urine levels, 52
Cortisone test, hyperparathyroidism, 49
Cranial nerves, examination, 33–35
Creatine kinase (CK, CPK), 83, 117, 179
Creatinine, 112
urine, 171
Creatinine clearance test, 167
Crosby capsule, 149
Crossmatching blood for transfusion, 105–106
Cryoglobulins, 119
Cryptococcal infection
antibody test, 17
CSF microscopy, 32
Crystals, urine, 165
Culture plates, 10
bacterial, 32
Culture, viruses, 13
Curettage, 9
Cushing's disease, 46, 51, 52, 59
Cushing's syndrome, 51, 55, 57, 58
Cyclic AMP (adenosine monophosphate), 113

parathyroid investigation, 50
Cyclosporin, 205
Cystic duct obstruction, 142
Cystine, urine, 170, 171
Cystogram, 169
Cystoscopy, 170
Cytology
bronchial brushings and washings, 74
gastroscopy material, 132
gynaecological, 197–198
sputum, 65
urine, 165
see also Fine needle aspiration (FNA) cytology
Cytomegalovirus medium, 12

Deafness
hearing tests, 29–30
malingering, 37
Death certificate and organ donation, 211
Death, investigating cause of, 211–213
Deep reflexes, 35
Definitive Synacthen test, 54
Dehydration, 90, 114
Dehydroepiandrosterone, 188
Denver tests, 41
11-deoxycortisol, 52
Depression, monitoring therapeutic drugs, 205
Dexamethasone suppression test, 53, 54–55, 59
Diabetes insipidus, 59
cranial and nephrogenic, differentiation between, 60, 116
Diabetes mellitus, 57, 144–148
blood sugar levels, 146
cholesterol levels, 112
pregnancy, human placental lactogen assay, 190
retinal examination, 33
Diabetic coma, prolonged, inorganic phosphate levels, 111
Diarrhoea, causes of, 157
Dicopac test, 127, 136
Differential agglutination test, 101
Differential white cell count, 92–93
Diffusing capacity, lung function, 71
Digoxin, 204
Dihyrotestosterone, 188
Dip innoculum transport outfits, 161, 164
Diphtheria
test for, 15–16
throat swab, 62–63
Dipslide, 161, 164
Dipspoon, 161, 164
Diquat, ingestion, 206
Direct antiglobulin test, haemolytic anaemias, 99
Direct laryngoscopy, 27
Diastolic blood pressure, 78
Discharges
infection, tests for, 11
urethral, 199–200
vaginal, 198–199

Discrimination, vibration and position
sense, 36
Dislocations, 177
Disseminated intravascular
coagulation (DIC)
screening, 97
thrombin clotting time, 98
Disseminated lupus erythematosus
(DLE), 103
two-stage prothrombin test, 95
Distraction tests, hearing, 29
Dizziness, malingering, 37
Donath-Landsteiner test, 99
Doppler ultrasound, 85
Double contrast radiography, 131,
155
Double gel diffusion test, 10, 17
Dressings, sterility of, 10
Drug monitoring, 203–208
addiction and drug abuse,
207–208
overdose and poisoning,
206–207
therapeutic drugs, 204–205
Drunkenness, 208
apparent, 206, 208
Dual energy X-ray absorptiometry,
176, 178
Duodenal aspiration tests, pancreatic
function, 143–144
Duodenal biopsy, 149
gastroscopy, 133
Duodenum
barium meal, 131
ulcer, pentagastrin test meal
findings, **135**
Dye excretion test, 167
Dying, tests related to, 209–213
Dynamic lung volumes and flow
volume, 68, 69–71
Dysphasia, 26

Ear lobe capillary blood, pH and gas
analysis, 72
Eating and drinking, tests related to,
123–151
Echocardiography, 85
E. coli, 128, 164
Ectopic ACTH, hormone secreting
tumour, 57
Electrical response audiometry,
30
Electrocardiogram (ECG), 79–**80**,
80, 81
exercise, 79
Electrocochlearography, 30
Electroencephalography (EEG), 38
brain death tests, 211
Electrolytes, 113–116
normal values, **113**
urine, 171–172
Electromyography (EMG), 41
Electron microscopy, viral and
rickettsial infections, 14
Electrophoresis
abnormal haemoglobins, 100
urine, 172
Elliptical surgical biopsy, skin, 8
Elliptocytes, 98
Emphysema

alpha, antitrypsin deficiency,
110
flow volume loops, 71
Empyema, 64
pleural fluid, 67
Encephalography, 39, 40
Endocervical scrape, 198
Endocrine system, 44–60
Endoscopic retrograde
cholangiopancreatography
(ERCP), 144
Endoscopy, arthroscopy, 178–179
Environment and the human body,
8–23
Enzymes, blood levels, 116–118
Epilepsy, therapeutic drug
monitoring, 204–205
Epinephrine, 55
Epithelial cells, urine, 165
Erb's sign, 50
Erythrocyte sedimentation rate
(ESR), 89
Erythrocyte transketolase activity,
126
Erythrocytes see Red blood cells
Erythropoietic porphyria, 157
Escherichia coli, 128
urine, 164
ESR, 89
Ethosuximide, 205
Euglobin lysis time (ELT), 97
Excision biopsy, 3–4, 196
breast, 196
salivary gland, 129
Exercise tolerance tests, 79
Exercise-induced asthma test, 72
Exophthalmic goitre, 49
Exophthalmos, 49
Extracellular fluid, 114
Extrinsic allergic alveolitis, 9–10
Eye swabs, 12–13

Facial nerve, examination, 33
Factor assay, 96–97
Faeces, examination of, 156–157
pancreatic function, 143
Fallopian tubes, patency, 186
salpingogram, 186
Familial cholinesterase deficiency,
117
Fantus, method of, 172
Fat in stools, 143
FE-CULT, 156
Female genital tract, tests relating to,
196–199
infertility, 185–186
Ferritin, 91
Fetal cells in maternal blood, 105
Fetal defects, 190–191
amniocentesis, 191, 192
genetic, tests for, 183
Fetal distress, assessment of, 192
Fetal haemoglobin, 100
Fetal heart monitoring, 192
Fetal lung maturity, 191, 192
Fetal material, sampling, 190–191
scalp blood examination, 190,
192
Fetus, intrauterine death, 96, 97,
189

Fibreoptics
colonoscopy, 154
gastroscopy, 132, **133**
oesophagoscopy, 130
Fibrindex, 96
Fibrinogen, 96, 118
Fibrinolysin, 97
Fibrocystic disease, sweat test, 143
Fibroid lung, 64
Field analyser, visual field testing, 28
Fine needle aspiration (FNA)
cytology, 5
breast, 195
liver, 141
lung, 75
pancreas, 148
prostate, 182, 185
salivary gland, 129
thyroid, 49
Flow volume loops, 70, **71**
Fluid balance, 115, 161
Fluid volumes, measurement of, 115
Fluorescent antibody technique, 103
Fluoroscopic screening, 20
barium swallow, 130
chest, 63
Folic acid, 127
Follicle stimulating hormone (FSH)
assay, 57
Follow-through barium examination,
131–132
Food poisoning, 128
Forced expiratory volume in 1
second (FEV₁), 69, **70**
Forced vital capacity, 70
Foreign bodies, 21, 22
bronchoscopy, 74
oesophagoscopy, 130
Fractures, 177
Franzen needle, 185
Free cortisol, urine, 52
Free T₃ index, 45, 46
Free T₄ index, 45, 46
Frei test, lymphogranuloma
venereum, 201
Frozen section, 4
breast, 195, 196
parathyroid, 50
thyroid, 49
Fructosamine, 148
Full autopsy, 212, 213
Functional brain scans, PET, 23, 39
Fungal infections, skin, 13

Galactosaemia, neonatal screening,
194
Gall bladder and bile ducts,
141–142
Gallium scanning, 23
Gamma globulin (IgG), 118
Gammaglobulin neutralization test,
108
Gammaglutamyl transferase, 117
alcoholics, 208
Gastric cancer, pentagastrin test
meal findings, **135**
Gastric secretion tests, 130,
134–136
Gastric ulcer
barium meal, 131

pentagastric test meal findings, **135**
Gastric washings, tubercle bacilli, 66
Gastrin, 136
Gastrocamera examination, 134
Gastrointestinal bleeding scan, 151
Gastroscopy, 132–133
Geiger counters, 23
Genetic fingerprinting, 182
  paternity, tests related to, 184
Gentamycin, 205
Gerhardt's test, 145
German measles, antibodies, 18
Glandular fever, 92, 98
  tests for, 101
Glaucoma, intraocular pressure, 29
Globulin, 118
Glomerular filtration rate, 167
Glossopharyngeal nerve,
  examination, 34
Glucagon, 149
  test, 58
Glucagonomas, 149
Glucose
  blood levels, 145–147
  CSF examination, 32
  in urine, 144–145, 162, 163
Glucose tolerance tests, 147–148
  intestinal malabsorption, 150
Glucose-6-phosphate
  dehydrogenase (G6PD)
  deficiency, 100
Glucostix, 146
Glutathione stability test, 100
Glycosylated haemoglobin, 147
Gonadal biopsy, 188
Gonadal endocrine function
  investigations, 187–188
Gonadotrophin releasing hormone
  tests, 58
Goniometry, 178
Gonococci, urethral discharge,
  199
Graves' disease, 47
Gravinex, 189
Griffiths' tests, 41
Grouping and crossmatching,
  bloods, 105–106
Growth hormone assay, 57, 158
Guinea pig test, 67
Guthrie test, 193–194
Gynaecological cytology, 197–198

Haemagglutination inhibition tests,
  189
Haemastix, 162
Haematocrit, 90
Haematology, 88–103
  see also Blood transfusion
Haematuria, 162, 165
Haemochromatosis, 91
Haemoglobin, 88–89
  abnormal, 98, 100
  carboxyhaemoglobin, 207
  glycosylated, 147
  haemoglobin S, 98
  haemolytic anaemias, 98
  lead poisoning, 207
Haemolysins, 99
Haemolysis, 99

Haemolytic anaemias, 88, 91
  acquired, 99
  investigations for, 98–101
  porphyrins in urine, 172
Haemolytic disease of the newborn,
  99, 104, 105, 107, 108
  routine tests for, 105
  severity, determining, 191
Haemolytic jaundice, 139
  laboratory test results, **140**
  serum bilirubin, 138
  urobilin and urobilinogen in urine,
  173
Haemolytic reactions, transfusions,
  107
Haemolytic streptococci, 63
Haemophilia, 94
Haemoptysis, malingering, 37
Haemorrhagic disorders, 93–98
Ham's test, 99
Haptoglobin, serum estimation, 98
Heaf test, 15
Hearing tests, 29–30
Heart, X-ray examination, 83
Heart failure, therapeutic drug
  monitoring, 204
Heart monitoring, 80, 81, **82**
  fetal, 192
Heart murmurs, phonocardiography,
  85
Heart scan, radioisotope, 84–85
Heat and cold, sensation to, 36
Heinz body test, 100
Helicobacter pylori antibodies
  and peptic ulceration risk, 132
Helisal rapid blood test, 132
HEMA-CHEK, 156
Heparin treatment
  APTT, 96
  clotting time, 94
Hepatitis, 101
  blood tests for, 16–17
Hepatoerythropoietic porphyria,
  157
Hepatolenticular degeneration, 112
Herbicidal toxins, ingestion, 206
Hereditary angioneurotic edema
  (HANE)
  complement C₁ esterase inhibitor,
  112
Heredity, tests related to, 183–184
Heriditary spherocytosis, 99
Herpes genitalis, 199
Hess's test, 94
High dose dexamethasone
  suppression test, 54
High-risk specimens, 12
Hippuric acid test, 139
Hirsutism, idiopathic, 188
Histamine test meal, 135, 136
Histology, 3–5
Histoplasmin test, 14
Histoplasmosis, 14, 17
HLA-B27 antigen, test for, 102
Hodgkin's disease, 83, 93
Hollander test, 135
Hookworms, 157
Hopkins Rod, 27
Human chorionic gonadotrophin
  (hCG), 188

pregnancy tests, 188, 189
  as tumour marker, 120
Human growth hormone secretion,
  57
  insulin tolerance test, 58
Human immunodeficiency virus
  (HIV), 201
Human papillomavirus, cervical
  cytology, 197
Human placental lactogen assay,
  190
Hyaline casts, urine, 165
Hydatid disease, 64
  antibody test, 18
  Casoni test, 14
Hydatidiform mole, 46, 188,
  189
17-hydroxycorticosteroid excretion,
  52
  in alternative dexamethasone
  suppression test, 54–55
5-hydroxyindoleacetic acid, urine,
  172
17-hydroxyprogesterone, 52
5-hydroxytryptamine (serotonin),
  urine, 172
Hyland LE test, 103
Hyland RA test, 101–102
Hyperkalaemia, 115
Hypernatraemia, 114
Hyperparathyroidism, 49, 111
Hypertension, 78
  retinal examination, 33
Hyperthyroidism, 45, 171
  special signs associated, 49
Hypoglossal nerve, examination,
  34
Hypogonadism, 187, 188
Hypokalaemia, 115
Hyponatraemia, 114
Hypoparathyroidism, 50
  blood calcium levels, 111
  calcitonin, 111
  cyclic AMP levels, 113
Hypopituitarism, 58, 188
  glucagon test, 58
  plasma cortisol, 51
Hypotension, 78
Hypothalamus, 34
Hypothyroidism, 45, 46
  congenital, 193–194
  plasma cortisol, 51

Ictotest, 138
Idiopathic hirsutism, 188
IgE, 9, 118–119
IgG, IgM, 118
Ileal biopsy, 149
Imaging techniques, 20–23
Immune paresis studies, 118
Immunofluorescent test for thyroid
  antibody, 48
Immunoglobulins, 118–119
Immunosuppression, drug
  monitoring, 205
In-vitro fertilization, pre-implantation
  genetic diagnosis, 184
Inborn errors of metabolism,
  neonatal screening, 193–194
Indirect laryngoscopy, 27

Infants
  haemolytic disease of newborn, 99, 104, 105, 107, 108, 191
  hearing tests, 29
  inborn errors of metabolism, 193–194
  rotavirus, 157
  temperature taking, 19
Infected materials, collecting, 11, 12
Infection, 8
  acute
    alpha antitrypsin, 110
    white blood count, 92
  drug monitoring, 205
  gallium scanning, 23
  in milk, 125
  tests for, 10–19
    blood tests, 16–19
    environmental, 10–11
    infections, 11–14
    skin tests, 11–16
    temperature, 19
Infertility, tests related to, 185–186
Influenza virus, tissue culture, 13
Inorganic phosphate, blood levels, 111
Insulin, 144–148
  anterior pituitary function combined test, 58
  serum, 148
Insulin test meal, 135
Insulin tolerance test, 58
  human growth hormone deficiency, 57
Insulin-induced hypoglycaemia stimulation test, 58
Intelligence quotient (IQ), 41
Intensive care patients, physiotherapy assessment, 179
International normalized ratio (prothrombin ratio), 95
Intestinal absorption, tests for, 149–150, 171
  intravenous glucose tolerance test, 148
Intestinal parasites, 157
Intraocular pressure, 29
Intrauterine death of fetus
  plasma fibrinogen, 96
  retained, DIC, 97
Intravascular haemolysis, haptoglobin estimation, 98
Intravenous cholangiogram, 142
Intravenous glucose tolerance test, 148
Intravenous short Synacthen test, 54
Intravenous urography, 168
Inulin clearance test, 167
Iron, 91
  deficiency, 90, 91
  serum, 91, 139
Iron saturation, 91
Iron-binding capacity, red blood cells, 91
Ischaemic heart disease
  cholesterol levels, 112
Ishihara charts, 27
Ivy's method, bleeding time, 94

Jaundice, 139
  alcoholic, 99
Joffroy's sign, 49
Joint fluid examination, 178
Joint mice, 178
Juvenile cirrhosis, 110

Kaolin cephalin time, 96
Kernig's sign, 30
17-Ketogenic steroids see Total 17-oxyogenic steroids
Ketones, tests for, 145, 162
17-Ketosteroids, 52
Ketostix, 162
Ketur Test, 162
Kidney disease, blood creatinine, 113
Kidney failure, blood magnesium levels, 111
Kidney investigations
  angiography, 169–170
  functional tests, 165–168
  intravenous urography, 168
  renal biopsy, 167–168
  scan, nuclear medicine, 169
  ultrasound, 169
Kidney stones, 171
Kleihauer test, fetal cells in maternal blood, 105
Klinefelter's syndrome, 186, 188
Klintex autoclave test paper, 10
Knee
  arthroscopy, 178–179
  jerk reflex, 35
Kveim test, 14

Laboratory investigations, 3–6
Labstix, 162–163
Lactate
  CSF examination, meningitis, 32
  fetal scalp blood, 192
Lactic dehydrogenase, 117
Language disturbance, tests for, 26
Laparoscopy, 150, 196
Laparotomy, 151
Large bore needle biopsy, liver, 140
Large intestine
  barium enema, 155–156
  barium follow-through examination, 132
Larynx
  laryngeal swab, tubercle bacilli, 66
  laryngoscopy, 27
Lassa fever, 12
Lead poisoning, 91, 207
  porphyrins in urine, 172
Lecithin level, fetal lung maturity, 192
Lee and White method, clotting time, 94
Legionnaire's disease, antibody test, 18
Legislation, autopsy and organ retention, 212
Leptospira antibody test, 18
Leucocytes see White blood cells
Leucocytosis, 92
Leucopenia, 92
Leukaemia, 92
  acute, 94

copper and caeruloplasmin levels, 112
  lymph node biopsy, 93
  white blood count, 92
Light, pupillary reaction to, 33
Limb paralysis, malingering, 37
Limited post-mortem, 212
Liquid based cytology, cervical scrape, 197
Lithium carbonate, 205
Liver biopsy, 140–141
Liver damage, 137–141
  acute
    AST levels, 116
    paracetamol overdose, **207**
Liver disease, 137–141
  cholesterol levels, 112
  gammaglutamyl transferase, 117
  haptoglobin, 98
  laboratory results, **140**
  plasma fibrinogen, 96
  porphyrins in urine, 172
  prothrombin ratio, 95
  thrombin clotting time, 98
Liver failure, amino acids in urine, 170
Liver function tests
  additional, 139–141
  interpretation, 139
  routine, 137–139
Liver imaging, 137
Low dose dexamethasone suppression test, 54
Lower motor neurone disease, tests for physiotherapy assessment, 180
Lower respiratory tract investigations, 63–75
Lumbar puncture, 30–31
Lumpectomy, 196
Lundh test, duodenal aspiration test, 144
Lung, fibrosis, FEV₁, 69, **70**
Lung function tests, 67–74
  postbasic tests, 72–73
Lung scans, 63–64
Lupus erythematosus 'cell preparation' test, 103
Luteinizing hormone (LH) assay, 56
Lymph node biopsy, 93
Lymph nodes enlargement, mediastinoscopy, 74
Lymphangiography, 83
Lymphogranuloma venereum, 201
Lymphoma, lymph node biopsy, 93

Macrocytic anaemia, 90
  see also Pernicious anaemia
Macrocytic red blood cells, 91
Macroglobulin (IgM), 118
Magnesium
  blood levels, 111
  urine, 171
Magnetic resonance imaging (MRI), 21
  bones, joints and tendons, 176, 176–178
  brain scan, 38, **39**, 56
  thyroid, 48
Malaria, 92

Male genital tract
  infertility, 186
  urethral discharge, 199
Malingering, 36–37
Mammography, 182, 194
Mantoux test, 15
Mass screening, inborn errors of
  metabolism, 193
Mean cell diameter, 90
Mean cell haemoglobin, 90
Mean cell volume (MCV), 90
  alcoholics, 208
Mediastinoscopy, 74
Mediastinotomy, 74
Mediterranean anaemia, 91, 100
  red cell osmotic fragility, 99
Medullary carcinoma, thyroid,
  calcitonin, 111
Membranes, tests for premature
  rupture, 193
Ménière's syndrome, 34
Meningeal irritation, 30
Meningism, 30
Meningitis, 30
  CSF examination, 31–32
Meningococci, meningitis, CSF
  stained film and culture, 32
Mental age, 41
Mental development tests, 41
Mental symptoms, malingering, 37
Mercury thermometers, 19
Mesothelioma, 211
  pleural needle biopsy, 75
Methaemalbumin, Schumm's test,
  101
Methaemoglobin reduction test, 100
Methicillin resistant *S. aureus*
  (MRSA), 11
Mice, joint, 178
Microbiology, 10–19
  blood tests, 16
  folic acid assay, 127
  sputum, 65
  urine, examination of, 163–164
Microcytic hypochromic anaemia, 90
  see also Iron: deficiency
Microcytic red blood cells, 91
Microscopy
  blood, wet films, 98
  CSF, cryptococcal infection, 32
  kidney, puncture biopsy, 167
  sputum, stained smear, 65
  urine, 164–165
  viral and rickettsial infections, 13
    electron microscopy, 14
Microspherocytes, 98
Micturating cystogram, 169
Middle ear deafness, 29
Midstream specimen of urine, 161,
  163
Milk, 124–125
Mini Wright peak flow meter,
  67, **68**
Miniature mass radiography, 64
Mobilizing, tests related to, 175–180
Moebius's sign, 49
Monila albicans, 199
Monoclonal IgG, 118
Monospot, 101
Monosticon, 101

Mouth, tests related to, 128–129
  palatal reflex, 35
MRSA, 11
Multiple myeloma, 171
  Bence-Jones proteins, 171
  ESR, 89
  urine, 171
Multitests, 162
Muscle fibre in stools, 143
Musculoskeletal system
  muscles, testing, 40–41
  physiotherapy assessment,
    179–180
  skeletal system, 176–179
Myelography, 40
Myocardial infarction, **80**
  C-reactive protein levels, 112
  chemical markers, 81–83
    alpha hydroxybutyrate
      dehydrogenase (aHBD),
      117
    CK isoemzyme, 117
    prothrombin ratio, 95
Myoglobin, 82
Myxoedema
  cholesterol levels, 112
  radioactive iodine tests, 47

Nasal cavities, foreign bodies, 22
Nasal swab, 62
Nasolaryngoscope, 27
Near patient testing, 5–6
Needle biopsy, 4–5
  see also Fine needle aspiration
    (FNA) cytology
Needle stick injuries, 12
Neonatal cholestasis, 110
Neonatal screening, inborn errors of
  metabolism, 193
Nephritis, 165
  acute, 112, 167
  chronic, 111, 112, 113
Nephrosis, copper and
  caeruloplasmin levels, 112
Nephrotic syndrome, 46–47
Nerve conduction tests, 40
Nerve deafness, 29
Nervous system, lesions, 177
Neuroblastoma, catecholamine
  excretion, 55
Neuromuscular system, 30–41
Neurone-specific enolase (NSE),
  121
Neutropenia, 93
Nitroblue tetrazolium (NBT), 103
Non-gonococcal urethritis, 199
Non-haemolytic transfusion
  reactions, 107
Norepinephrine, 55
Normoblastic showers, 98
Nose, investigations, 61–62
  foreign bodies, 22
  nasal swab, 62
Nuclear medicine, 22–23
  bone scan, 176
  brain scan, 38
  gall bladder scan, 142
  gallium scanning, 23
  gastrointestinal bleeding, 151

heart scan, 84–85
kidney scan, 169
liver scan, 137
lung scan, 63
thyroid scan, 47
  see also Radiation exposure:
    monitoring; Radioisotope assays
Nucleated red cells, 98
5-Nucleotidase, 117
Nutrition, 124–128
NyoCard, C-reactive protein assay,
  113

Obstructive airways disease, FEV$_1$,
  69, **70**
Obstructive jaundice, 111, 139
  clotting time, 94
  laboratory test results, **140**
  serum bilirubin, 138
  urobilin and urobilinogen in urine,
    173
Occlusive arterial disease, 85
Occulomotor nerves, examination,
  33
Occult blood test, faeces, 156
Oedema, 114
  artificial, malingering, 37
Oesophageal varices, 130
Oesophagitis, test for, 129
Oesophagoscopy, 130
Oesophagus, tests related to,
  129–130
Oestradiol, gonadal endocrine
  function investigations, 187,
  188
Oestradiol–17b, ovarian function,
  187
Oestrogen excretion, placental and
  fetal function, 190
Oestrogens, total non-pregnancy,
  187
Olfactory nerve examination, 33
Optic discs, examination, 33
Optic nerve examination, 33
Oral cytology, 128–129
Oral glucose tolerance test, 147
Organ donation
  and brain death, 211
  tissue typing, 102
Organisms and parasites, stools,
  156–157
Organs, post-mortem retention of,
  212
Osmolality, 59, 115
Osteomalacia, 111
Osteomyelitis, 177
Osteoporosis, 178
  radiological quantification, 176,
    178
Otoscopy, 29
Ovarian biopsy, 186
Ovarian function, tests of, 187
Overnight dexamethasone
  suppression test, 54
Ovulation, tests for, 186
17-Oxosteroids, 52
Oxygen therapy, long-term
  assessment, 73
11-Oxygenation index, 53
Oxytocin, 59

Packed cell volume, 90
Pain
  malingering, 37
  sensation to, 36
Palatal reflex, 35
Pancreas, 142–149
Pancreatic disease
  gammaglutamyl transferase, 117
  pancreatic and related tumours,
    148–149
Pancreatic function tests, 143–144
  insulin secretion tests, 144–148
  pancreatic juice secretion,
    143–144
Pancreatic polypeptide, plasma,
  149
Pancreatitis, tests for, 142–143
Papilloedema, 33
Paracentesis, 150
Paracetamol overdose, 206–**207**
Paralysis of limb, malingering, 37
Paraquat, ingestion, 206
Parasites
  in blood, 92
  in stools, 156–157
  urine, 165
Parathormone, 50
Parathyroid gland investigations,
  49–50
  blood calcium levels, hyperplasia
    and tumour, 111
Paratyphoid, Widal reaction for, 16
Paroxysmal nocturnal
  haemoglobinuria, 99, 101
Partial heart block, **80**
Partial pressures, blood gases, 73
Pasteurized milk, 125
Patellar clonus, 35
Patch tests
  allergies, 9
  tuberculin sensitivity, 15
Paternity, tests related to, 184
Pathological fractures, 177
Patient preparation, 2–3
Paul-Bunnell test, 101
Peak flow rate (PFR), 67–**68**, 69
Pelvic carcinoma, lymph node
  involvement, 83
Pelvic examination, female infertility,
  185
Pelvimetry, 189
Pentagastrin test meal, 130,
  134–**135**
Peptic ulceration risk, *H. pylori*
  antibodies, 132
Percutaneous (transhepatic)
  cholangiogram, 142
Perimeter and field analyser tests,
  28, 56
Periostitis, 177
Peripheral nerves, 40
Peritoneum, 150–151
Pernasal swab, 62
Pernicious anaemia, 91, 93, 103,
  136
  alcohol and histamine test meal
    findings, 136
  bleeding time, 94
  mean cell volume, 90
  pentagastrin test meal, 134, **135**

vitamin BU12u deficiency,
  126–127
pH, 73–74
  fetal scalp blood, 192
  urine, 161
Phaeochromocytoma, 55
Phenistix, 163
Phenylalanine, blood test, 163, 193
Phenylketone, detection in urine,
  163
Phenytoin, 204–205
Phonocardiography, 85
Phosphatase test, pasteurized milk,
  125
Phosphokinase (CPK), 83
Phosphorus (inorganic phosphate),
  111
Physiotherapy assessment,
  179–180
Pituitary fossa, enlarged, 177
Pituitary gland, 44, 46, 51, 56–60
Pituitary hormones, 56
Placental and fetal monitoring,
  189–193
Plantar reflex, 35
Platelet antibody formation, 94
Platelet count, 93–94
Platelets, 88
Platinum loop, eye swab, 12–13
Pleural effusion, 64
  laboratory examination, 66–67
Pleural needle biopsy, 75
Pneumonia, 65
  antibodies in primary atypical, 19
  sputum, microscopy, 65
Pneumothorax, 65
  following FNA of lung, 75
Point of care testing, 5–6
Poisoning, 206
Poliomyelitis virus, tissue culture, 13
Polychromasia, 91, 98
Polycythaemia, 89, 90
  haematocrit, 90
  porphyrins in urine, 172
Polymyositis, 102
Porphyria, 172–173
Porphyrins
  in faeces, 157
  and related substances in urine,
    172–173
Portable cardiac monitor, **82**
Position sense, 36
Positron emission tomography
  (PET), 23
  brain studies, 39
  heart imaging, 85
  oesophageal tumour, 130
  thyroid imaging, 47
Post-coital test, 186
Posterior pituitary function
  assessment, 59–60
Postmortem, 212–213
Postpartum haemorrhage, low
  serum prolactin, 57
Potassium, 113, 115
  in urine, 172
Ppomas, 149
Pregnancy, 188–193
  alpha-fetoprotein, 119, 120, 192
  cholesterol levels, 112

copper and caeruloplasmin levels,
  112
herpes genitalis, 199–200
plasma fibrinogen, 96
protein-bound iodine, 47
tests for, 188–189
vaginal discharge, 199
Pregnanetriol, 52, **53**
Pregnosticon, 189
Preimplantation genetic diagnosis,
  184
Premature rupture of membranes,
  tests for, 193
Preparation of patient, 2–3
Prepuerin, 189
Prepurex, 189
Prick tests, allergies, 9
Primary atypical pneumonia,
  antibodies, 19
Primary hypothyroidism, 45, 46
PRIST (Paper RadioImmunoSorbent
  Test), 9
Proctoscopy, 153–154
Progesterone, gonadal endocrine
  function investigations, 187
Progressive multistage exercise test,
  72, 73
Prolactin assay, 57
Prolactinoma, 56, 57
Prostate, 185
  hypertrophy, 166, 185
  tumours, 182, 185
  carcinoma, euglobin lysis time,
    97
Prostatic specific antigen (PSA),
  185
Protein
  CSF, 32
  serum, 118–119, 139
  urine tests for, 162, 173
Protein electrophoresis, 118
Protein selectivity, 167
Protein-bound iodine (PBI),
  46–47
Prothrombin consumption test,
  96
Prothrombin and proconvertin test,
  95
Prothrombin ratio, 95
PSA, 185
Pseudohypoparathyroidism
  calcitonin, 111
  cyclic AMP levels, 113
Pseudomembranous colitis, 157
Psychometry, 41
Puerperal infection, 193
Pulmonary angiography, 64
Pulmonary embolism, 64
Pulmonary tuberculosis, 65, 66
Pulse oximetry, 73, 81
Pulse pressure, 78
Punch biopsy, skin, 8
Pupil reflexes, 33
Purulent pleural fluid, 67
Pus, 11
  cells in urine, 164
Pyelonephritis, 164
Pyloric stenosis, 131
Pyogenic meningitis, CSF
  examination, 31–32, 32

Pyruvic acid, vitamin B, deficiency, 125–126
Pyruvic tolerance test, vitamin B, deficiency, 126

Queckenstedt's test, 31
Quick's one-stage test, 95

Radiation exposure
monitoring, 22–23
white cell count, 92
Radioactive iodine tests, 47
Radioallergosorbent (RAST) test, 9, 119
Radioimmunoassays, 182
human chorionic gonadotrophin, 189
pregnancy tests, 189
TSH, 46
Radioisotope assay, 22–23
folic acid, 127
red cell survival, 101
scans, see Nuclear medicine
Schilling test, 127, 136
thyroid function, urine excretion method, 47
Radioisotopes, radiation monitoring, 22–23
RAST (Radio AllergoSorbent Test), 9, 119
Reaginic antibody (IgE), allergies, 9, 119
Recalcification time, 94
Rectum and colon, visual examination, 153–155
Recurrent laryngeal nerve, 34
Red blood cells, 88
appearance, 91, 207
cell mass, 90
count, 89
osmotic fragility, 99
survival, 100–101
in urine, 165
Reducing substances in urine, 173
5-alpha-reductase deficiency, 188
Reflex actions, 34–35
Refraction tests, 28
Reiter protein complement fixation test, 200, 201
Reiter's disease, 102
Relapsing fever, 92
Renal angiography, 169–170
Renal failure, blood magnesium levels, 111
Renal investigations
angiography, 169–170
function tests, 165–168
intravenous urography, 168
renal biopsy, 167–168
scan, radioisotope, 169
ultrasound, 169
Renal stones, 171
Renin-angiotensin system, 78
Request for investigation, 3
Respiratory acidosis, 73
Respiratory centre test, brain death, 210–211
Respiratory distress, 73
Respiratory system
foreign bodies, 22

lower, investigations, 63–75
test done by surgeon or physician, 74–75
upper, investigations, 61–63
Respiridone, 205
Reticulocyte count, 90–91
Reticulocytosis, 98
Retrograde cystography, 169
Retrograde pyelogram, 168–169
Retrosternal goitre, 48
Rhesus immunization, human placental lactogen assay, 190
Rhesus type, 104
Rhesus-negative women, antenatal blood tests, 104–105
Rheumatic fever
C-reactive protein levels, 112
ESR, 89
Rheumatoid arthritis, 101, 101–102
physiotherapy assessment, 180
tests for, 101–102
Rhinoscopy, 61–62
Rickets, 111, 177
Rickettsiae, tissue culture, 13
Ringworm, diagnosis of, 13
Rinne's test, 29
Romberg's sign, 36
malingering, 37
Rose-Waaler test, 101
Rose's test, 101
Rothera's test, 145
Roundworms, 157
Rubella antibodies, blood test, 18

Salivary gland, tests related, 129
Salmonella group, food poisoning, 128
Salpingogram, 196
Sangur Test, 162
Sarcoidosis, Kveim test, 14
Scans, see Nuclear medicine
Schick test, diphtheria, susceptibility to, 15–16
Schilling test, 127, 136
Schistosomiasis
antibodies, blood test, 18
organisms in stools, 157
Schizophrenia therapeutic drug monitoring, 205
Schumm's test, 101
Scintillation counters, 23
Scleroderma, 102
Scrape and smear, oral cytology, 129
Scratch tests, allergies, 9
Screening criteria, neonatal screening, 193
Scurvy, 127, 177
Secondary aldosteronism, 52
Secretin test, duodenal aspiration tests, 144
Self-examination, breast, 194
Self-monitoring, blood sugar, 146–147
Semicircular canal tests, 34
Seminal fluid examination, 186
Sensation, testing, 36
Septic abortion, 193
Septic arthritis, 178

Septic meningitis, CSF examination, 32
Septicaemia, 16
Serum hepatitis, 16–17
Settle plates, 10
Sex chromatin examination, 183
Sexing, fetal, 190, 191
Sexually transmitted diseases, 199–201
Shave biopsy, skin, 9
Sheep cell agglutination test, 101
Sialography, 129
Sickling, tests for, 98
Sight
loss of, malingering, 37
testing, 27–29
Sigmoidoscopy, 154
Silicosis, 65
Simmond's disease, 59
Single photon absorptiometry, 176
Single-photon emission computerized tomography (SPECT), 85
Sinogram, 22
Sinuses, X-ray examination, 62
Sjögren's syndrome, 102
Skeletal muscle damage, AST levels, 116
Skeletal system, 176–179
Skin, 8
fungal infections, 13
Skin biopsy, 8–9
Skin conditions
fungal, 13
malingering, 37
Skin scrapings, 13
Skin tests
allergies, 9
infection, 14–16
Skull lesions, 177
Sleeping sickness, 92
Slide tests, pregnancy, 189
Slit sampler, 10
Small intestine, 149–150
biopsy, 149
follow-through examination, 131
Sodium, 114, 115
in urine, 172
Sodium chloride, dietary, 114
Spalding's sign, 189
Specific gravity, urine, 161
Specimens, 3–5
high-risk, 12
labelling, 3
Spectroscopy, methaemalbumin, 101
Speech tests, 26–27
Spherocytosis, hereditary, 99
Spinal accessory nerve examination, 34
Spinal block, complete, cysternal puncture, 31
Spinal lesions, 176
Spinal reflexes, 35
brain death tests, 211
Spinal tumour, Queckenstedt's test, 31
Spirochetes, 92, 200
Spirometer, 69, **70**

Spontaneous hypoglycaemia, 146, 147
Spore strips, 10
Sputum
  collection techniques, 65
  laboratory examination, 65–66
Stanford-Binet tests, 41
Staphylococcal antibodies, 19
Staphylococcus aureas, 11
Staphylococcus carriers, nasal swabs, 62
Staphylococcus pyogenes, 128
Static lung volumes, 71, **72**
Stereoradiography, foreign body localization, 21
Sterile pyuria, 164
Sterility of dressings, 10
Sterilized milk, 125
Steroid excretion test, 53
Steroids, 50
  blood tests for, 51–52
  urine tests for, 52–53
Stick or strip tests, urine, 161
  bilirubin, 138
  blood, 162
  glucose or ketones, 144–145, 162
  protein, 162
Still's disease, 101
Stimulation and suppression tests, 53–55
Stimulation tests, endocrine system, 44
Stomach, barium meal, 131
Stomach and intestines, tests related to, 130–136
Stomach washout, poisoning, 206
Stools, 143, 156–157
Streptococci
  carriers, 63
  streptococcal ASO (antistreptolysin 'O' titre), 18
  throat swabs, 63
Streptokinase resistance test, 98
Streptokinase treatment, 98
  Euglobin lysis time, 97
Stuart's transport medium, 12
STYCAR (Sheridan Tests for Young Children and Retards), 41
Subarachnoid haemorrhage, 30, 31
Subluxations, 177
Substances of abuse, 208
Sugar, urine tests for, 144–145, 162
  chromatography, 173
Superficial reflexes, 34–35
Suppression tests, endocrine system, 44
Supraregional Assay Service (SAS), 182
  tissue enzyme studies, 183–194
Swabs, testing for infection, 11
Sweat test, fibrocystic disease, 143
Synacthen (ACTH) test, 53–54
Syphilis, 200
  blood tests for, 200–201
  confirmatory test, 201
  CSF examination, 31, 32
Systemic lupus erythematosus (SLE), 103
  two-stage prothrombin test, 95
Systolic blood pressure, 78

T-tube cholangiogram, 142
Tapeworms, 157
Target cells, 91
Teeth, 128
Temperature, 19
  artificial, malingering, 37
  and brain death tests, 211
Ten-day rule, 196
Tendon reflexes, 35
Tenogram, 178
Test types, sight testing, 28
Testosterone and other androgens, 188
Tests, special tests and investigations, 1–2
Tetany, 50, 110–111, 111, 115
Thalassaemia *see* Mediterranean anaemia
Theophylline, 204
Therapeutic drug monitoring, 204–205
Thermocouple, testing autoclave function, 10
Thermography, breast, 194
Thoracoscopy, 74
Threadworm, 157
Throat swab, 62–63
Thrombin clotting time, 98
Thrombocytopenic purpura, 93, 94
Thromboplastin generation test (TGT), 97
Thrombotest, 95
Thyroglobulin, 46
Thyroglobulin antibody test, 48
Thyroglobulin sensitized sheep cells, 48
Thyroid binding globulin (TBG), 46
Thyroid complement fixation test (TCFT), 48
Thyroid function tests, 45–47
Thyroid investigations, 45–49
  autoimmune disease, 48, 103
Thyroid precipitin test, 48
Thyroid scan, 47
Thyroid stimulating hormone (TSH), 45, 46, 193–194
Thyrotoxicosis, 45, 46, 47
Thyrotropic hormone, Simmond's disease, 59
Thyrotropin releasing hormone (TRH), 45
Thyroxine (T₄), 45
Tine test, 15
Tissue culture, 13
Tissue enzyme studies, 182, 183–194
Tissue, examination of, 3–5
Tissue sections, sex cromatin examination, 183
Tissue space fluid, 114
Tissue type, HLA antigens, 102
Tomography, chest, 63
Tonometer, intraocular pressure, 29
Total 17-oxyogenic steroids, 52
Touch preparation, oral cytology, 128
Touch, sensation to, 36
Toxaemias of pregnancy, 192

Toxic and infective hepatitis, 139, **140**
Toxic nodular goitre, 47
Toxoplasma antibodies, 19
Transaminases, 116
Transfer factor, lung function, 71
Transfusion reactions, investigation, 107
Transport media, samples, 11–12
Treponema pallidum, 200
Trichina antigen test, 15
Trichomonas medium, 12
Trichomonas vaginalis, 197, 198–199
Trigeminal nerve, examination, 33
Triglycerides, 111, 119
Triiodothyronine (T₃), 45, 46
Triple diagnosis, breast lump, 195
Troponin T, 82
Trousseau's sign, 50
Trucut needle biopsy, 4
  breast, 195
  liver, 141
Trypanosomes, 92
Trypsin test, stools, 143
Tubercle bacilli
  sputum, laboratory examination, 66
  urine, 161, 164
Tuberculin skin reactions, 15
Tuberculin-tested milk, 124
Tuberculosis, 65
  bones and joints, 178
  ESR, 89
  lymph node biopsy, 93
  pleural needle biopsy, 74
  urinary tract, 164
Tuberculous meningitis, CSF examination, 31, 32
Tumour markers, 119–121, 185
Twelve-hour urine collection, 161
Twenty-four hour fetal function, 190
Twenty-four hour urine collection, 160–161
  amino acids, 170
  calcium and magnesium levels, 171
  chloride, 171
  dexamethasone suppression test, 54, 55
  lead and coproporphyrin, 207
  placental and fetal function, 190
  porphyrins in urine, 172–173
  proteins, 173
  steroid hormones, 50–51
  total non-pregnancy oestrogens, 187
  urobilin and urobilinogen, 173
Two-stage prothrombin test, 95
Typhoid
  carrier state, test for, 16
  white cell count, 92
  Widal reaction for, 16
Typhus fever, 13

UHT milk, 125
Ultrasound, 20
  abdomen, 137
  aneurysms, 83
  Doppler, 85

kidney, 169
  pregnancy, 190
  thyroid, 48
Undescended testes, 188
Undulant fever, 16
Unnatural causes of death, 211
Upper alimentary tract investigations, 128–129
Upper respiratory tract investigations, 61–63
Upper third vaginal wall scrape, 198
Uraemia, 166
Urea clearance test, 166–167
Urea, concentration in urine, 173
Urethral discharge and sexually transmitted disease, 199–200
Uric acid (urate), 120
Urinalysis, 160–170
Urinary infection, detection of hidden, 164
Urinary tract, radiology of, 168–170
Urine excretion method, radioactive iodine, 47
Urine tests, 160–173
  bilirubin, 137–138, 163
  collection, 160–161
    see also Twenty-four hour urine collection
  cytology, 165
  excreted substances, 170–173
    alcohol, 208
    cannabis, 208
    catecholamines, 55
    lead and coproporphyrin, 207
    glucose and ketones, 144–145, 162
  gonadal endocrine function investigations, 187
  haematuria, 162, 165
  laboratory examination, routine, 161
  liver function tests, 137–138
  microbiology, 163–164
  microscopy, 164–165
  osmolality, 59
  phenylketonuria, 163
  placental and fetal function, 190
  red cell survival, 101
  renal function tests, 165–168
  steroids, tests for, 52–53
  toxaemias of pregnancy, 192
  urinalysis, 160–170
  urine amylase (diastase), 143
  urobilogen, 138, 163, 173
  ward or clinic examination, 161–163

Uristix, 162
Urobilin, 138
  haemolytic anaemias, 101
Urobilinogen, 138, 163, 173
Urobilogen, 138, 173
Urogenital system, foreign bodies, 22
Uterine curettings, 186, 196–197
Uterine swabs, 193

Vagina, gynaecological cytology, 198
Vagus nerve, testing integrity of, 34, 135
Van den Bergh test, 138
Vanillylmandelic acid, 55
Vasculiti, ESR, 89
Vasoactive polypeptide, pancreatic, 149
Vasopressin (antidiuretic hormone) assay, 59
  stimulation test, 60
Venereal disease reference laboratory slide test, 200
Ventricular fibrillation, **81**
Ventriculography, 40
Vestibular tests, 34
Ví test, 16
Vincent's angina, 63
Vipoma, 149
Viral hepatitis A, C, D, E, 17
Viral and rickettsial infections, 13–14
Virilism, 17-Oxosteroids, 52
Virus transport medium, 12
Viscometry, 89–90
Visual field testing, 28
Vitamin C
  ascorbic acid saturation test, 127
  tests for glycosuria, false-negatives, 145
Vitamin D excess, blood calcium levels, 111
Vitamin deficiencies, 125–128
  A, 125
  B₁, 125–126
  B₁₂, 126–127, 136
  C, 127
  D, 127–128
  K, 128
Voice assessment, 26
von Graef's sign, 49

Walking test, 6 minute, 72
  portable oxygen assessment, 73
Wassermann reaction, 200, 200–201
Water deprivation test, 59

Water dilution and concentration test, 166
Water and electrolyte balance, 114
Weber's test, 29
Wegener's disease, 102
Weil's disease, leptospira antibodies, 18
Westgren method, ESR, 89
Wet film, 98
White blood cells, 88
  in urine, 164
White cell count, 92
  differential, 92–93
Widal reaction for typhoid and paratyphoid, 16
Wilson's disease, 112
Wintrobe method, ESR, 89
Wood's glass, ringworm, diagnosis of, 13
Wounds, infection, tests for, 11
Wright peak flow meter, 67, **68**
Written consent, 2

X-ray examinations, 20
  abdomen, 137, 168
  bones, joints and tendons, 176–178
  cardiovascular system, 83–84
  chest X-rays, 63–65
  foreign body localization, 21, 22
  gall bladder and bile ducts, 141–142
  of gut, 155–156
  mammography, 182, 194
  pituitary gland, 56
  pregnancy, 189
  radiation monitoring, radioisotopes, 22–23
  salivary gland, 129
  sinuses, 62
  teeth, 128
  thyroid enlargement, 48
  urinary tract, 168
  uterus, tubes and ovaries, 196
  see also Radiation exposure: monitoring
X-xylose excretion test, 150
Xanthochromia, CSF, 31
Xeroradiography, breast, 194

Ziehl-Neelson stain, sputum, 66
Zinc, 120
Zollinger-Ellison syndrome, **135**, 136